THE COMPLETE
BRAIN
EXERCISE BOOK
Train Your Brain!

THE COMPLETE
BRAIN
EXERCISE BOOK
Train Your Brain!

Improve Memory, Language, Motor Skills & More

+

A Health & Diet Plan with 125 Recipes

Dr. Fraser Smith, BA, MATD, ND

Robert ROSE

For complete cataloguing information, see page 370.

Disclaimer
This book is a general guide only and should never be a substitute for the skill, knowledge and experience of a qualified medical professional dealing with the facts, circumstances and symptoms of a particular case.

The nutritional, medical and health information presented in this book is based on the research, training and professional experience of the author, and is true and complete to the best of his knowledge. However, this book is intended only as an informative guide for those wishing to know more about health, nutrition and medicine; it is not intended to replace or countermand the advice given by the reader's personal physician. Because each person and situation is unique, the author and the publisher urge the reader to check with a qualified health-care professional before using any procedure where there is a question as to its appropriateness. A physician should be consulted before beginning any exercise program. The author and the publisher are not responsible for any adverse effects or consequences resulting from the use of the information in this book. It is the responsibility of the reader to consult a physician or other qualified health-care professional regarding his or her personal care.

This book contains references to products that may not be available everywhere. The intent of the information provided is to be helpful, however, there is no guarantee of results associated with the information provided. Use of brand names is for educational purposes only and does not imply endorsement.

The recipes in this book have been carefully tested by our kitchen and our tasters. To the best of our knowledge, they are safe and nutritious for ordinary use and users. For those people with food or other allergies, or who have special food requirements or health issues, please read the suggested contents of each recipe carefully and determine whether or not they may create a problem for you. All recipes are used at the risk of the consumer. We cannot be responsible for any hazards, loss or damage that may occur as a result of any recipe use. For those with special needs, allergies, requirements or health problems, in the event of any doubt, please contact your medical adviser prior to the use of any recipe.

Design and Production: Daniella Zanchetta/PageWave Graphics Inc.
Editors: Sue Sumeraj and Tina Anson Mine
Copy editor: Kelly Jones
Proofreader and indexer: Gillian Watts
Nutrient analysis: Magda Fahmy
Illustrations (p.13, 15–19, 96–99, 116): Kveta/threeinabox.com
Other illustration & photo credits: p. 33 Happy/annoyed faces (source) © iStockphoto.com/MuchMania; pp. 40, 41, 42 Owls (source) © iStockphoto.com/kidstudio852; p. 64 Picnic basket © iStockphoto.com/IvonneW; p. 65 Beach party © iStockphoto.com/mediaphotos

The publisher gratefully acknowledges the financial support of our publishing program by the Government of Canada through the Canada Book Fund.

Published by Robert Rose Inc.
120 Eglinton Avenue East, Suite 800, Toronto, Ontario, Canada M4P 1E2
Tel: (416) 322-6552 Fax: (416) 322-6936
www.robertrose.ca

Printed and bound in USA

1 2 3 4 5 6 7 8 9 CKV 23 22 21 20 19 18 17 16 15

*This book is dedicated to my family,
who make it possible and who
make it all worthwhile.*

Contents

Introduction

Turn on subscription television anytime from midnight to six o'clock in the morning and you'll see a number of promotions for exercise systems to make the body perform better. A drive through most communities will reveal at least a few health clubs and various fitness, yoga and martial arts centers. This is great, because the body craves movement and exercise. But as we age, there is another part of our bodies that needs to be used, stretched and strengthened: our brain, the part of us that houses our memories and thoughts and controls our bodies. We often take for granted our brain's functions and reliability, or simply hope that it won't decline too quickly with age. This is a mistake, because experience and emerging science on the topic of cognitive abilities (thinking and brain performance) clearly demonstrate that the brain responds to work. Training the brain yields changes to its performance.

The adage "use it or lose it" is true when it comes to our mental resources, but there is an important further detail. As we get older, we must avoid the trap of simply repeating behaviors and skills that we mastered long ago. To be young, we must act young — we must acquire and practice new skills, develop new understanding and create new experiences. Novelty literally wakes up the brain and gives it the input it needs for optimal performance.

We live in an age of computer-based (and increasingly mobile) brain training. Although some mental tasks do seem to improve with computer training, the net value may not be consistent among individuals and the total benefit is still unclear. In this book, I present the perspective that any type of brain exercise ought to encourage the use of a variety of aspects of our intelligence, especially those that are underdeveloped or even dormant. That means doing and experiencing a variety of activities in different environments. That means using your hands as well as your head and having experiences in the real world, not in a pixelated screen environment on a computer.

Although computer-based brain training is a wonderful resource, this book takes a more holistic approach. I hope it will provide you with some very useful "how to" instructions so you can live, work, eat, play and love to the best of your ability throughout your life.

— *Fraser Smith, BA, MATD, ND*
Lombard, Illinois

The 4 Steps of the Complete Brain Exercise Program

1 Train more than just memory. Most brain exercise books focus on preventing and treating memory loss due to aging and disease. This book not only covers this type of memory training but also offers exercises that will help preserve or possibly improve your mental speed, visual acuity, language acquisition, sensory growth and motor skills. We often overwork parts of our brain, based on our work or hobbies, and neglect others. Not only does this lead to untapped potential, but the repetitive way in which we use our brains as we get older is the very opposite of what we need. By stretching our mental abilities and, most important, using a variety of different aspects of our intelligence, we stand a better chance of maintaining our cognitive (thinking) abilities.

2 Prevent and repair losses. Recovery of lost brain function is another common priority of brain exercise programs. This book covers not only recovery strategies but also ways you can prevent these losses in the first place, even when they are the result of a neurological disease.

3 Feed your brain with a healthy diet. The relationship between brain health and diet is touched on as an afterthought in most brain exercise books. In these pages, diet and nutrition are front and center, with detailed brain-food lists, menu plans and delicious recipes.

4 Have fun and grow at the same time. This book contains plenty of serious, in-depth scientific information, but it is entertaining as well as informative. The games are just as fun as those you will find in other brain puzzle books, but they are more sharply focused on interactive activities that enable you to assess your brain health and witness its growth as you work through the exercises.

Part 1
More Than Memory

• •

Aging Naturally

Everyone ages; it's a fact of life. This is easier to ignore in our younger years, when we are still growing, changing and maturing. But eventually it dawns on all of us that our bodies, such as they are, were not made to last forever.

What We Know about Aging

Although we can continue to make new cells as we get older, cell division becomes less efficient and starts to develop some problems.

The causes of aging are only partially understood now, in the early 21st century. We know that our cells' ability to divide and create healthy new cells is limited, and eventually they can't replace themselves. Once old cells have undergone enough wear and tear, they cease functioning normally. The only cells that seem to reproduce endlessly (as far as scientists have been able to observe) are certain cancer cells, which lose all relationship to normal function and whose normal growth-control mechanisms have been destroyed.

You might be wondering, "If cells have a built-in shut-off valve, how has the human race been able to pass on genes and cellular information and survive from generation to generation?" The answer is that sexual reproduction allows for two people to combine their genes to make an entirely new organism, starting from square one. When this happens, the cellular clock is set to zero and the brand-new person has the opportunity for many, many cell divisions as their body grows. In childhood (aside from some inborn genetic diseases and, unfortunately, some cases of cancer in the very young), cells grow quickly and do so easily. Organs and other tissues grow fast — but according to a plan. Although we can continue to make new cells as we get older, cell division becomes less efficient and starts to develop some problems.

As we age, cell division is limited by one factor in particular. When a cell is undergoing division, it must first copy its own genetic material (the chromosomes, or your body's genetic blueprints), then align the two copies so that it can split itself in half to create a brand-new cell. The "pulleys" that align the chromosomes are called telomeres. These proteins start off at a certain length in our youth and shorten over time. By the time we reach old age, our telomeres have shortened significantly and will eventually stop working.

FAQ

Q. *Will technology allow us to live longer?*

A. It's likely that scientific advances will extend the human lifespan. It's arguable that, one day, many people could live to be 120 years old if they use preventive medicines, undergo surgical and medical interventions, and adhere to a way of living that addresses the determinants of health, such as optimal nutrition, sleep, exercise and so on. It doesn't seem so far-fetched when you think of the possibilities inherent in the use of tissue grafts — such as those that use umbilical cord stem cells (regenerative cells harvested from the umbilical cord of a baby immediately after birth, which are frozen for future use). Although still experimental, there have been impressive reports about the injection of stem cells into the central nervous system to help stroke victims. There are various sources of stem cells and ways to deliver them; it is a new and complex field. The great hockey player Gordie Howe, who suffered a debilitating stroke in 2014, was injected with stem cells when his son, a physician, took him to a center that performs this very new therapy. A few months later, his speech had returned and he was playing ball hockey with his grandchildren. Perhaps the healing abilities of this great athlete asserted themselves over time, but the rate of his recovery astounded his family and friends. Serious research into stem cell treatments for neurological diseases, such as multiple sclerosis, is ongoing.

Everyday Life Affects Cells

Normal living takes its toll on our cells' ability to reproduce themselves. The various toxins and reactive chemicals that our cells are regularly exposed to can create damage that we simply can't repair. our DNA is definitely susceptible to this kind of harm.

Oxygen is a good example of an everyday factor that can damage cells under the right conditions. The oxygen molecule can take unstable forms that react with other chemicals — just look at a rusty nail or rusty gate to see what oxygen can do. Oxygen is essential to human life and enters our cells all the time. But it can also react with our cell components, including DNA, and damage them. We have natural defenses against this, but eventually the body takes a hit from the damage caused by oxygen and other reactive compounds.

As DNA, cell components and important hormones and other body chemicals become imbalanced and damaged, the body undergoes disturbances in function. In spite of this, we are incredibly adaptable. Our organs are able to continue to function at less than full capacity, and the rest of the body can compensate, to a degree, for a weak organ. But these compensations — such as the retention of water in someone with heart failure, or the making of concentrated urine by someone who is dehydrated — come with a price. Eventually, adaptability erodes, degeneration accelerates and the body can no longer pull off the miraculous balancing act that we call life.

Normal Brain Function

Human life and body functions depend on the brain. When it is healthy, well nourished and functioning properly, it ensures communication between all the body's systems and is the home of thoughts, memories and creativity. To understand how the brain ages naturally, it is valuable to understand how a normal, healthy brain works. The more we learn about the different tasks our brain performs, and how we use different brain areas to accomplish those tasks, the more the concept of exercising the brain begins to seem a necessity.

Brain Basics

The brain is an extremely complex structure made of tissue and nerves and it controls everything we do, from voluntary actions (such as walking) to involuntary actions (such as breathing). The brain is responsible for communicating moment by moment with all other parts of the body through the central nervous system (CNS) and the peripheral nervous system (PNS). The brain is also responsible for managing our emotions and thoughts, and for nurturing our short-term and long-term memories.

Scientists are slowly discovering its secrets, but in many ways the brain is still a new frontier, and aging-related diseases continue to challenge neurologists to fully understand them. However, there is no need to take a course in neuroanatomy to grasp the structures and functions of the brain that relate to aging-related diseases. It is intriguing to know how our brains function normally so we can see how they sometimes do not function so well as we age.

Neuron Function

The adult brain contains between 80 and 100 billion cells. Each cell has about 100,000 connections to other cells. Known also as neurons, these cells fire an electrochemical signal (a small electrical current) along their lining, or membrane, until this signal reaches the tip of one of the branches of another cell. There it causes the release of a chemical compound that attaches to the next neuron in the chain, leading to a new signal. These chemicals are called neurotransmitters.

Neuron Function

Each neuron has a cell body, which maintains the life of that cell, as well as specialized parts that include an axon and dendrites. The axon sends signals to other neurons, usually thousands of them. The dendrites receive signals from other neurons. The communication between two neurons, known as a synapse, is done by chemicals known as neurotransmitters.

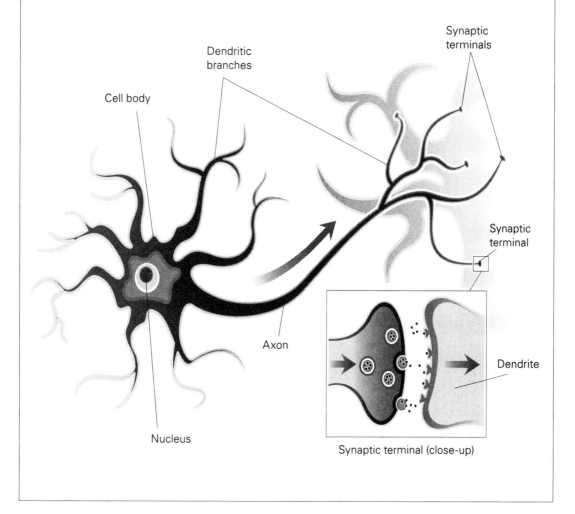

Synaptic terminals

Dendritic branches

Cell body

Synaptic terminal

Axon

Dendrite

Nucleus

Synaptic terminal (close-up)

Kinds of Neurotransmitters

The disruption of dopamine production in the brain is a causal factor in Parkinson's disease.

Neurotransmitters can be excitatory (prompting a neuron to fire) or inhibitory (preventing a neuron from firing). Some of the major excitatory neurotransmitters are the chemical monoamines, including epinephrine, norepinephrine, histamine, serotonin and dopamine. The disruption of dopamine production in the brain is a causal factor in Parkinson's disease. Some of the major inhibitory neurotransmitters are serotonin and gamma-aminobutyric acid (GABA). Other neurotransmitters include acetylcholine and amino acids.

- **Acetylcholine**
- **Amino acids:** Gamma-aminobutyric acid (GABA) and glycine glutamate aspartate
- **Monoamines:** Epinephrine, norepinephrine, histamine, serotonin and dopamine
- **Neuropeptides:** Oxytocin, endorphins and vasopressin

Anatomy of the Brain

The parts of the brain are typically grouped by location into the forebrain, midbrain and hindbrain. The forebrain is a region with three distinct components: the cerebrum, thalamus and hypothalamus. The hypothalamus is joined by some other specialized structures that generate emotional responses to make up the limbic system. The midbrain contains the tectum and tegmentum; the hindbrain contains the cerebellum, pons and medulla. A vital part of keeping the body's basic systems (such as breathing) operating is the brain stem, which can be described as the midbrain plus the pons and medulla. All of these parts of the brain interact through a series of networks and feedback loops.

Forebrain

The cerebrum, thalamus and hypothalamus make up the forebrain. The pituitary gland is connected to the hypothalamus and secretes hormones that regulate homeostasis, or equilibrium, among the various body systems and the brain.

Cerebrum

Also known as the cerebral cortex, the cerebrum is the largest part of the human brain and is associated with higher brain function, such as thought and action. The cerebral cortex is composed of two hemispheres, right and left, and they are

Parts of the Brain

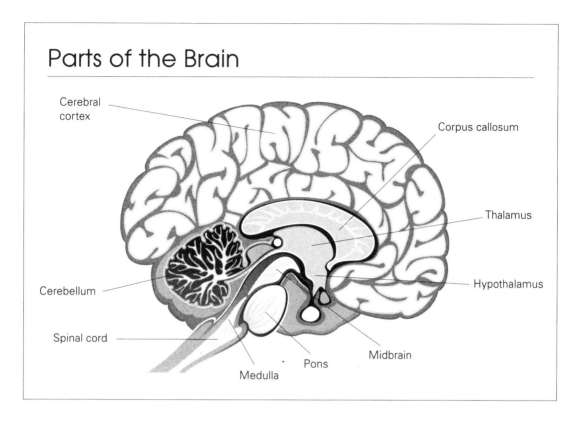

Cerebral cortex

Corpus callosum

Thalamus

Hypothalamus

Cerebellum

Spinal cord

Midbrain

Pons

Medulla

connected by the corpus callosum. The right hemisphere is typically associated with creativity, holism and pattern recognition, and the left hemisphere is associated with logic and reasoning. The cerebral cortex also has nerve cells that control muscle movement. Many of our impulses to move originate there. We also use much of this part of the brain for memory function. How we store memories is still unknown. In some neurological diseases, such as Alzheimer's disease, these functions of the cerebrum are disturbed.

Thalamus

The thalamus acts as a processing center for the sensory information coming into the brain. The information gathered from various parts of our body, such as our hands, eventually passes through the thalamus en route to other brain centers. The spinal cord carries signals and actual neurons (some of which are 3 feet/90 cm long) that transmit information from the brain down to and from the sensory nerves up to our central nervous system. The thalamus is a kind of switching center that intercepts information from the body. In some neurological diseases, such as stroke (depending on where blood supply to the brain was interrupted), the thalamus is damaged and the senses become confused.

The information gathered from various parts of our body, such as our hands, eventually passes through the thalamus en route to other brain centers.

Cerebral Lobes

The cerebral cortex is further divided into four lobes:

- *Frontal lobe:* Associated with the "higher functions" of the human mind, such as complex thinking, appreciation of art, making plans and the finer aspects of communication

- *Parietal lobe:* Associated with hearing, speech and some aspects of controlling the body

- *Occipital lobe:* Receives sensory input from the eyes and relays it to other parts of the brain for interpretation

- *Temporal lobe:* Important for hearing and speech

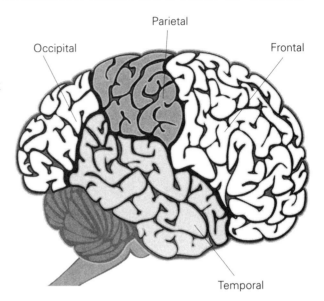

Occipital · Parietal · Frontal · Temporal

Hypothalamus

The hypothalamus is responsible for hormone production. These hormones govern body temperature, thirst, hunger, sleep, moods, sex drive and the release of other hormones. The hypothalamus is one of several glands, including the pituitary gland, that interact within the endocrine system. This interaction is extensive. For example, secretion of the thyroid gland hormone is triggered by thyroid-stimulating hormone (TSH), which comes from the pituitary gland, which is under the control of the hypothalamus. In some neurological diseases, such as tumors that destroy portions of the hypothalamus or pituitary gland, endocrine function can be lost or increase and become unbalanced.

In some neurological diseases, such as tumors that destroy portions of the hypothalamus or pituitary gland, endocrine function can be lost or increase and become unbalanced.

Limbic System

The limbic system, often referred to as the emotional brain, is found within the cerebrum. This system contains the thalamus, hypothalamus, amygdala and hippocampus. The amygdala responds to threats by generating feelings of anxiety and emotional energy, the fight-or-flight response. The hippocampus is absolutely critical to learning and helps to "write" memories into our brain. The hippocampus actually sprouts new neurons, and the faster we learn, the more it can regenerate.

Executive Function

The prefrontal cortex is the executive of the brain, responsible for planning, judging, decision making and assigning tasks. Let's take a simple example — imagine you are in the kitchen making a new recipe. The prefrontal cortex arranges your actions logically: first you assemble your utensils, then you gather your ingredients, then you blend and cook the ingredients. You cannot execute all these tasks at one time, so the prefrontal cortex organizes them and enables you to complete them sequentially. In some neurological diseases, the prefrontal cortex loses this executive ability, and thinking becomes confused.

Brain–Body Feedback Loop

The three main communication systems in the body — cardiovascular, immune and endocrine — are governed by the brain, which instigates the circulation of hormones that feed back signals to the brain in a loop. How does this work? Using the thyroid system as an example, the hypothalamus sends thyrotropin-releasing hormone to the pituitary gland to create more thyroid-stimulating hormone (TSH). When the thyroid successfully makes more thyroid hormone and blood levels of the hormone rise, both the pituitary and the hypothalamus are inhibited — and, for a time, less thyroid hormone is produced.

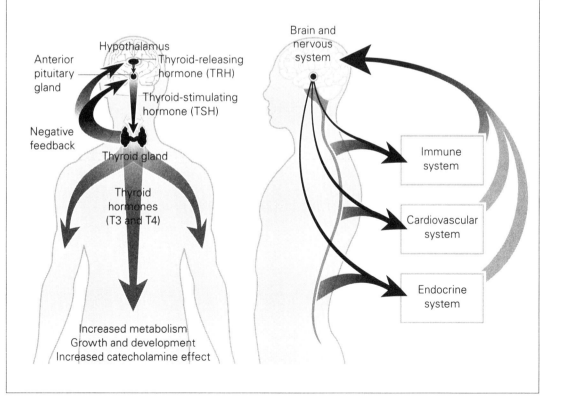

Hypothalamus

Anterior pituitary gland

Thyroid-releasing hormone (TRH)

Thyroid-stimulating hormone (TSH)

Negative feedback

Thyroid gland

Thyroid hormones (T3 and T4)

Increased metabolism
Growth and development
Increased catecholamine effect

Brain and nervous system

Immune system

Cardiovascular system

Endocrine system

Midbrain

The midbrain is a relay center for vision and hearing information. The midbrain includes the tectum and tegmentum, which in turn includes the substantia nigra. The neurotransmitter dopamine is generated in the substantia nigra. This neurotransmitter is used in the regulation of movement. When there is a deficiency of dopamine, as in the case of Parkinson's disease, movement becomes stiff, uneven and difficult. Dopamine is also involved in motivation, pleasure, desire and reward systems in the brain.

Hindbrain

The hindbrain is responsible for basic vital life functions, such as breathing, heartbeat and blood pressure. The hindbrain is made up of the pons, medulla and cerebellum. The first two structures are also known as the brain stem, which merges with the upper portion of the spinal cord. The pons is a bridge that connects the medulla to the spinal cord and governs the autonomic system, including digestion, body temperature and heart rate. This part of the brain is common to many other living organisms, including all animals. The brain stem is involved in cardiovascular system control, respiratory system control, pain-sensitivity control, alertness, awareness and consciousness. In some neurological diseases, such as traumatic head injury, damage to the brain stem can be life-threatening.

Cerebellum

The cerebellum is a part of the hindbrain but bears some structural resemblance to the cerebrum, with two hemispheres and a cortex. The cerebellum is involved with the regulation and coordination of movement, posture and balance. The cerebellum also acts as a source of learning, memory and control for coordinated movements. When a dancer learns a complex dance routine, the cerebellum is involved. The cerebellum not only ensures the smooth operation of the motor system but is also involved in the overall thought-processing system of the brain. In some neurological diseases, such as Wernicke-Korsakoff syndrome (brought on by long-term excessive alcohol consumption and deficiency of vitamin B_1), the cerebellum loses control of motor functions.

Cerebellum as Executive Assistant

The cerebellum is like a mini-brain located at the rear of the brain. While it may not be the site of your highest and most abstract thinking, your brain wouldn't work without it. The cerebellum coordinates movement patterns and many other functions. Whether you're an elite gymnast learning a complicated mat routine or a regular person driving a car or doing your job, the cerebellum helps execute and coordinate complex muscle movements. It also assembles information and helps you make and act on decisions. As your brain receives sensory information, the cerebellum helps present relevant information to the higher thinking parts of the brain (just as a good assistant puts vital work in front of an executive based on a schedule or priority list). The higher centers of your brain can then send rapid signals to other parts of the brain. The good news is that the cerebellum is neuroplastic, which means it can respond to training and become stronger and more supple.

Peripheral Nervous System

The peripheral nervous system (PNS) consists of the nerves and ganglia outside of the brain and spinal cord. The main function of the PNS is to connect the central nervous system (CNS) to the limbs and organs, essentially serving as a communication relay going back and forth between the brain and the extremities. Unlike the CNS, the PNS is not protected by the bones of the spine and skull, or by the blood–brain barrier, leaving it exposed to toxins and mechanical injuries.

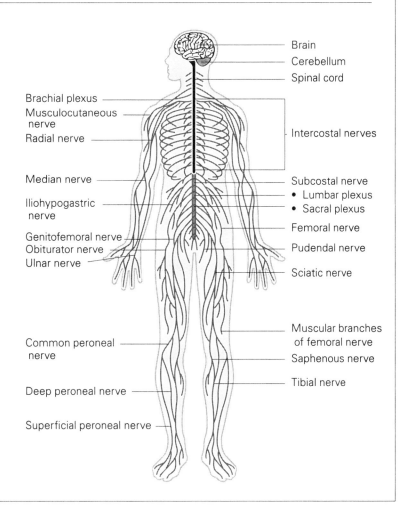

Brain
Cerebellum
Spinal cord

Brachial plexus
Musculocutaneous nerve
Radial nerve

Intercostal nerves

Median nerve

Subcostal nerve
• Lumbar plexus
• Sacral plexus

Iliohypogastric nerve

Femoral nerve

Genitofemoral nerve
Obiturator nerve
Ulnar nerve

Pudendal nerve

Sciatic nerve

Common peroneal nerve

Muscular branches of femoral nerve
Saphenous nerve

Tibial nerve

Deep peroneal nerve

Superficial peroneal nerve

Key Neurologic Terms

Atherosclerosis: a condition characterized by medium-sized arteries that have developed a layer of plaque that can obstruct the vessel or lead to a blood clot.

Atherosclerotic plaque: an outgrowth in the inner lining of the blood vessel that is composed of cholesterol, dead white blood cells, proteins and eventually calcium. Plaques can block arteries and stiffen their walls.

Central nervous system: a system composed of the brain and spinal cord, where information from the senses is transmitted to the brain, thinking and learning occurs, and control signals of muscles originate.

Chronic: a condition that spans a length of time. The exact criteria depend on the condition, but by definition, months or years (or decades).

Cognition: a term referring to the mental processes involved in gaining knowledge and comprehension. These processes include thinking, knowing, remembering, judging and problem solving.

Dementia: a process in which thinking, memory and the control of behavior erode into what is usually a permanent state of disability. Dementia has various degrees of severity. The disease is progressive but can develop slowly. This is not to be confused with delirium, which is a temporary loss of orientation to place and people and can result in uncontrolled or even violent behavior.

Ischemia: a term referring to the phenomenon in which the blood supply and therefore the oxygen supply to a tissue are interrupted. Ischemic events that last more than a few minutes typically lead to cell death. Ischemic events in the heart are often termed myocardial infarction, and in the brain, stroke (although there are several variants).

Neurology: the diagnosis and treatment of diseases of the nervous system.

Neuroplasticity: the phenomenon whereby the brain can relearn certain skills and remap, or rewrite, information and memories to new areas of the brain. This is related to the ability of the brain to spawn new cells or remodel existing connections — often in the hippocampus, a brain region critical to learning and memory that can actively grow even later in life.

Pathology: the study of the causes, processes and outcomes of disease. Pathology can be directed at the study of cells, the components of cells (such as the nucleus and DNA, or deoxyribonucleic acid), tissues and organs, as well as the effects of disease on overall functions in the body.

Traumatic brain injury: damage to the brain from a physical force, which can lead to loss of or lowered consciousness and long-term changes in personality, mood and cognitive function. It is not a degenerative change in the sense that Alzheimer's disease is, but chronic, progressive issues in thinking and mood can occur that will intensify if not treated.

Impaired Brain Function

The brain is exceedingly complex, and scientists learn more about it all the time. Even relatively small regions of the brain, such as the cerebellum, have distinctive microstructures and functions that are very different from other parts of the brain. When one part of the brain is damaged, there are a number of predictable effects — and some surprising ones.

Aging and Dementia

As the brain ages, various levels of impaired function can result. A dramatic, and unfortunately common, example of impaired function is dementia. In this condition, thinking, memory, mood and learning are all severely affected. Alzheimer's disease is a well-known type of dementia. It robs its victims of the ability to learn and, eventually, erases their most important memories. Isolated healthy pockets of brain tissue may continue to function normally, but the overall cognitive (thinking) power of a person with dementia is greatly reduced.

Mild Cognitive Impairment

A milder but pervasive type of brain aging is also seen in older adults and is often accepted as an inevitable part of life. Physicians call this condition "mild cognitive impairment" and most people think it is a result of the normal aging process.

There are many examples of older individuals who have lost their cognitive abilities but don't suffer from dementia. Learning, reflexes, recall and decision making can slow down measurably in the time between our early twenties and our early fifties. Young people have a definite speed advantage — just watch them at play and you will see that they are at their peak physical and mental ability.

However, scientists have also proven, by examining both case histories and research results, that people can maintain their mental speed as they age. In fact, people can compensate for slight declines in mental speed with greater efficiency in thinking, experience or wisdom. Unfortunately, many older people do not take action to help their brains maintain peak performance. This is often understandable: people who are ill and in pain may find it difficult to engage in activities that would enrich their learning, and people with mobility issues or who are socially isolated may lack the stimulation we all need. However, the lack of brain stimulation almost guarantees that they will begin to see their mental acuity decline — even if they don't have a progressive illness such as Alzheimer's disease.

Premature Aging

Many things can contribute to premature aging, including premature aging of the brain. One powerful factor is nutritional status, or making sure your body gets the nutrients it needs. The repair and regeneration of our cells depends on having the right building blocks at hand.

FAQ

Q. *What are the best age-fighting nutrients?*

A. To help maintain brain function, you need the right components in your diet. In this case, that means consuming the right proteins, fatty acids, vitamins and minerals to support the greatest possible amount of repair to aging cells. In addition to these essentials (plus carbohydrates, which your body also needs), a variety of health-enhancing compounds found in plant foods, such as bioflavonoids, enhance brain health.

Did You Know?

Free Radicals

Electrons help form chemical bonds between atoms. A free radical is a compound that is trying to take an electron from, or give an electron to, another molecule. When an electron is ripped away from a molecule, such as a protein, by a reactive free radical, it damages the donor molecule. Certain forms of oxygen are well-known free radicals.

The Dangers of Free Radicals

When your nutrient intake is good enough to keep you alive but is not optimal, the body can be more susceptible to the damage that everyday life dishes out. Free radicals are a common example that is easy to understand (see box, at left).

Our cells and their components, including our genes, are susceptible to free-radical damage. This phenomenon is known as oxidative stress, and it's a fact of life. The power plants in our cells, called the mitochondria, use oxygen to generate energy, and some "collateral damage" is expected as a result.

Fighting Free Radicals

The good news is that the body makes powerful enzymes that act as shields against free radicals. These enzymes can actually break some of them down and render them relatively harmless. Vitamin C and many plant-based compounds also act as sacrificial molecules that "soak up" free radicals and prevent damage. When you are nutritionally depleted and/or under assault by free-radical generators (see box, below), oxidative stress can run rampant in the body.

Free-Radical Generators

Free radicals are naturally present in cells. But some behaviors and environmental factors can deliver extra free-radical compounds to the body. These compounds make biochemical demands on the body and cause cellular damage. Some examples are:

- Smoking — this hits the vascular system and lung tissue hard and depletes the body's stores of antioxidants, such as vitamin C
- Air pollution
- Toxins in food and water
- Some medications, in excess
- Burnt food, including grilled food

Stress and Aging

Stress is another factor that can accelerate aging. Stress is actually the body's natural reaction to life events. Most people are familiar with the acute stress response — commonly called the fight-or-flight response. When something startles or endangers you, your body kicks into high gear. Blood rushes to your muscles to enable a quick getaway or a fight, your reflexes quicken and your heart rate soars.

What many people don't realize is that when this initial excitement wears off, the body is supposed to return to a state of normal balance. And that can definitely be the case if the stressor (the event that encourages the fight-or-flight response) doesn't last. After all, being chased by a wild animal or having a near miss on the highway is a temporary event.

Chronic Stress

Dr. Hans Selye, the great scientist and "father" of stress research who developed his theories in the first half of the 20th century, found that human bodies make larger amounts of the hormone cortisol when they experience prolonged stress. Modern scientific

Human bodies make larger amounts of the hormone cortisol when they experience prolonged stress.

studies have reinforced that fact over and over again. As a result of excess cortisol, the immune system weakens, digestion slows down and blood pressure goes up. In the long term, stress stops being adaptive and starts hurting us.

A little stress is good; in fact, life should challenge us. But prolonged, unrelenting stress, such as staying in situations where we feel trapped, can poison our bodies with stress hormones, which leads to premature aging.

Although we can't always easily change our circumstances, there are many things we can do to alter our stress response. Techniques such as mindfulness and mind–body relaxation can alter both our physical state and our mental state. Spending time with friends or family and exposure to natural settings can help restore our feelings of well-being. In some cases, direct interventions by a psychologist or psychotherapist, such as cognitive behavioral therapy, can help us rewrite our perception of events — to learn new responses to our challenges.

Use It or Lose It

If you spend decades doing the same work, pursuing the same hobbies and visiting the same places without learning anything new, your brain can lose its capacity to learn the way it once could.

The old adage "If you don't use it, you'll lose it" is particularly true in relation to the brain. When you don't exercise or challenge this vital organ, the effects of time and aging can overtake you quickly. Problem solving, processing speed and thinking can all go downhill.

Another pitfall is repeating your usual behavior patterns. The brain is good at learning and replaying the same recorded behaviors over and over. This makes people efficient at things like driving a car or performing routine tasks. But if you spend decades doing the same work, pursuing the same hobbies and visiting the same places without learning anything new, your brain can lose its capacity to learn the way it once could.

Neuroplasticity

Neuroplasticity is the brain's ability to change, adapt and remodel in response to needs. An excellent example of this is when a person loses brain tissue as the result of a stroke but learns to walk again. Amazingly, with the help of therapy, other parts of the brain can learn to control the act of walking. Neuroplasticity is also the reason why the hippocampus — a small area in the center of the brain that controls new memories, associations and learning — can actually regenerate if you stimulate it enough.

New Cells, Better Function

Fortunately, the human brain has an amazing ability to create new connections. For some time, scientists believed that people developed a finite number of brain cells by the end of childhood, then lost them slowly over time. The story went that, in old age, our cells diminished and our fate was to become mentally weaker. We certainly could not reset the clock and grow new brain cells. But modern studies have shown that this is exactly what can happen. There are limits to our regrowth potential, but people can and do forge new brain cells later in life.

There are limits to our regrowth potential, but people can and do forge new brain cells later in life.

FAQ

Q. *How can I encourage my brain to make new connections?*

A. Creating new brain cells requires several factors working together. First, healthy blood circulation and proper nutrition are paramount. Second, the brain can't be under attack by any aggressive and/or progressive disease. Third, you can't repeat yesterday's patterns. You must learn new things in order to keep the brain active later in life. That means learning new concepts as well as having novel experiences. The brain needs to be needed — to stay healthy, it must have new connections to work out in response to new information.

Lifestyle Changes

Physical, mental and emotional determinants of health need to be addressed in order to build new connections in your brain. Good-quality sleep is a must to spur neuroplasticity. Enjoyable social interactions are necessary, too — very few people thrive as hermits. Movement and exercise also play a role because they not only feel good but also encourage the brain to release growth factors, such as brain-derived neurotrophic factor (BDNT). "Neurotropic" literally means "brain-nourishing." These spur new connections and "wiring" between brain cells, which can stimulate the growth of new cells.

Stay Active

People who stay busy and engaged can remain productive and amazingly resilient into their nineties.

While aging is to some degree inevitable, it does not have to be what we think of as "normal" aging in our society (in other words, loss of brain function). Active seniors can maintain their youthful zeal and mental sharpness by simply staying busy and feeling needed in retirement. These people never really "retire" or withdraw from life.

Any stimulating and fulfilling work that keeps the mind engaged to an older age is beneficial; some professions tend to see people working into their eighties and beyond. Politicians, artists, scientists, actors and professors are common examples of people able to maintain active mental lives in their disciplines — especially when the physical demands of their work are not intense and they simply keep going beyond the average retirement age. People who stay busy and engaged can remain productive and amazingly resilient into their nineties.

Multiple Intelligences

The concept of multiple intelligences is a useful one to consider in the context of brain health. The renowned psychologist Howard Gardner developed the theory that intelligence is not just a single entity but rather the sum of a number of different areas of intelligence. He originally proposed seven such categories and others have since been added, though the general concept is still credited to Dr. Gardner.

Linguistic and mathematical intelligences are different from kinesthetic intelligence (which involves movement, physical

Type of Intelligence	Example
Bodily/kinesthetic	Executing a complicated gymnastics maneuver
Interpersonal	Understanding someone else's point of view and their emotional reaction to a situation
Intrapersonal	Gaining insight into why you feel a certain way about a situation
Logical/mathematical	Solving a mathematical equation
Musical/rhythmic	Composing a song
Verbal/linguistic	Articulating your thoughts clearly
Visual/spatial	Figuring out directions to a destination

coordination and strength) and social intelligence (being "people savvy"). We are all endowed with varying degrees of these intelligences, which work together to help us solve life's problems. We are all intelligent in different ways and develop these aspects of our minds differently, based on our interests and the activities we choose to pursue.

The table on page 26 illustrates seven examples of the types of tasks multiple intelligences can help you perform.

Building Mental Strengths

The idea of multiple intelligences is important when creating a brain fitness program. By assessing your strengths and weaknesses (see box, at right), you can go out of your way to do exercises — mental or otherwise — that build up brain capacity in areas where you are not as naturally astute. By extending and expanding your intelligences, you spur the development of neuroplasticity and stave off aging.

How Exercises Boost Brain Power

Sometimes as you age, you start to impose limitations on yourself. You might say, "It's too late to learn a new language." You might also make it an all-or-nothing proposition, saying, "I can't go back to college and do it all over again." Fortunately, learning doesn't have to be that complicated and time-intensive. It is really about using your brain and assigning yourself new tasks and challenges. By doing this and stretching your intelligence, you'll stay quick. There are so many ways to work out your brain, and all you need is willingness and a plan.

Learning doesn't have to be that complicated and time-intensive. It is really about using your brain and assigning yourself new tasks and challenges.

We Can Rebuild It

Remember *The Six Million Dollar Man*, played with steely determination by Lee Majors? With the help of 1970s TV show technology, he was rebuilt and could perform "better, stronger, faster!" Sometimes we wish we could do that mentally to combat that slow feeling that can develop as we age. It can feel like we are searching through an enormous attic filled with memories and experiences, while younger people see things in a less convoluted way.

It's true that the brain's processing speed can slow down as we age. Both biological and structural issues can cause this to happen. But it can also occur if we settle into years of the same routines, work and pastimes. We may be quick and efficient at those particular things, but we are not giving our brains a proper workout when we replay mental scripts that we have rehearsed for decades.

FAQ

Q. *Why are new routines important for healthy brain function?*

A. The ability to execute rehearsed mental functions is important. We need to be efficient at routine tasks and make difficult or complicated ones second nature to achieve success in many areas of life — our skills as drivers, cooks, cleaners and employees depend on this. However, life inevitably presents challenges to us, in the form of new information, new situations or unusual configurations of familiar situations. Without this new input, our brains stagnate. In order to keep up with this new input from our environment, we have to be able to think fast enough. Challenging our mental capacity with new routines ensures we will be able to continue adapting to new information.

Did You Know?

Filtering Information

The brain screens incoming information and ignores what is unnecessary. For example, if you are sitting in the food court at a busy mall, your brain will not attempt to process every one of the many conversations happening around you. But the brain will focus on important information if it comes up. Imagine you're still in the food court but someone says, "They just robbed the jewelry store." Your brain will likely orient itself toward that conversation.

Stimulating Growth

What are we doing when we exercise the brain? To answer this question, we have to look at psychology and learning theory and understand how the brain responds to incoming information.

Automatic Responses

New information arrives in the brain as sensory input. For example, you hear someone say your name and ask a question. The region of the brain responsible for auditory information must process this, then route the message to an area of the brain that controls higher reasoning.

Once your brain has registered and processed incoming information, it may trigger an automatic response. For example, imagine you live around the corner from a popular tourist attraction. For the hundredth time, someone pulls up beside you and asks for directions to the attraction's parking lot. Your mind (and your mouth) automatically spits out the answer, like a reflex: "Just go down the street, turn right at the light and the entrance is on your right." Many of the answers we give people at our jobs fall into this category, such as "That warranty is only for parts, not labor, sir" or "We offer that course only in the spring semester."

Processing New Data

Things change when the brain encounters a novel situation or when incoming stimuli do not "play the tape" associated with some previously learned skill or behavior. In this case, the issue is routed to the brain's higher learning and thinking centers. The executive parts of our brain — the forebrain and, specifically, the prefrontal cortex — have to decide how to respond.

New information may come in the form of a mental task that requires us to think spatially and tap into our visual processing. A good example of this is when you have to give directions in an area that's not as familiar as your own street. You need to think through the landmarks and the layout of the neighborhood, so the process is not as effortless as directing someone in a place you see every day. Alternatively, new information may require the brain to search through long-term memories. Or it may require auditory processing, such as saying the name of a place you have previously learned.

Short-Term Memory

Short-term memory also plays a role in dealing with new information. Certain operations require you to hold new information, such as a telephone number, in your immediate consciousness. For example, think of the last time you asked someone for a telephone number. If you did not write it down immediately, you probably had to repeat it to yourself until you dialed it.

We also have a type of short-term sensory memory that allows us to recall images, sounds or sensations that we experienced seconds before.

FAQ

Q. Will frequent mental workouts really boost my brain's agility?

A. Yes! The more you work out the task-oriented areas of your brain and the connections between them, the fitter they will become. To build them up, you need regular exposure to challenging tasks and novel situations. These force you to use your brain to a higher capacity than you would if you relied on previously learned strategies. Remember, however, that too much exercise can be just as problematic as too little. Overtraining, especially by performing repetitive exercises on a computer or smartphone, provides diminishing returns.

Creating a Brain Exercise Routine

Dividing brain exercises into categories, such as sensory processing or motor learning, helps you stimulate different types of brain function. Start by choosing a variety of exercises from several categories. This type of holistic approach works because the various parts and functions of the brain are interdependent.

Think of your routine as similar to one you would follow when working out at a gym. You wouldn't want to strengthen only your arms and end up with weak legs that can't support you when you lift heavy objects. Similarly, having well-developed leg muscles won't make you a good runner unless your cardio-vascular and pulmonary systems are in top shape, too. You need a variety of exercises to strengthen all areas over time.

FAQ

Q. *Don't these exercises overlap a bit?*

A. Yes, there are somewhat arbitrary distinctions between the different exercise categories. In everyday life, the brain uses multiple pathways to process information and create action. For example, using muscles requires a great deal of sensory input. Similarly, the brain's visual and language systems are closely linked because words on a page or screen (or emotions on the face of a person speaking) are combined in the task of using language. Dividing the exercises into categories is helpful for making sure you get a well-rounded workout.

Assessing Areas to Work On

Targeting your exercise program to the areas most in need of improvement is a good strategy. From the following nine areas, pick the two that need the most work and make those exercises your highest priority.

Skills	Category
How fast you think, solving problems	Mental Speed Warm-Up Exercises (page 33)
Directions; noticing things, colors, details in a room or in outfits; remembering what people look like	Visual-Spatial Intelligence Exercises (page 49)
Vocabulary, speaking, language	Language Growth Exercises (page 68) and Language Acquisition Exercises (page 149)
Using information provided by the senses (sight, hearing, touch, taste and smell), recognizing things	Sensory Processing Exercises (page 80)
Coordination, learning new physical skills	Motor Learning Exercises (page 95)
Remembering names, tasks and details	Memory Augmentation Exercises (page 118)
Getting to sleep, falling asleep and having a restful sleep	Sleep and Rest Exercises (page 131)
Moving and building strength, flexibility and good circulation to the brain, heart and the rest of the body	Sports and Recreation Exercises (page 136)
Feeling generally at peace with oneself and others, feeling the ability to create and contribute, and feeling loved and cared for	Social Support and Emotional Health Exercises (page 141)

Start Small

For the first week, begin by doing one or two exercises per category. It may not sound like a lot, but it can feel surprisingly intensive because some of these exercises require quite a bit of new brain activity. Research indicates that practicing a skill repeatedly strengthens it. Persistence (not overtraining) produces results.

Add More

Every week, add two new activities from one of the categories, choosing a different category each week. Try to choose one repetitive activity (such as a game) and one experiential activity (doing something new), if possible. A sample schedule might look like this:

Week 1: Two new Sensory Processing Exercises (page 80)
Week 2: Two new Motor Learning Exercises (page 95)
Week 3: Two new Language Growth Exercises (page 68) or Language Acquisition Exercises (page 149)
Week 4: Two new Mental Speed Warm-Up Exercises (page 33)
Week 5: Two new Visual-Spatial Intelligence Exercises (page 49)

Alternate between the two exercises over the course of the week. For example:

Monday: exercise A
Tuesday: exercise B
Wednesday: exercise A
Thursday: exercise B

Friday: exercise A
Saturday: exercise B
Sunday: day off

Once you have built up a reasonable set of exercises, practice them for a few weeks, then switch them up. Every few weeks, switch them up again. Practice may make perfect, but the point is not just to score well in these exercises but to keep the brain out of a dull routine.

Track Your Progress

Consider doing a self-evaluation using an online tool about once a month. From time to time, take a month off from a particular category of brain training, then do an evaluation. It will tell you if you have consolidated the gains you have made, and whether your exercise regimen is providing long-term improvements.

Sometimes an evaluation may reveal that you have become good at doing a specific activity without really improving the underlying brain function. For example, you might perform well during a specific memory exercise or game but still be forgetful in most areas of your life. This is a critical issue for all brain training. But don't be discouraged — keep working at it. It is reasonable to modify your activities and use the ones that yield the best results. Remember that performing a variety of mental workouts and having real, not just simulated, experiences is the best strategy.

Part 2
Brain Strength Training Exercises

. . . .

Mental Speed Warm-Up Exercises

Mental speed is a difficult thing to measure, although that's exactly what some scientists do. In general, the speed at which our brains process information and make decisions speeds up from childhood to adulthood and then holds steady until late middle age. At that point, it typically begins to decline, but how rapidly and how greatly varies among individuals.

Exercise 1: Count Quickly

Step 1
Examine the diagram at right. Count the happy and annoyed faces as quickly as you can.

Step 2
Examine the diagram again. How many of the faces are noticeably larger than the others?

Step 3
Examine the diagram again. Of those larger faces, how many of them are happy and how many are annoyed?

What does this exercise accomplish?
You are being asked to process two different types of visual information and make comparisons (size and emotional expression). This requires processing based on geometry but also interpretation of the expressions. You are creating subcategories by counting happy versus annoyed faces within the "noticeably larger" category of faces.

To work quickly, the brain must operate and coordinate various subcenters, which it is quite good at. Engaging in activities that help us balance these different brain activities can support some aspects of mental speed. But there are other factors, too, such as the health of our brain's circulation and the amount of gray matter (neurons) and white matter (the connectors that neurons send out to touch each other) in the brain. That's why physical health and good nutrition are also key.

Exercise 2: Mental Math

Step 1

While shopping for groceries, look at the price of two similar products and compare the amount (weight or volume) or count of the contents listed on the packaging.

Step 2

See how quickly you can mentally calculate the unit cost for each product (cost divided by amount or count).

Step 3

Check your work. Does your calculation match the product's unit cost, which is included on the product's price tag on the shelf (it appears in a smaller font than the price)? No cheating! Look at the products and the large-font prices first — and ignore the unit cost. (Step back if you need to, to make the smaller font harder to see.)

Bring a small pad of paper and a pen or golf pencil with you to record your answer. If someone can time you, that's even better. If you are repeating this exercise three times a week, it is a good excuse to buy fresh produce that will provide nutrients that support the brain.

What does this exercise accomplish?

This mental arithmetic exercise is simple but important, because many of us have no need to do these calculations on a daily basis — and when we do, we usually pull out our smartphones and use the calculator. Using a calculator allows our arithmetic skills to weaken. Doing this exercise will strengthen your math skills.

Exercise 3: Sort Different Types

Step 1

While you're out of the room, have an assistant remove two items from each of five types of canned or packaged food (soups, canned fruit, etc.) from your pantry, then mix up the 10 packages and set them out on a table for you.

Step 2

Come into the room and sort the foods into pairs by type while your assistant times you.

What does this exercise accomplish?

You are strengthening your ability to categorize similar objects by physically sorting them under time pressure.

Exercise 4: Spell Backward

Step 1

Listen carefully as an assistant says a name out loud to you (for example, the name of a well-known celebrity or politician).

Step 2

Spell the first name and last name of the person backward, out loud, while your assistant times you. (If you would rather do this exercise on your own, look at the first full name you recognize in a news story online or in the paper. Look away and spell it backward, out loud, while you time yourself.)

What does this exercise accomplish?

When you do this exercise, you must first recall the name, then use your auditory memory to spell it backward. If you have mentally pictured the name spelled out, then you are using your visual memory, too.

Exercise 5: Interpret Instructions

Step 1

Pick an electronic device (such as a DVD player, a smartphone or a digital audio player) that has a function you have never learned to use. This might be an automated recording feature or a way to change the appearance of the screen.

Step 2

Find the instructions for turning on and using this function — they can be written in a print or electronic manual or embedded in the Help menu on the device.

Step 3

Carefully read the instructions through once.

Step 4

Go back and reread the instructions. This time, visualize what you are going to do, step by step.

Step 5

Go back and reread the instructions a third time, this time just skimming them and relying on your mental image of what you need to do. If you like, use your hands to rehearse the movements.

Step 6

Perform the task using your mental step-by-step picture. Refer to the instructions only if you need to.

What does this exercise accomplish?

This is not a memory test or even a speed test. This exercise works your brain by having you process sensory inputs and create a mental model based on them. You then turn this model into physical actions. You are interpreting written words, using your short-term memory and processing the information in the instructions.

Exercise 6: Name That Color

Step 1

Create a chart with five columns and five rows. You can create one using a computer and printer, or just draw it on paper using pens or markers. If an assistant can prepare this exercise for you, even better.

Step 2

Write the name of a color (pink, orange, blue, red, etc.) in each square of the chart. For most of the names, write the word in a different color than it says; for example, write the word "orange" in blue.

Step 3

Put the chart away for two weeks without looking at it.

Step 4

Look at the chart. As quickly as you can, say the *colors* you see, not the words that are written.

What does this exercise accomplish?

In this game, the brain's executive function must override very rapid messages from its visual center. We recognize words by sight all the time, such as on signs — Stop, Caution, Sale or Open House, for example. When you see the word "blue," you will want to say that word quickly. In order to say the color the word is written in, rather than the word itself, you must perceive the color and identify the name of it before your higher thinking centers can override your impulse to say the word as spelled.

pink				

Exercise 7: Do a Perceptual Sort

Step 1

Choose a room in your house that you can be alone in. Take a good look around for 10 minutes.

Step 2

Leave the room. Stay out of visual and auditory range so that you can't see or hear what is happening in the room.

Step 3

Have an assistant move 10 objects in the room. The changes should be obvious enough that you can see them easily (you won't notice that a lamp was moved $\frac{1}{2}$ inch/1 cm). Have the assistant call you back into the room when done.

Step 4

Note the changes, giving yourself about five minutes to find them all. You can look randomly around the room or divide the room into sections and examine them one by one. Alternatively, you can divide the room by category of object (such as floors, walls, furniture, lamps, art, tables, cabinets or books) and examine each to see what has changed.

What does this exercise accomplish?

By searching for changes, you are comparing sensory information against a mental map you have of the room. This exercise challenges both memory and mental processing speed, two functions that are naturally related.

1. ....

2. ....

3. ....

4. ....

5. ....

6. ....

7. ....

8. ....

9. ....

10. ....

Exercise 8: Reason and Visualize

Step 1

Time yourself as you unravel this brainteaser. Your sock drawer contains **24 white socks** and **30 black socks**. The lights in your room are off, so you cannot see the color of the socks. What is the minimum number of socks you must grab to ensure that you have one matching pair?

....

Step 2

Check your solution in the answer key (page 48).

What does this exercise accomplish?

By imagining the outcome of this puzzle, you must visualize the socks and use reasoning to come to the correct conclusion.

Exercise 9: Add It Up

Step 1

Do the following calculation in your head (without using a pen and paper or a calculator):

Start with 500.
Add 50.
Add 550.
Add 150.
Add 1000.
Add 75.
Add 275.
Add 25.

=
....

Step 2

Write down your answer.

Step 3

Check your solution in the answer key (page 48).

What does this exercise accomplish?

You are doing simple addition but you have to maintain your concentration and use your short-term memory to avoid simple errors at each step.

Exercise 10: Perspective #1

Step 1

Examine the illustration below.

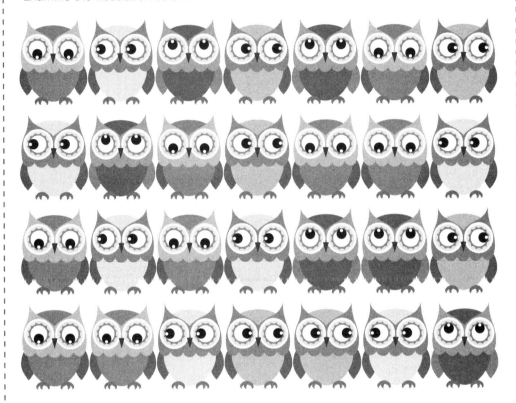

Step 2

From left to right, top to bottom, call out the direction the eyes are looking from *your* perspective (down, up, left or right) while an assistant times you.

Step 3

Repeat the exercise until you can do it in 30 seconds without any errors.

Step 4

Keep practicing until you can do it in 15 seconds without any errors.

What does this exercise accomplish?

This exercise requires rapid processing of visual information, followed by determination of the spatial orientation of the eyes in the picture, leading to a verbal expression ("down," "up," etc.). This links the thinking involved in visual and spatial interpretation with verbal expression.

Exercise 11: Perspective #2

Step 1

Examine the illustration below.

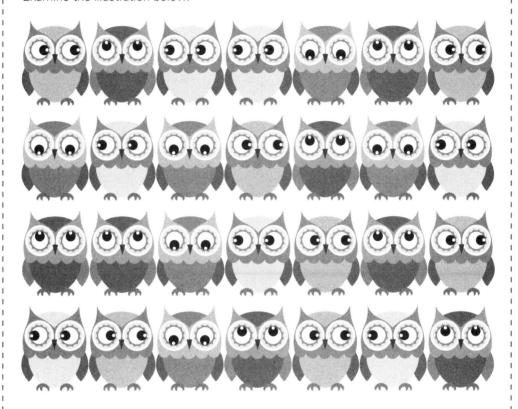

Step 2

From left to right, top to bottom, call out the direction the eyes are looking from *the owls'* perspective (down, up, left or right) while an assistant times you.

Step 3

Repeat the exercise until you can do it in 30 seconds without any errors.

Step 4

Keep practicing until you can do it in 15 seconds without any errors.

What does this exercise accomplish?

As with Exercise 10: Perspective #1, this exercise requires rapid processing of visual information, followed by determination of the spatial orientation of the eyes in the picture, leading to a verbal expression. This links the thinking involved in visual and spatial interpretation with verbal expression. In this case, you must shift your point of view and put yourself in the place of the owls in the illustration, which means your brain must rotate the image.

Exercise 12: Perspective #3

Step 1

Examine the illustration below.

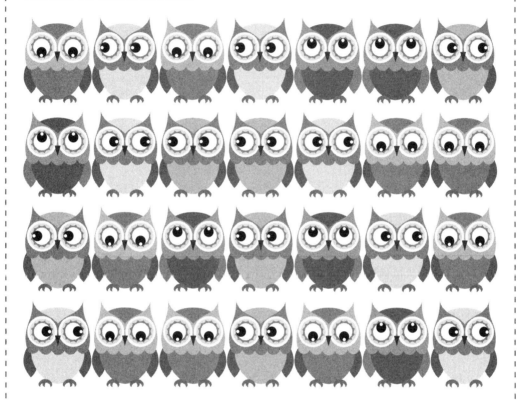

Step 2

From left to right, top to bottom, call out the direction the eyes are looking from *your* perspective (down, up, left or right) while pointing in the opposite direction (for example, say "down" while pointing up). Have an assistant time you.

Step 3

Repeat the exercise until you can do it in 30 seconds without any errors.

Step 4

Keep practicing until you can do it in 15 seconds without any errors.

What does this exercise accomplish?

This exercise is similar to Exercise 10: Perspective #1, but it adds a psychomotor component. It requires you to think twice about the visual and spatial information you have gathered, then physically express this information through pointing.

Exercise 13: Read Slowly

Step 1

Read the following text carefully:

Can you find the the mistake?
1 2 3 4 5 6 7 8 9

Step 2

Write down your answer.

....

Step 3

Check your solution in the answer key (page 48).

What does this exercise accomplish?

This exercise is about slowing down and thinking about each of the words and numbers you see. The brain tends to read ahead, filling in or omitting repeated items so that the writing makes sense.

Exercise 14: Try a New Scent

Step 1

Next time you go to work (whether it's in an office or at home), take along a bottle of a pleasant-smelling essential oil or botanical extract (such as lavender, vanilla or citrus).

Step 2

Choose a repetitive daily task that you do without a lot of thought (such as filing, reading a standard report or folding laundry). The best timing for this exercise is during some routine part of your day. Just before starting the task, take out the essential oil and inhale the scent deeply.

Step 3

Focus on the scent as you perform the task. Bring your attention fully to what you are experiencing. If you are not reading, closing your eyes may help you concentrate.

What does this exercise accomplish?

Repetitive tasks require little thought. With new sensory input from the scent, you wake up your brain.

Exercise 15: Opposite Writing #1

Step 1

Place a pen and a piece of paper on a table in front of you.

Step 2

If you usually write with your right hand, pick up the pen with your left hand (or vice versa).

Step 3

Write five words that you know how to spell correctly.

What does this exercise accomplish?

By using your nondominant hand to write, you engage the motor cortex on the opposite side of your brain from the one you usually use. At the same time, your brain also processes visual information as you read and coordinates your hand movements. Writing a word that you already know how to spell ensures that your brain activity will flip to the opposite side.

Exercise 16: Opposite Writing #2

Step 1

Place a pen and a piece of paper on a table in front of you.

Step 2

Close your eyes. If you usually write with your right hand, pick up the pen with your left hand (or vice versa).

Step 3

Keeping your eyes closed, write five words that you know how to spell correctly.

What does this exercise accomplish?

This exercise achieves many of the same outcomes as Exercise 15: Opposite Writing #1, but your brain also has to use information from your fingers and hand to guide them in making letter shapes without visual cues.

Exercise 17: Memory Game #1

Step 1

Open two decks of cards and create pairs of identical cards (such as both aces of clubs, etc.).

Step 2

Remove four of the pairs that you've made and arrange the eight cards randomly on a table, face up.

Step 3

Flip the cards over so they are face down.

Step 4

Flip over one random card, then immediately try to find its match, one card at a time.

Step 5

Continue to turn over identical pairs, seeing how many you can do without making a mistake. If you turn over the wrong card, turn it face down again and continue trying to find the match for the original card.

What does this exercise accomplish?

This simple exercise builds your very short-term memory, or "working" memory. Good observation of the flipped card helps to solidify the short-term memory.

Exercise 18: Memory Game #2

Step 1

Open two decks of cards and create pairs of identical cards (such as both aces of clubs, etc.).

Step 2

Remove five of the pairs that you've made and arrange the ten cards randomly on a table, face up.

Step 3

Flip the cards over so they are face down.

Step 4

Flip over one random card, then immediately try to find its match, one card at a time.

Step 5

Continue to turn over identical pairs, seeing how many you can do without making a mistake. If you turn over the wrong card, turn it face down again and continue trying to find the match for the original card.

Step 6

Continue to add more pairs of cards to this exercise as your proficiency increases.

What does this exercise accomplish?

Much like Exercise 17: Memory Game #1, this exercise helps work your short-term memory.

Exercise 19: Memory Game #3

Step 1

Open two decks of cards and create pairs of identical cards (such as both aces of clubs, etc.).

Step 2

Remove five of the pairs that you've made and arrange the ten cards randomly on a table, face up.

Step 3

Flip the cards over so they are face down.

Step 4

Walk away from the table and let five minutes pass.

Step 5

Flip over one random card, then immediately try to find its match, one card at a time.

Step 6

Continue to turn over identical pairs, seeing how many you can do without making a mistake. If you turn over the wrong card, turn it face down again and continue trying to find the match for the original card.

Step 7

Continue to add more pairs of cards and add more time away in Step 4 as your proficiency increases.

What does this exercise accomplish?

This exercise requires you to rely more on your longer-term, rather than short-term, memory.

Exercise 20: Organize Your Work Space

Step 1
Go to the place where you accomplish work, be it your actual place of employment or a room in your house where records are kept and bills are paid.

Step 2
Make a list of the basic tasks that go on in this area.

....

....

....

....

Step 3
Categorize the various surfaces, drawers and objects in the area: what tasks do they support? Some, such as the phone, will support all. Others, such as a calculator, are for specific functions.

Step 4
Assess how readily you can find something when you need it. Does your filing cabinet and/or computer filing system need an overhaul? If so, create a simple system that will help you find documents easily. You can apply the same organization principles to files and folders on a computer as in a paper filing system. Create a logical hierarchy of files within smaller folders within larger folders and/or drawers. For example, a drawer might be for "Household Business"; a large hanging folder might say "Mortgage"; and smaller folders might hold "Payment History" and "Original Mortgage Agreement."

Step 5
Clear your work area. Organize or file the items that are lying around, and minimize any clutter.

What does this exercise accomplish?
This exercise creates a physical and structural environment that helps your brain group tasks and process them in an efficient manner. It's important to create a work environment that feels natural, or "user-friendly," but one that is also somewhat neat and orderly. Keep it simple — if you can't figure out where an invoice or memo should go when you are not busy, it will be hard to find it when you are!

Mental Speed Warm-Up Exercises Answer Key

Exercise 8: Reason and Visualize (page 39)

Three. You could be lucky and make a match with the first two socks. But if the first two socks you grab do not match (one is black and the other is white), then the next sock you take out is guaranteed to pair up with one or the other.

Exercise 9: Add It Up (page 39)

2625.

Exercise 13: Read Slowly (page 43)

The word "the" appears twice in the sentence.

Visual-Spatial Intelligence Exercises

These exercises focus more intensively on the use of visual-spatial intelligence, which requires your brain to make sense of visual perception inputs and also requires action on those images. One recurring skill that is used in many visual-spatial operations (as exercises or in real life) is rotating an image — imagining it in three different dimensional positions. A certain amount of memory may also be involved regarding structures, rotations or more complex routes (such as following directions). Some people seem to be naturally adept at this; others find such tasks very confusing. If you are in the latter category, this is probably a good area to practice.

Exercise 1: Which Way?

Step 1

Examine the diagram at right. Reading from left to right, top to bottom, name the direction in which each arrow is pointing while an assistant times you.

Step 2

Repeat the exercise until you can do it in 30 seconds with no more than one error.

What does this exercise accomplish?

This exercise requires rapid processing of visual information with the added step of turning that information into a verbal expression (stating the direction out loud).

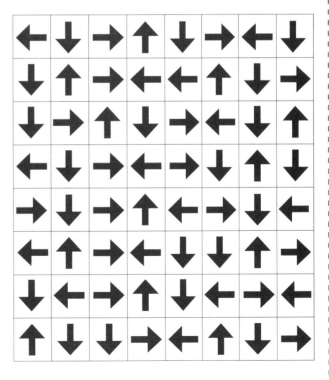

Exercise 2: Tic-Tac-Toe

Step 1

Draw an empty three-by-three grid on a piece of paper.

Step 2

With an opponent, take turns playing tic-tac-toe. Instead of the traditional x's and o's, use either b's and d's, or p's and q's, to mark the squares (see example, below). If one player writes the wrong letter (in other words, the opponent's letter), the opponent gets to keep that square. No changing!

What does this exercise accomplish?

Like traditional tic-tac-toe with x's and o's, this game requires you to visualize potential moves that you or your opponent could make — in other words, you are visualizing a potential pattern. Using letters other than x and o helps make this a little more novel for those who have played tic-tac-toe before and may be able to play without really having to think (which defeats the purpose here).

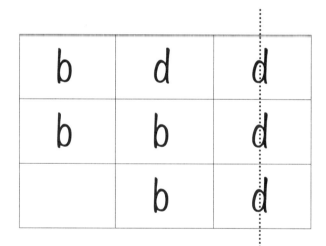

Exercise 3: Map Recall

Step 1

Study a printed map closely.

Step 2

Have an assistant cover up one of the street names on the map. See if you can recall it.

Step 3

Study the map again.

Step 4

Choose a starting point and an ending point on the map. Pick an unfamiliar but safe and navigable part of town. Write out the directions on a piece of paper.

Step 5

Study the directions carefully.

Step 6

Put away the directions in your wallet or bag.

Step 7

Go to your starting point and start making your way toward your ending point without referring to the map or your directions.

Step 8

When you reach your destination or start to feel lost, take out the map and your directions. (If you are driving or riding a bike, pull over to a safe place first.) Did you get to your destination? If so, did you get there by following your directions, or did you wind up taking a different route? If you didn't reach your destination, how close are you?

Step 9

As you improve at this task, create routes that have more turns and more complex directions.

Caution

If this exercise causes confusion while driving or makes you feel unsafe or anxious, skip it. Nothing is more important than road safety. Choose safety over being right when doing this activity — if you need to turn in a different direction than you planned because it's the safe, legal or defensive thing to do, do so.

What does this exercise accomplish?

This activity requires memorization of the layout of the map and an understanding of the directions. As you travel along your route, you must process incoming visual information and relate it to the image of the terrain that was imprinted on your brain while you studied the route. Depending on the number of turns it takes to reach your destination, the use of rotational thinking might also be important here.

Exercise 4: Read with One Eye

Step 1

Choose a piece of reading material. Have a friend assist you by being the audience.

Step 2

Cover up one eye and read a paragraph aloud.

Step 3

Explain to your assistant the essence of what you have just read.

What does this exercise accomplish?

This exercise involves standard reading comprehension but adds the challenge of visual input coming from only one eye. The change in perspective that occurs for those who have two healthy eyes can be quite dramatic. The change from binocular to monocular vision requires your brain to adapt and, in a sense, do two things at the same time.

Exercise 5: Rotation Task

Step 1

Visit www.cambridgebrainsciences.com/play/rotation-task.

Step 2

Read or watch the video instructions for the test.

Step 3

Take the test. Practice rotating one of the images in your mind and note the orientation of some of the squares in relation to those in the other image. Compare the two: if you rotate the first one, does it look like the second one?

What does this exercise accomplish?

A lot of very complex things are happening in your brain when you do this exercise. The part of your brain that manipulates mental imagery of new visual sensory input has to work hard. The brain searches for angles and "sidedness" of objects.

Exercise 6: Pick a Color

Step 1

Assemble the materials you'll need for this exercise. You need fresh grapes and multicolored plastic sword-shaped picks (the kind used to skewer fruit in cocktails).

Step 2

Insert three different-colored picks into one grape, making sure they radiate outward at roughly the same angle. (The picks should look like a tripod the grape can stand on.) Insert a fourth pick, in a different color from the other three, through the top of the grape.

Step 3

Pick up the grape with the picks in it. Examine the configuration of the picks closely.

Step 4

Repeat Steps 1 through 3 with a fresh grape and new picks. Place the picks in a different color order than you did with the first grape.

What does this exercise accomplish?

This activity helps your brain understand chirality, or handedness. This involves perceiving and understanding the 3-D orientation of the colored picks around the central object.

Exercise 7: Make a Pizza

Step 1

Assemble the ingredients you'll need for this exercise. You need one prebaked pizza crust (or a homemade one, if you prefer), 2 cups (500 mL) shredded mozzarella cheese, 1 cup (250 mL) prepared pizza sauce, 8 circular slices pepperoni, 8 thin round slices carrot, 8 strips green bell pepper and 8 pitted black olives. (You can substitute other toppings, but they should be roughly similar in shape and size.)

Step 2

Arrange the crust on a pizza pan or baking sheet and place it in front of you on a table. Sit down in front of it, with the toppings at hand. Remain seated for the rest of the exercise.

Step 3

Spread the sauce on the crust.

Step 4

Sprinkle the cheese evenly over the sauce.

Step 5

Visualize the pizza cut into eight slices. Mentally make one vertical cut and one horizontal cut, then two diagonal cuts to create the eight slices. Don't cut the pizza yet! Just imagine it.

Step 6

Imagine placing one each of the pepperoni slices, carrot slices, pepper strips and olives on the first slice at the top of the pizza. (If the pizza were a clock, you would place the ingredients on the slice at 12 o'clock.)

Step 7

Repeat Step 6, mentally moving counterclockwise to the next slice. Imagine each topping in the same place on that slice as it was on the previous one.

Step 8

Repeat Step 7 until you complete all eight slices.

Step 9

Mentally observe your pizza. Are the slices roughly symmetrical and similar in size?

Step 10

Mentally observe your pizza again. Are the toppings in the same configuration for each slice?

Step 11

Finish assembling the pizza in front of you and bake it according to the package directions on the crust until it's golden and the cheese is bubbly. Enjoy eating the results.

What does this exercise accomplish?

This activity asks you to form a mental image of the slices and to arrange toppings in a certain spatial configuration. Because you are seated in one position during the exercise, you will find that the slice closest to you (at the 6 o'clock position) is the hardest to make. This is an example of how rotation, which seems simple in theory, can be rather taxing for some of us!

Did You Know?

Video Games for the Brain

Echochrome is a fascinating, brain-stimulating game that requires the player to imagine rotating various objects. It is available on Sony PlayStation; for more information, visit www.playstation.com/en-us/games/echochrome-ps3.

Minecraft is also a brain-building game. In this game, the player builds various objects out of blocks. You can choose to make it a visual and geometric game rather than a combat game if you wish. You can access the free demo at https://minecraft.net.

Exercise 8: Pack Your Groceries

Step 1

Shop for some healthy brain foods (see page 160) at a store that hands out large brown paper shopping bags (they should be about 18 inches/45 cm deep). Or bring your own to any grocer. Buy at least two full bags of food, making sure the items are varied in size and shape.

Step 2

When you get home, set the bags on a table.

Step 3

Take the contents of one bag out and place them on the table.

Step 4

Repack the empty bag as efficiently as you can, adding items from another full bag. Try to pack in as much as you can — but no going over the rim of the bag or squishing!

Step 5

Repeat this game when you shop each week, to improve your packing skills. It will not only keep plastic bags out of the environment but will also provide a recurring mental challenge. Eventually you should be able to pack more efficiently than the person bagging items at the store.

What does this exercise accomplish?

When you repack the bag, you use sight and, to a lesser degree, touch to ascertain the size and orientation of objects. Your mental image of the geometry of these things — and your mental image of the capacity and space inside the bag — helps you choose where to position different items. It is a 3-D visual-spatial puzzle.

Exercise 9: Build a Model

Step 1

Go to a hobby store and buy a model to build. Keep it simple, especially if you're not a model-building enthusiast. Pick a shape that interests you, such as a car, train, plane, boat or building.

Step 2

At home, in a quiet place where you can concentrate, set out the model components and adhesive on a work surface.

Caution

If the adhesive emits noxious fumes, make sure you properly ventilate the area, take breaks and take extra vitamin C that day. Stop immediately if you become dizzy, disoriented or nauseated.

Step 3

Following the instructions in the box, build the model. Read each step carefully, put down the instructions, then carry out the step from memory.

What does this exercise accomplish?

You may never have built models before, or you might not have done it since childhood. Either way, your brain takes a written instruction and converts it into a mental image. It then applies the image to the task of making a three-dimensional object. This exercise is more enriching if you visualize each step before you do it.

Exercise 10: Do a Jigsaw Puzzle

Step 1

Lay out the puzzle pieces on a table.

Step 2

Study the picture of the completed puzzle on the front of the box.

Step 3

Find a corner piece (with two adjacent flat edges) and look for adjoining pieces.

Step 4

Complete the outer frame of the puzzle first, then build the interior from that point.

What does this exercise accomplish?

Everyone is familiar with this childhood activity, but it's a terrific workout for spatial memory and reasoning skills. You concurrently use the picture on the box, the shapes of the interlocking pieces and small image details to guide you in putting it all together. Your short-term memory holds the picture of the completed puzzle, and you use your ability to examine close-up details to put the pieces into place so they match this mental picture.

Did You Know?

Free Brain Games

Happy Neuron offers lots of brain-building exercises (the website asks for your email to register, but playing is free). There are a number of visual-spatial games as well as other mind-strengthening activities. Visit www.happy-neuron.com/brain-games/visual-spatial.

Exercise 11: Memorize a Map

Step 1

Choose a map that is detailed and contains country names.

Step 2

Pick a country that you are not familiar with (one that is not surrounded by water).

Step 3

Ask an assistant to time you. For 60 seconds, study the names and positions of the countries to the north, south, east and west of your chosen country.

Step 4

Turn the map over so you can't see it and wait for 60 seconds.

Step 5

On a piece of paper, write down the name of your chosen country and circle it. Assume that north is at the top of the page, above the name you wrote down.

Step 6

Write the names of the surrounding countries in their correct locations around your circled country. An example would look like this:

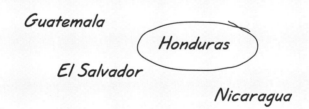

What does this exercise accomplish?

This exercise requires you to process visual information, then understand, recall and express the spatial relationships between the countries you see on the map.

Exercise 12: Map It Out #1

Step 1

With a piece of paper and a pencil in hand, head to a small park or a friend's yard — either should be a place where you don't spend a lot of time. The area should be small enough that you can scan it easily with your eyes.

Step 2

Visually scan the overall terrain.

Step 3

Mentally divide the area into quadrants.

Step 4

Walk all around the area. In each quadrant, observe the landmarks — large trees, picnic tables, swings, flowerbeds and so on — and mentally take note of where they are located. Are they in the center of the quadrant? To one side?

Step 5

Stop walking. Without looking back at the terrain, draw a map of the area on your paper, dividing it into the quadrants you visualized in Step 3. Include as many landmarks in each quadrant as you can.

Step 6

Retrace your steps and refresh your memory.

Step 7

Stop walking. Without looking back at the terrain, add more detail to your map.

Step 8

Repeat Steps 6 and 7 until you think your map is thorough.

Step 9

Walk around the area again, comparing what you see with the map you created. Is your map complete and accurate?

What does this exercise accomplish?

This activity requires a certain amount of memory for visual information, but ultimately it requires you to be observant. Some people can take in a huge amount of information visually (think of an interior designer or home renovation expert); others notice just a few things.

Exercise 13: Map It Out #2

Step 1

With a piece of paper and a pencil beside you, drive to a part of town that is not familiar.

Step 2

Choose a starting point. Begin driving, making four turns (right or left, as you wish). As you drive, take mental note of street names.

Caution

Continue to pay close attention to the road as you drive. Never write notes or draw while you are driving.

Step 3

Pull over and park in a quiet place where you can write.

Step 4

Using your paper and pencil, draw a map of the route you followed from the starting point, including street names and locations where you made turns.

Step 5

Check your work against a printed or online map. Is your map as complete as you thought?

What does this exercise accomplish?

This exercise requires your recall of a series of visual-spatial tasks and experiences. That recall will likely be easier for those with a good sense of direction.

Exercise 14: Describe a Painting

Step 1

Go with an assistant to an art gallery of any size. This exercise is a good excuse to go out with a friend.

Step 2

Find a painting that includes figures or scenes that are easy to describe. Realistic paintings are easier to describe than abstract ones.

Step 3

Study the painting for 30 seconds.

Step 4

Turn your back to the painting. Describe the painting in detail to your assistant.

Step 5

Reexamine the painting.

Step 6

Turn your back to the painting again. Add additional details to your description (such as "the prince is wearing the sword on his right hip").

What does this exercise accomplish?

This activity requires attention to detail and more intense use of visual perception. Art is a way of communicating, and artists include details in a painting for a reason. This is a good way to practice widening your visual perception.

Exercise 15: Spot the Differences

Step 1

With a notebook and pencil in hand, visit a department store that has rows or stacks of shirts produced by several different designers. Men's dress shirts work well for this exercise because they are superficially similar.

Step 2

Choose three different brands so you can compare three different designers. Make sure the brands you choose have more than one style/pattern of shirt.

Step 3

Write the designers' names in your notebook.

Step 4

Examine the first designer's shirts for 30 seconds. Make notes under his or her name about the details of the shirts (such as the types of collars, buttons, stitching and so on).

Step 5

Repeat Step 4 with the second designer's shirts.

Step 6

Repeat Step 4 with the third designer's shirts.

Step 7

With your notebook open, review your notes as you reexamine each brand of shirts again. Were there subtle elements that you missed?

What does this exercise accomplish?

This exercise helps boost your visual discrimination skills. It requires you to pay attention to fine details. This skill comes easily to some people, while others may be surprised by how much they missed.

Exercise 16: Expand Your Colors

Step 1

Start paying close attention to the outfits you wear on a daily basis.

Step 2

Write down the colors of your outfits each day for one week (such as "Monday: blue and orange" or "Tuesday: green, white and blue").

Step 3

Add one color you don't usually wear to your outfit each day for one week. You can create new outfits that combine a greater number of colors than you typically wear by incorporating a more complex tie or adding a multicolored scarf. (Ask a trusted friend for advice if you are worried about your fashion or color sense.)

What does this exercise accomplish?

When you add more hues to your outfits, you use the part of your brain that sees and interprets color. You may already do this very well and need little practice, while others may need more encouragement to work out the changes.

Did You Know?

Mazes and Connect the Dots

You know those puzzle books you see on newsstands (especially in airports)? They are inexpensive, portable and packed with excellent brain-building games. Look for ones filled with maze games and connect-the-dots puzzles to build your visual-spatial skills. You can also find many free printable versions online.

Exercise 17: Name That Animal

Step 1

Assemble the supplies you'll need for this exercise. You need a piece of opaque paper, scissors and a wildlife-themed book with lots of large pictures of different animals in it.

Step 2

Cut a 1-inch (2.5 cm) square hole out of the paper.

Step 3

Have someone else place the paper over a random picture in the book, then hand you the covered picture.

Step 4

Examine what you see through the hole. Can you identify the animal from this small square of detail?

Step 5

If not, move the paper to a different spot on the picture. Can you identify it now?

Step 6

Continue moving the paper around the picture and getting more glimpses of the animal until you can correct identify it.

What does this exercise accomplish?

For this exercise, you tap into the visual and mental skills your brain uses to fill in missing parts of an image. By seeing the small portions, you get clues to the complete picture. A small piece might connect to the mental image you have of that animal (for example, if you see part of a tusk, you might be able to connect that with your mental image of an elephant). This exercise requires memory power as well, because you can actively look at only one small area at a time. You can play this game with all sorts of images. Animals are a good choice because people are familiar with so many of them. You can also try using photo albums of family or places you've visited a few times.

Exercise 18: Visual Memory #1

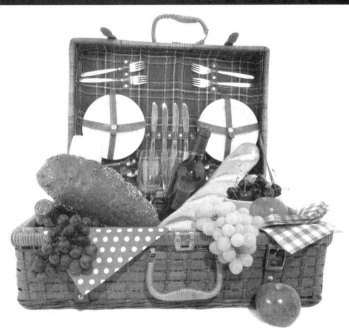

Step 1

Closely examine the picture at right for 30 seconds.

Step 2

Cover the picture completely so you can't see it.

Step 3

Write down 10 details about the picture that you remember.

1. ....

2. ....

3. ....

4. ....

5. ....

6. ....

7. ....

8. ....

9. ....

10. ....

Step 4

Uncover the picture. How accurate were your memories?

What does this exercise accomplish?

Visual memory is the ability to convert a very short-term sensory memory into short-term knowledge about the environment around you. Pure sensory memory lasts just a second, but it can be converted to short-term memory, where we conjure up or imagine what we just saw. A different part of the brain is now involved — it is no longer a purely sensory experience. To do well in this type of exercise, you must simultaneously engage your perception skills and pay attention to details as you purposefully examine the image.

Exercise 19: Visual Memory #2

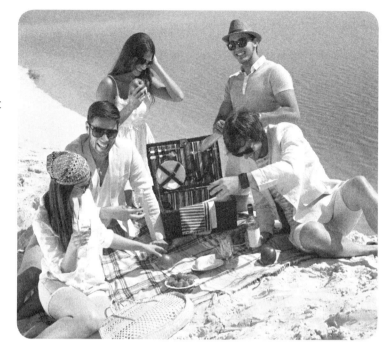

Step 1

Closely examine the picture at right for 30 seconds.

Step 2

Cover the picture completely so you can't see it.

Step 3

Write down 10 details about the picture that you remember.

1. ....

2. ....

3. ....

4. ....

5. ....

6. ....

7. ....

8. ....

9. ....

10. ....

Step 4

Uncover the picture. How accurate were your memories?

What does this exercise accomplish?

This exercise gives you more time to study the picture than Exercise 18: Visual Memory #1, but is not necessarily easier. The picture in Exercise 18 is a close-up shot of a set of objects (mostly foods), whereas this picture is less well defined and has more subtle shading that requires a little more inspection.

Exercise 20: Check Your Blind Spot

Step 1

Cover your right eye completely. With your left eye only, stare at the image on the right, below. Focus on the cross with the circle around it.

 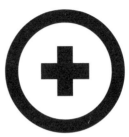

Step 2

Lean forward and backward so that your eyes are at different distances from the image. Notice that, at certain distances, the cross on the left side seems to vanish.

What does this exercise accomplish?

This exercise makes it clear that the visual information we see as reality is actually put together from different sources. At points where one eye is "blinded," your brain takes information from the opposite eye. But the image is perceived as continuous, complete information, not as a one-sided experience — until you mask one eye.

Exercise 21: Visual Retention Test

Step 1

Study the image at right for 10 seconds and then cover it up.

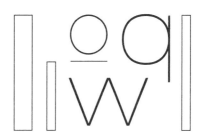

Step 2

Wait 30 seconds and then look at the four choices below. Which one matches the design from Step 1?

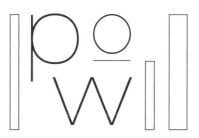
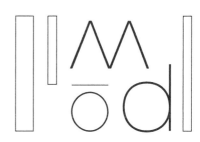
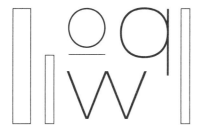
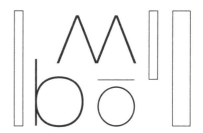

Source: Images based on the Benton Visual Retention Test, developed by Dr. Arthur Benton.

Step 3

Uncover the original image from Step 1 and compare it with your selection. If you chose incorrectly, can you now see which one is the same?

What does this exercise accomplish?

This exercise tests your memory of complex visual structures, which requires your brain to understand the angles, rotations and overall geometry of the original image and then compare it to a selection of four images. (Note: The Benton Visual Retention Test is also used diagnostically to help unmask brain issues that could arise from various conditions, such as a brain injury. This diagnostic aspect is beyond the scope of this book.)

Language Growth Exercises

We are surrounded by words all day long. We talk, we listen, and our audio environment, be it news programs or radio, exposes us to a deluge of speech. So why practice language? The reason is that our typical way of speaking and hearing, while amazing in itself, tends to use well-trodden brain pathways that we laid down when we were young children. Doing more focused and extensive language exercises causes some vital centers of our brain to light up and work harder. Moreover, learning new languages can stimulate vital brain structures such as the hippocampus, the memory index-maker of the brain.

For readers who write or read often as part of their work (such as teachers, writers, editors, professors, etc.), some of these exercises might be less important. But they are good workouts for most of us.

Exercise 1: Read and Summarize

Step 1
Choose a passage in a book or magazine that is about one page long. The book or magazine can be printed, in an online browser or on a tablet. The passage can be fiction or nonfiction, on any sort of topic.

Step 2
Read the passage.

Step 3
Reread the passage.

Step 4
Close the book, magazine, browser or tablet so you can't see the passage.

Step 5
Write a one-paragraph summary of what you read.

Step 6
Put your summary aside for at least one hour.

Step 7
Reread the passage and evaluate how well your summary captures the main points.

Step 8
If you like, have an assistant read your summary, then read the passage and compare the two.

What does this exercise accomplish?
When you write the summary, you create a new way to tell the story, which employs your language skills. This activity not only works the many brain centers needed for reading, it also uses memory and higher centers of the brain (like the prefrontal cortex) to interpret a story and make sense of things.

Exercise 2: Read and Conclude

Step 1

Choose an opinion-based article in a printed magazine or on an online news site. Some good places to search are *Time*, *Newsweek*, *Maclean's*, *The Economist*, *The Atlantic* and *Harper's Magazine*.

Step 2

Read the article.

Step 3

Close the magazine or browser so you can't see the article. Wait for 20 minutes.

Step 4

Write down the main conclusion of the article, such as "According to the author, shale oil is not sustainable because of the short life of shale wells and the need for perpetual financing to open new ones."

What does this exercise accomplish?

By reading, then summing up the main point of an opinion piece, you practice your comprehension of the written language and the linguistic skills you need to restate the conclusion. This requires some short-term memory use as well and can help boost the function of that area of the brain.

Exercise 3: Learn Foreign Words

Step 1

Visit a website or choose a book that's written in a foreign language that interests you, but one that you do not speak.

Step 2

Examine the text and identify five words you want to learn.

Step 3

Using a dictionary or researching online, study the meanings and pronunciations of the five words.

Step 4

Practice pronouncing the words and memorize their meanings.

Step 5

Write down the words and their meanings. Set aside your notes and wait for 24 hours.

Step 6

The next day, try to recall and say all five of the words.

Step 7

Compare what you remembered with what you wrote down.

What does this exercise accomplish?

This exercise involves learning new vocabulary information and engages the language centers of the brain. Your brain establishes new patterns and new associations as you learn the new words.

Exercise 4: Learn a Foreign Phrase

Step 1

Visit a website or choose a book that's written in a foreign language that interests you, but one that you do not speak.

Step 2

Examine the text and choose a phrase that pertains to a common situation or request — an everyday phrase such as "How are you this evening?" or "Where is a good restaurant around here?"

Step 3

Using a dictionary or researching online, study the meaning and pronunciation of each word in the phrase.

Step 4

Practice pronouncing the phrase and memorize its meaning.

Step 5

Teach the phrase to someone else or use the phrase with a friend who already speaks that language.

What does this exercise accomplish?

This activity works similar skills and parts of the brain as Exercise 3: Learn Foreign Words. The bonus is that it forces you to link the words together into the more complex overall meaning of the phrase.

Exercise 5: Learn Five Synonyms

Step 1

Pick an English word — one that pops into your head or one chosen at random from a newspaper or magazine.

Step 2

Using a printed or online thesaurus, look up five synonyms (words with similar meanings) for your chosen word.

Step 3

Write down the word and its five synonyms. Try to use these words in conversation in the weeks that follow this exercise.

★
....

1. ....

2. ....

3. ....

4. ....

5. ....

What does this exercise accomplish?

This is a way to expand your vocabulary, encoding new knowledge about word meanings into your long-term memory.

Exercise 6: Learn Five Antonyms

Step 1

Pick an English word — one that pops into your head or one chosen at random from a newspaper or magazine.

Step 2

Using a printed or online thesaurus, look up five antonyms (words with opposite meanings) for your chosen word.

Step 3

Write down the word and its five antonyms. Try to use these words in conversation in the weeks that follow this exercise.

★ ....

1. ....

2. ....

3. ....

4. ....

5. ....

What does this exercise accomplish?

Like Exercise 5: Learn Five Synonyms, this exercise expands your vocabulary. In this case, comparing words that have opposite meanings helps you to learn and remember the words.

Exercise 7: Build New Vocabulary

Step 1

Find a printed dictionary (if you don't own one, your local library will have a great big one).

Step 2

Open to a random page.

Step 3

Scan the words on the page until you encounter one you don't know.

Step 4

Read and memorize the meaning and pronunciation of the word.

Step 5

Share this new word with a friend.

What does this exercise accomplish?

This exercise encourages vocabulary expansion, which tends to involve the left hemisphere of the brain.

Exercise 8: Do a Play-by-Play

Step 1

Plan ahead to watch a sporting event on television or online. Pick a sport you are familiar with and understand.

Step 2

Enlist the help of an assistant who is also a fan of the sport.

Step 3

Phone the assistant when the game begins and sit in front of the television.

Step 4

Turn down the volume so you can't hear the announcers on the broadcast.

Step 5

As the game commences, act as the announcer. Describe to your assistant, in as much detail as possible, the action and plays that occur. Don't worry about missing information — you won't have all the views at once. Continue for up to 20 minutes.

What does this exercise accomplish?

Watching a game on a screen and describing it to someone over the phone requires you to absorb visual information, interpret it and turn it into descriptive language very quickly. A fast-moving game, such as hockey or football, will require more verbal agility than a slow-moving one such as baseball or golf — but there are benefits to describing either.

Exercise 9: Use Your Hands

Step 1

Line up a friend or family member who will listen to you tell a story.

Step 2

Recall a story you know well, such as something that happened to you or that you witnessed. It should take a couple of minutes to tell.

Step 3

Tell the story to your audience, using your hands as much as possible. Make gestures, outline shapes and point out directions of elements in your story.

What does this exercise accomplish?

By using your hands as you speak, you coordinate physical activity with verbal activity. This exercise stimulates two separate control centers of the brain and they work together (the prefrontal cortex, which controls movement, and the left frontal lobe, which controls speech).

Exercise 10: Rhyme Time

Step 1
Write a list of
five random words.

Step 2
For each of your five words, write five more words that
rhyme with it.

1. ....

2. ....

3. ....

4. ....

5. ....

What does this exercise accomplish?
This is a simple linguistic warm-up exercise, but it requires you to mentally scan your
vocabulary and use your mental representation of like sounds to generate the list.

Exercise 11: Write a Poem

Step 1
Think about an idea or feeling that
you want to express.

Step 2
Research poetry styles to determine
which you'd like to try. There are many
excellent resources on the Internet
that offer poetry-writing how-tos, such
as www.creative-writing-now.com/
how-to-write-poetry.html. Libraries are
another great resource — you can look
at a book of poems and try to copy the
style of the one you like best.

Step 3
Write your poem.

Step 4
Put the poem away where you can't
read it. Wait 24 hours.

Step 5
Take your poem out and reread it.

Step 6
Ask a supportive person in your life
to read the poem and tell you what it
means to him or her.

What does this exercise accomplish?
This exercise is a great way to work out
the language center of the brain. When you
write poems, you have to fit words into a
specific structure, which makes the brain
follow rules. It also stimulates creative
expression of your thoughts in words.

Exercise 12: Write a Short Story

Step 1

Choose a topic, situation or period of history that interests you.

Step 2

Read about the nuts and bolts of short story writing. Books and websites — such as www.letswriteashortstory.com/5-steps-to-write-a-short-story — can help.

Step 3

Set aside some uninterrupted time and begin writing your story.

Step 4

Take time to complete your work. Keep going, and don't give up if you have some unproductive days.

Step 5

When you are finished writing, editing and proofreading your story, ask a supportive friend to read it, then discuss your friend's impressions of it.

Step 6

Put away the story for one week, then reread it. Thinking about your friend's impressions of the story, see if you can reread it with a fresh perspective. If one week is not enough (writers sometimes need distance from their creations), take two weeks.

What does this exercise accomplish?

Story writing is both a creative endeavor and a way to exercise your language skills. In this exercise, you use language to relay the actions, thoughts, feelings and dialogue of the characters in your story. You place the language in a certain order — chronological or otherwise — and you choose words carefully. Working your brain in this way builds your overall linguistic intelligence.

Exercise 13: Find the Fallacy

Step 1

Study up on the nature of logical fallacies. There are lots of books on the theories of argumentation and informal logic. There are also helpful websites, such as https://owl.english.purdue.edu/owl/resource/659/03.

Step 2

Once you are familiar with the types of logical fallacies, it's time to practice. Buy a newspaper and look at one of the letters to the editor. This approach is more effective than reading comments on web-based news stories, which are chock-full of logical fallacies and insulting and inflammatory remarks. (They make for colorful reading but are not very helpful.)

Step 3

Read the letter and analyze the argument of the writer. Are there any logical fallacies, such as ad hominem, ad populum or straw-man arguments?

Step 4

As you do your review, make notes about where the fallacies are.

Step 5

As this exercise becomes easier, listen to the arguments on an intelligent TV news or topical show where speakers are given ample time to outline their logic. Repeat your critical review process of these arguments in real time. You can also use this kind of review to analyze logic employed in newspaper editorial board editorials and syndicated columnists' opinion pieces.

What does this exercise accomplish?

This is a tough but helpful workout for your language skills. You must interpret and assemble the meanings of the words and think through the concepts they outline on an abstract level. This requires reasoning skills but is tied in tightly with the linguistic capabilities of the brain.

Exercise 14: Notice Dialect

Step 1

Watch a YouTube video of a speaker, possibly a famous person, who has a discernible accent that is different from your own.

Step 2

Replaying the video as necessary, repeat what the speaker says and write down two or three words that you and the speaker pronounce very differently.

Step 3

Say these words out loud and listen to yourself. See if you can detect exactly how your pronunciation differs from the pronunciation of the speaker.

Step 4

Repeat this exercise using video clips of a speaker from a different region of your own country. They will not have a foreign accent but they may speak a regional dialect that is easy to understand but different than yours.

What does this exercise accomplish?

This workout builds your brain's ability to understand the nuances of language — those of others as well as yours. We do this automatically and can often tell intuitively if someone is not from "around here" (wherever that might be). But we often don't really listen to what those differences are. This is an intensive listening exercise that will improve your powers of observation as well.

Did You Know?

Increase Dialect Awareness

If you want to raise your awareness of how differences in speech are quite distinct but sometimes escape your conscious awareness, watch a few minutes of a dialect coaching website (such as www.rachelsenglish.com) or YouTube video. Hearing even regional differences in English pronunciation and word usage is very interesting.

Exercise 15: Tongue Twisters

Step 1

Look up a tongue twister in a book or online. The website www.fun-with-words.com has many language practice resources, and there is a whole page of tongue twisters to try.

Step 2

Choose a new tongue twister every day for a week and practice saying it. For example, try "Do brain exercises for life; besides, it's not size but exercise that brains require."

Step 3

Choose increasingly difficult tongue twisters as you improve your accuracy. When previously challenging tongue twisters start to roll off your tongue, pick longer ones or those with phonemes (sounds/pieces of words) that are more difficult for you.

What does this exercise accomplish?

Reciting a tongue twister is a way of working on your brain's speaking powers while simultaneously reading and processing words on a page or screen.

Exercise 16: Make a Metaphor

Step 1

Learn what a metaphor is if you are unfamiliar with the term. It is a figure of speech in which you link two words or phrases in order to make a comparison, but the sentence is not literally true. An example would be: "Brain exercise is a gym membership for the mind." Your brain is not literally going to the gym, but both are forms of exercise, making them easy to compare.

Step 2

Pick a situation, place or familiar story, then consider another example that is similar in some important detail. Create your metaphor.

Step 3

Create a new metaphor every day for a week.

Step 4

Share your metaphors with a supportive friend and see if they make sense.

What does this exercise accomplish?

In this exercise, you use both language and the parts of your brain that process comparisons and create analyses. You challenge your linguistic skills when you think carefully about the meanings of the words.

Exercise 17: Make a Simile

Step 1

Learn what a simile is if you are unfamiliar with the term. It is a comparison of two words or phrases using the words "like" or "as." An example would be: "Brain exercise is like lifting weights."

Step 2

Pick a situation, place or familiar story, then consider another example that is similar in some important detail. Create your simile.

Step 3

Create a new simile every day for a week.

Step 4

Share your similes with a supportive friend and see if they make sense.

What does this exercise accomplish?

Like Exercise 16: Make a Metaphor, this activity challenges your vocabulary and your use of descriptive language.

Exercise 18: Create Alliteration

Step 1

Learn what alliteration is if you are unfamiliar with the term. It is a series of words in which most of the words start with the same letter or sound.

Step 2

Describe something using a phrase made up of alliterative words. Perhaps something like this: "Besides boosting brain function, a brain-busting workout bestows other big, beautiful benefits."

Step 3

Create a new sentence using alliteration every day for a week.

Step 4

Share your alliterative sentences with a supportive friend and see if they make sense.

What does this exercise accomplish?

This fun activity gives your vocabulary a workout and strengthens your sense of the sounds of words.

Exercise 19: Its/It's Practice

Step 1

Review or memorize the difference between "its" (the possessive, or "belonging to it") and "it's" (the shortened form of "it is").

Step 2

Without looking at the definition above, write five sentences using "its" or "it's."

Step 3

Review them to see if you are correct.

What does this exercise accomplish?

It may be a short one, but this grammar review is a very good opportunity for you to memorize a grammatical rule that many people cannot use well.

Exercise 20: Don't Say "Uh"!

Step 1

Think of a topic you want to give a speech about. Limit yourself to about three minutes of speaking.

Step 2

Write out your speech. Start with why you think the topic is important, then state your position. Next, give three reasons that support your position. Summarize and restate your position as a conclusion.

Step 3

Read through your written speech.

Step 4

Recite the speech to an assistant or into a recording device (so you can hear yourself later). Start with a perfect score of 10/10 and subtract one point for each time you say "uh" or "um" or pause for longer than 2 seconds. What was your score?

What does this exercise accomplish?

This is a verbal fluency workout for your brain — and it is harder than most people may think. We naturally pause when we speak, and we often dangle words or use delayers such as "uh" and "um." Giving a fluent, clear speech is quite challenging.

Sense Compensation

When a person loses a sense (such as sight or hearing), that loss may be difficult or even traumatic initially, but over time, the person's other senses will begin to feed the brain more information and stimulation. The human brain will attempt to compensate for and adapt to almost any challenge.

Sensory Processing Exercises

The sensory system is the key to waking up the brain. We depend on sensory input to trigger many of our thoughts and movements. Babies are dependent on touch and use sight as a tool to orient themselves in their environments. As adults, we sometimes find ourselves in environments with few options for sensory enrichment, or those that provide very repetitive sensory input.

Exercise 1: Catch a Wave

Step 1

If you don't live near the beach, purchase a CD of ocean sounds. There are many of these on the market; most contain quiet music along with the sound of gentle waves. If you're lucky enough to live near the ocean, go to a quiet stretch of beach and sit on the shore.

Step 2

Close your eyes and focus on listening to the waves. Concentrate on their rhythm.

Step 3

Become aware of your breathing relative to the waves. Let your breathing be regular and rhythmic like the ocean (though it will probably not be at the same pace).

Step 4

Focus on your breathing for 15 minutes.

What does this exercise accomplish?

This exercise induces a meditative state. The key is the repetitive and reassuring sound of the waves. There is something calming and primal about moving water, so listening to waves is an excellent tool for creating a sensory-rich experience for your brain.

Exercise 2: Learn to Paint

Step 1

Sign up for a beginner painting class at a local recreation center or buy a good painting-instruction book for beginners.

Step 2

Buy the necessary supplies.

Step 3

Set up a place in your home where you can paint without worrying about stains or mess, and where it is easy to store your supplies. If you are painting subjects outside your home, pack a case that allows you to transport your supplies.

Step 4

Begin painting. Practice, practice, practice.

What does this exercise accomplish?

Many people take up painting as a hobby, often later in life. There are good reasons for this. Painting is a sensory-rich, creative endeavor. It also requires some degree of coordination and skill (depending on what style of painting you pursue). The use of colors, including choosing and blending them, is one source of that sensory information. The application of the paint to the canvas, paper or other surface is another. The shapes or images you create stimulate your mind. This is the kind of rich sensory nourishment that the brain craves.

Did You Know?

Pottery Is Brain Work

Another brain-strengthening, sensory-boosting hobby is pottery. There are plenty of places to take up this creative pursuit: local studios and recreation centers often offer classes. Touching and manipulating the clay is a fun, rich experience for the senses. You will be learning a new skill, which is vital for keeping your brain active and preventing mental stagnation.

Exercise 3: Enjoy Aromatherapy

Step 1

Run warm water into your bathtub; it should be warm enough to be relaxing but not overly hot. Don't overfill the tub. The water should be just deep enough to provide a warming soak.

Step 2

Add a few drops of a relaxing essential oil to the water. Lavender and citrus oils work best for providing relaxation.

Caution

If you have sensitive skin, make sure to choose an essential oil your skin will tolerate.

Step 3

Get into the tub and soak for 15 minutes. Slow down and calm your breathing.

Step 4

Become aware of the scent of the essential oil. Focus on it. See what memories, if any, it brings up or what it makes you think of.

What does this exercise accomplish?

The benefits of this sensory experience are well known. The sensation of being in water is powerful because every person floated in the womb at the beginning of life; the experience as an adult is restorative. Adding a botanical aroma is important in this exercise because olfaction (the sense of smell) brings information into the brain at a point that is situated very close to the centers for emotion. The sensory information from aromas can get to these emotional centers faster than it can to the higher centers of the cerebral cortex, where we interpret or think about information. Smelling something calming while sitting in a comfortable bath is a rich experience for your senses and stimulates the emotional areas of the brain.

Exercise 4: Relaxing Massage

Step 1

Book an appointment with a massage therapist in a professional, clean, relaxed environment.

Step 2

Ask the therapist to give you a relaxing massage.

Step 3

As you enjoy your massage, focus on the different aspects of the experience. What area is the therapist working on? Does the massage feel different on the neck than on the lower back? How much pressure is the therapist using? Are any areas tender? (If so, don't hesitate to communicate this.) Is the therapist using aromatherapy and/or music to further relax you? Are you able to slip into a neutral state where you are not thinking about much?

What does this exercise accomplish?

It goes without saying that a relaxing massage will feel good. The nervous system is hardwired to crave touch. By fulfilling this need, you feed your brain a great deal of sensory information that you might be lacking if you do not often experience this type of sensory input. Massage is also a great stress reliever.

Exercise 5: Therapeutic Massage

Step 1

Book an appointment with a massage therapist in a professional, clean, relaxed environment.

Step 2

Ask the therapist to give you a therapeutic massage that involves multiple techniques. This might involve relaxing techniques as well, but it will combine those with a variety of other massage techniques — such as muscle stretching, gentle vibration delivered to knotty or tense muscle areas, or skin rolling — to achieve therapeutic results.

Step 3

Pay attention to details of the different techniques. If the therapist works deeply and separates muscles a bit or rolls the skin and lifts it, how does that feel? What does it make you remember? How do you feel afterward? Loose-jointed? Relaxed? Happy? Tired?

What does this exercise accomplish?

As you learned in Exercise 4: Relaxing Massage, the human nervous system needs touch to thrive. By fulfilling this need, you support the brain and nervous system. In this instance, there are more varieties of sensory input to explore. The stretching of your muscles or the sensation of skin rolling sends tons of stimulating information to the brain.

Exercise 6: Indulge in Watsu

Step 1

The word "Watsu" is short for "water shiatsu." Shiatsu is a type of therapeutic massage that uses gentle pressure to stimulate acupressure points. Watsu is done in warm salt water, because it helps the patient float almost weightlessly.

Step 2

Call and ask the practitioner about their rates, training and setup. If you have mobility issues, inquire about the accessibility of the facility. If you cannot swim, ask how buoyant the saltwater will make you, if the therapist will offer flotation devices and how he or she will supervise your treatment to ensure your safety. Make an appointment for a treatment if you are comfortable.

Step 3

Experience the treatment. How do you feel floating freely or gliding along the water? Does the wavelike pattern restore you or put you to sleep? What is going through your mind during the treatment? Is there a point at which your thinking slows down and you forget about your next stop during a busy day? What is your emotional state when the treatment is over?

Step 4

When the treatment is finished, wait for a while before driving home. (Better yet, have a friend pick you up.) Some people find Watsu elevating, while others may find it disorienting or even sedating.

What does this exercise accomplish?

Aquatic bodywork is a feast for your senses. As you know, immersion in water is a powerful sensory experience. Adding the power of therapeutic touch and the sensation of floating stimulates multiple sensory pathways. People often experience significant benefits from this therapy, including enhanced relaxation and a reduction in pain, stiffness and other complaints.

Did You Know?

Watsu Basics

During a Watsu treatment, a therapist guides the patient through a series of gentle motions, such as rocking and drifting, and offers an acupressure treatment while the patient floats in water. Many patients fall asleep or emerge in a state of deep relaxation. Visit www.watsu.com to learn more about this technique, and click on the "Search Practitioners" link to find a practitioner near you.

Exercise 7: Try Acupuncture

Step 1

Learn a bit about acupuncture. It is a practice used in traditional Chinese medicine. It involves inserting a sterile, very thin, very strong needle into a specific point of the body. These points are aligned along energy pathways that are associated with specific functions and/or organs. Acupuncture points are often located near multiple nerves and can easily transmit powerful signals to the brain.

Step 2

Find a qualified acupuncturist. This individual should be licensed by the state or provincial authority that issues licenses to health-care professionals in your area. Some naturopathic doctors, chiropractors, physiotherapists, osteopaths and conventional physicians perform acupuncture.

Step 3

Request a consultation and treatment.

Step 4

Experience the treatment. Communicate clearly with your practitioner and make sure he or she knows how you are feeling throughout the visit.

What does this exercise accomplish?

Acupuncture is a sensory therapy and much more. It is a potent, sophisticated type of treatment that has been used for thousands of years. It introduces very powerful sensory information to your body, which conveys it to your brain via the spinal cord.

Exercise 8: Experience Acupressure

Step 1

Learn the ins and outs of acupressure. It is also derived from traditional Chinese medicine, like acupuncture, but touch and pressure are used instead of needles to stimulate specific points on the body. Shiatsu is the Japanese form of this therapy. Acupressure is not always licensed as strictly as acupuncture but there is no issue around needle safety.

Step 2

Find an acupressure or shiatsu expert in your area. Look for an established clinic with a solid track record — good online reviews or word-of-mouth recommendations are the best indicators of quality. You might want to start by talking to an acupressure practitioner who works in the office of another medical practitioner, such as a naturopath, a chiropractor, an osteopath or a conventional physician.

Step 3

Request a consultation and treatment.

Step 4

Experience the treatment. Communicate with your practitioner before, during and after the treatment. Share how you are reacting to the treatment and what you need.

What does this exercise accomplish?

Acupressure treatments are rich sensory experiences. When acupressure points, especially sensitive ones, are pressed with the thumb or finger, your brain receives a large amount of sensory input. Special receptors for touch, pressure and stretch in the skin, muscles and the tissues in between will send the brain a wealth of information.

Exercise 9: Relax with Reflexology

Step 1

Learn about the techniques and benefits of reflexology. It is a form of manual therapy in which the hands stimulate points on the feet. It can be relaxing, and many people who use it report other wellness-enhancing benefits.

Step 2

Find a qualified reflexologist. Start by looking for a well-trained massage therapist who is licensed by the state or province. Ask if he or she has training in reflexology as well.

Step 3

Set up a consultation and treatment.

Step 4

Experience the treatment. Does it relax the overworked muscles in your feet? Are you experiencing an overall feeling of relaxation? Make sure the reflexologist knows all the important facts about your medical history, such as arthritis or problems with circulation or nerves in your feet.

What does this exercise accomplish?

The feet are incredibly well supplied with nerves, and rather large areas of the brain are assigned to process sensory input from them (this is true of the hands and face, too; they get extra attention from the brain). A reflexology treatment stimulates specific points on your feet and not only relieves tension and pain but can also deliver a lot of information to your sensory cortex (the part of the brain that reads what is going on in various parts of the body).

Exercise 10: Sensory Processing

Step 1

Buy an ultrasonic toothbrush if you don't have one. If you have had extensive dental work, check with your dentist before attempting this exercise.

Step 2

Read the instructions for using the toothbrush.

Step 3

Brush your teeth according to the instructions. The brush head uses fine vibrations instead of friction to "brush" the teeth. You'll find you just have to gently run the brush along the gum lines and tooth surfaces instead of sweeping it back and forth as you would have to do with a manual toothbrush.

What does this exercise accomplish?

An ultrasonic toothbrush is a new sensation for many people (and an effective tool for good dental hygiene). By using a new tool and method to brush your teeth, and experiencing the new sensations that go with that, you give your brain new input instead of routine input. It's an excellent brain-building activity and can have a positive impact on your smile at the same time.

Exercise 11: Wear a Different Fabric

Step 1

Take a look at the garments in your wardrobe. What types of fabrics are they made from? Are they mostly cotton, wool or synthetics?

Step 2

Take a closer look at the texture of the fabrics, and feel them with your hands. Do they have smooth finishes? Are they fleecy? Are they flat like ironed cotton?

Step 3

Find a fabric in your wardrobe that has a texture you don't wear often. You may need to go out and purchase something a little different. For example, if you wear mostly cotton, what would a wool garment feel like?

Step 4

Wear this less familiar fabric for a day. Make sure it comes into contact with your skin. Focus on the sensation of the fabric on your body.

What does this exercise accomplish?

The skin's sense of touch is very sensitive and can distinguish subtle differences. We often settle into the same wardrobe with the same look, made from the same materials — and feel the same all the time as we go about our lives. This exercise is a way to introduce new sensations to your skin, nerves and brain. The sense of touch can become deadened when exposed to the same stimuli all the time, and a new fabric's input can stimulate your brain and nervous system in a positive way.

Exercise 12: Listen Up

Step 1

Take an inventory of the styles of music you typically listen to.

Step 2

Consider a type of music you don't usually listen to. Make sure it's one that you are open to. In other words, it should be different but not offensive to your beliefs or inappropriate in your home environment (if you have children, they should be able to listen to it).

Step 3

Purchase an album or find a radio station that plays this new type of music.

Step 4

For a week, listen to several songs in this genre every day.

Step 5

After a week, instead of returning to your usual musical tastes, find another genre to explore.

What does this exercise accomplish?

Music is a sensory buffet, with harmonies, melodies (such as vocal or instrumental solos), rhythms and lyrics wrapped up together. We all have a favorite style, and after a while we start listening to songs passively, only hearing some of what they have to offer. When you pick a different style of music, you give your brain novelty, which is an important cue for stimulation and new learning.

Exercise 13: Chill Out

Step 1

Set two large towels, side by side, on the floor in front of a comfortable chair.

Step 2

Place a small basin on one of the towels; it should have a capacity of about 6 gallons (23 L) and should be a shape that accommodates your feet comfortably.

Step 3

Fill the basin with ice water. It's better to make several trips with a pitcher of water, because the filled basin will be heavy and awkward to carry.

Step 4

Set a timer for one minute. Immerse your feet in the ice water and start the timer.

Step 5

Remove your feet from the ice water and rest them on the adjacent towel for three to five minutes, until the circulation has fully returned to your feet. (If it does not or you experience pain, do not continue with this exercise.)

Step 6

Repeat Steps 4 and 5 two more times. (Again, if you begin to experience pain, do not continue with this exercise.)

Step 7

Remove your feet from the ice water and dry them well.

What does this exercise accomplish?

This exercise is actually a type of hydrotherapy, using water and temperature to stimulate your body and improve circulation. The direct application of cold, the sensation of immersion in water and the alternation of room temperature and cold all provide strong sensory signals to your brain.

Caution

Don't attempt this exercise if you have a circulatory or other health issue that prevents you from immersing your feet in cold water.

Exercise 14: Go Barefoot

Step 1

Pick a day to walk outside early in the morning. Make sure the temperature is well above freezing (pleasantly cool is just fine).

Step 2

Pick a grassy area, such as your front lawn or a nearby green space, that is clean, safe and free of animal waste, broken glass and sharp objects.

Step 3

Shortly after dawn, while the grass is still dewy, go to your chosen place.

Step 4

Remove your shoes and socks and walk barefoot on the dewy grass for five minutes. Change up the way your feet touch the grass. Stand and plant your feet firmly, making yourself aware of how the surface of your foot makes contact with the grass and earth. Then walk around the area normally for a while. You can also try walking on your toes, then on your heels.

What does this exercise accomplish?

The surfaces of your feet are very well connected to areas of the brain (see page 87 for more on reflexology). They contain lots of nerves and sensory receptors, which pick up information about their environment. A barefoot walk is a natural experience that's rich in sensory stimulation. The barefoot walking itself, on a natural and sometimes uneven surface, activates small muscles and nerves in your feet and ankles and sends even more information to your brain.

Exercise 15: Taste Something New

Step 1

Think about the types of foods and the dishes that you typically eat.

Step 2

Write down a list of cuisines that are not part of your typical diet. If you need ideas, refer to a dining guide, a food website or the food section of the newspaper. There you'll find restaurant reviews and recommendations that cover a wide variety of interesting international cuisines.

Step 3

Choose a restaurant that serves an unfamiliar cuisine you would like to try. The only caveat is to make sure it is appropriate for you — in terms of dietary restrictions, spiciness tolerance and so on. If you don't have those sorts of restaurants nearby, you can try cooking a new and different recipe at home.

Step 4

Go to the restaurant and enjoy a meal.

What does this exercise accomplish?

The senses of taste and smell are primal and powerful, but they are often blunted from exposure to the same foods day in and day out. When you dine on something different — such as a dish that contains unfamiliar spices, flavors or ingredients, or that is cooked using a different technique — you take in a whole lot of new sensory information.

Exercise 16: Go to the Zoo

Step 1

Find a zoo in your area and plan a visit.

Step 2

Pick a day when the zoo is not likely to be crowded. Avoid heavily promoted days, such as a free-pass Saturday for non–zoo members, when you will spend more time lined up to get into the parking lot than on the zoo grounds themselves.

Step 3

Explore! As you go from exhibit to exhibit, focus on the new sights and sounds around you. Are there different odors? What do the habitats of the animals look like? Do the animals seem different close up and live, compared to what you see in pictures?

What does this exercise accomplish?

This exercise provides a living, breathing, novel experience with multiple sensory stimuli. Our minds and senses crave this type of input. An accredited and humane zoo offers you the chance to see many different species in enclosures that mimic their natural homes. And while it is an artificial environment maintained by humans, a zoo allows you a way to connect with animals and nature.

Exercise 17: Experience Art

Step 1

Find an art gallery in your area.

Step 2

Visit the gallery on a quiet day when you can explore without distractions.

Step 3

If you find it difficult to focus on works of art solo, join a tour led by a knowledgeable guide. Remember: Hands off! This sensory exercise is for the eyes, not the hands. You don't want the sensory experience of alarm bells sounding to mar a perfect afternoon.

What does this exercise accomplish?

This is a visual sensory tour in which you absorb the colors, geometry, lighting and other techniques artists use to communicate ideas and feelings. Not only can great art show off technical expertise but it is also a form of communication that stimulates the visual input area of your brain.

Exercise 18: Dress in the Dark

Step 1

Lay out the clothes you are going to wear for the day in a familiar place. You should know the room layout well.

Step 2

Close your eyes and change into the new outfit. Don't peek unless you absolutely can't find a piece of clothing or if you feel like you are about to fall.

What does this exercise accomplish?

By closing your eyes and getting dressed, you rely on touch and your sense of your limbs' position in space — instead of relying on visual input. Your fingers are capable of taking in a lot of information as you dress and handle the clothes. The key is to slow down and pay close attention.

Caution

Do not attempt this exercise if you have poor balance or are at higher risk of falling.

Exercise 19: Take a Ride

Step 1

Find an amusement park that has an excellent safety record and a good reputation. This is a fun exercise to try when you're on vacation.

Step 2

Choose five different rides that offer a variety of sensory experiences. They may include music, different directions of motion, different structures of cars or seats, etc.

Step 3

Go on the rides. As you experience them, try closing your eyes, then keeping them open. Does the ride feel different with your eyes closed? Try listening to the sounds of other people on the ride and compare them to the noises you are making, if any.

What does this exercise accomplish?

This is a very intense type of sensory workout. It stimulates your brain using sensations of movement, speed and rotation, as well as the perception of sights and sounds. Roller coasters and other rides may not be for everyone, but they can be a powerful break from the deadening sensory routines that we confine our brains to in everyday life.

Caution

Only do this exercise to your comfort level, and avoid it entirely if you have any medical restrictions, such as a heart condition, that prevent you from going on rides.

Motor Learning Exercises

Movement is essential to our neurological development as infants. Even in the womb, we are very active during the early weeks of pregnancy. Movement is not only a complex choreography of muscles and joints, but also a symphony of brain activity. Some brain cells move large muscles; others dampen those signals to prevent jerky or overly spastic muscles.

Learned and coordinated muscle movement requires the cerebellum, and we process a lot of sensory information as we move. Our brain is constantly receiving information about where our body and its limbs, trunk and head are in three-dimensional space. Less consciously, our muscles must coordinate so that pairs or groups of muscles that oppose each other (those that bend the knees and those that straighten them, for example) know when to relax and when to fire. Movement exercises don't just work muscles; they give the brain a lot to do. The synchronization of brain and body is important and requires practice.

Movement exercises don't just work muscles; they give the brain a lot to do. The synchronization of brain and body is important and requires practice.

Did You Know?

In Utero Learning

By the eleventh week of gestation in the mother's uterus, a fetus can suck its thumb. Some movements begin even earlier!

Exercise 1: Cross Crawl #1

Step 1

Stand with your feet firmly planted, shoulder-width apart, arms at your sides.

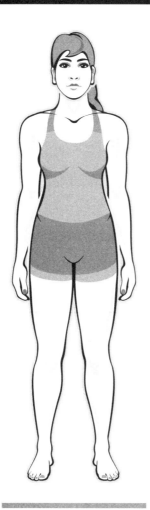

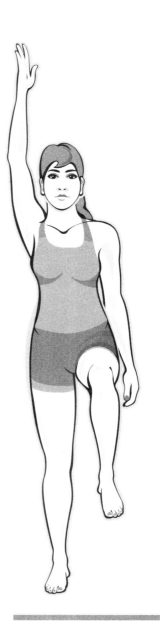

Step 2

Simultaneously raise your right arm high over your head and lift your left leg, bending it at the knee and bringing your knee up as high as you can in front of you.

Step 3

Keeping your core muscles tightened to support your body and balance, simultaneously lower your right arm and left leg to the starting position. Just as your left foot returns to the floor, repeat Step 2 using the opposite limbs (your left arm and your right leg move in unison).

Step 4

Do 50 repetitions of Steps 2 and 3, developing a marching rhythm as you progress.

What does this exercise accomplish?

This exercise stimulates your brain and spinal cord as they control your muscle coordination. By practicing these motions, you are repeating movement patterns you started making as an infant when you first learned to crawl and then as you learned to walk. Retracing these developmental movements can help your brain reinforce coordinated side-to-side motions across a stable body core.

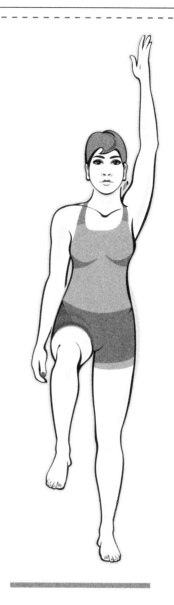

Did You Know?

Crawling Is Vital

As infants, our nervous systems begin to develop control over our bodies using a cross-crawling motion. A baby's eyes lock on to something, then move toward it. Initially, crawling involves a simultaneous primary movement in which the opposite arm and leg move in sync while the core muscles of the trunk and abdomen stabilize the body. When babies first try this move, they slide onto their bellies, but as they gain strength, they can lift up, pick up speed and move quickly across the floor. This cross-crawling motion is an important milestone in learning to walk, because one leg must learn to be stable as the other leg swings. This is a primitive movement and many other animals do it; some, such as reptiles, often use a cross-crawl as their primary motion.

Exercise 2: Cross Crawl #2

Step 1

Get down on all fours. Make sure you're wearing comfortable clothes and kneeling on a surface that is gentle on your knees. Keep your head in a neutral position, looking at the ground just in front of your shoulders rather than craning your neck up.

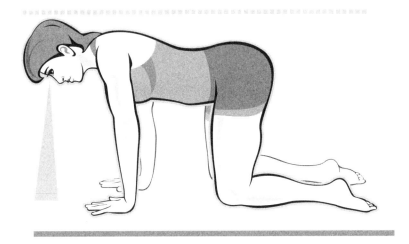

Step 2

Simultaneously raise your right arm in front of you and stretch your left leg out behind you until they are parallel to the ground. Point your arm and hand straight ahead and extend your leg fully behind you, pointing your toe. Keep your back parallel to the ground and your core muscles tightened to support your body.

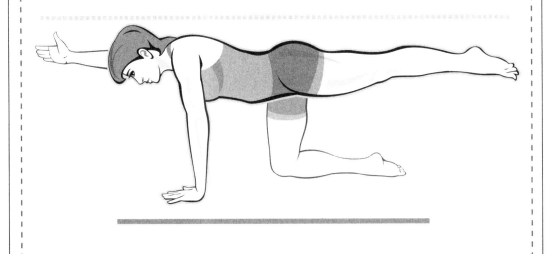

Step 3

Simultaneously return your right hand and left knee to the starting position. Repeat Step 2 using the opposite limbs (your left arm and your right leg move in unison).

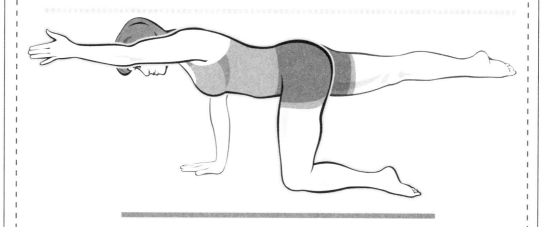

Step 4

Do 20 repetitions (10 per side) of Steps 2 and 3, developing a rhythm as you progress.

What does this exercise accomplish?

Like Exercise 1: Cross Crawl #1, this is a wake-up call for the nervous system. This version places your body in a horizontal position and is even more similar to the crawling movement you mastered as a baby.

Caution

Avoid this exercise if you have knee problems or difficulty getting up and down; in that case, stick with Exercise 1: Cross Crawl #1.

Exercise 3: Cross Crawl #3

Step 1

Get down on all fours. Make sure you're wearing comfortable clothes and kneeling on a surface that is gentle on your knees. An open grassy area works well, given the distance you need to cover. You might want to do this in a private yard or explain to others what you are up to. They may offer to help you look for a lost item in the grass if you haven't explained your brain exercise program to them!

Step 2

Fix your eyes on an object about 30 feet (9 m) away from you. Ask an assistant to time you.

Step 3

Crawl toward the object, keeping your eyes locked on it.

Step 4

Turn around and crawl back to the place you started.

Step 5

Repeat Steps 3 and 4 for three minutes.

What does this exercise accomplish?

As in the previous crawling exercises, you are reliving developmental activities you did as a baby. In this motor and nervous system activity, your eyes lead the way, making it almost identical to a baby's crawling experience.

Caution

Avoid this exercise if you have knee problems or difficulty getting up and down; in that case, stick with Exercise 1: Cross Crawl #1.

Exercise 4: Alternating Movements

Step 1
Sit comfortably in a chair with your hands resting on your thighs.

Step 2
Turn your left palm so it is facing up.

Step 3
Move your right hand so that it is hovering over your left palm. Ask an assistant to time you.

Step 4
Tap your left palm with your right palm, then quickly turn your right hand over and tap your left palm with the back of your right hand. (Your left hand has not moved from its place on your thigh.)

Step 5
Repeat Step 4 for 30 seconds, developing a rhythm as you progress.

Step 6
Repeat Steps 1 through 5 on the opposite side. Your right hand will be resting, palm side up, on your thigh, while your left hand taps.

What does this exercise accomplish?
In this exercise, you work the cerebellum area of your brain. This task requires coordinated alternating movements. In fact, physicians use this exercise and variations of it to test patients' cerebellar function.

Exercise 5: Muscle Awareness

Step 1

Sit comfortably in a chair with your hands resting on your lap.

Step 2

Close your eyes.

Step 3

Visualize your right biceps muscle.

Step 4

Slowly contract your right biceps muscle. Tighten it, but do not curl your arm. Try to leave the surrounding muscles as loose as possible. By focusing your mind on your right biceps muscle, you'll find this easier.

Step 5

Hold the tension in your right biceps muscle for 10 seconds.

Step 6

Slowly release.

Step 7

Repeat Steps 3 through 6 with your left biceps muscle.

Step 8

Repeat Steps 3 through 6 with your right triceps muscle.

Step 9

Repeat Steps 3 through 6 with your left triceps muscle.

What does this exercise accomplish?

When you tighten each muscle separately in this exercise, you are practicing mental control over muscles as well as isolating their contractions. At the same time, you keep the surrounding muscles as relaxed as possible. In our daily routines, we often activate many muscles at once when we don't need to, often as part of a repetitive pattern. This exercise in moving just one muscle at a time helps reestablish the finer aspects of controlled movement versus the awkward recruitment of an entire muscle group.

Exercise 6: Heels and Toes

Step 1

Walk across a room, balancing just on your heels. If you have trouble balancing, spread your feet farther apart to enhance stability.

Step 2

Turn around and walk back across the room, balancing just on your toes.

Step 3

Do three repetitions of Steps 1 and 2.

What does this exercise accomplish?

This exercise allows you to isolate different muscle groups and tests the strength of just some of the muscles you typically use to walk. It is partially a balance exercise as well. If you have arthritis or poor balance, walk beside a bed or couch that you can hold on to, or avoid this exercise altogether.

Exercise 7: Learn a New Stroke

Step 1

Go to a pool and get in at the end where you feel comfortable. If you are not a strong swimmer, the shallow end works just fine. (A public pool with a lifeguard on duty is always a safe bet.)

Step 2

Try a new, less familiar swimming stroke. For example, if you typically do the front crawl, try the backstroke.

Step 3

Swim using this stroke until you are ready to get out. Never do it to the point of exhaustion; always make sure you can navigate your way back to the edge of the pool.

Step 4

Each time you return to the pool for a workout, use this stroke, increasing the length of your swim.

Step 5

Take note of when this stroke becomes a coordinated, smooth motion that you don't have to think about. How long did it take to become a natural movement?

What does this exercise accomplish?

Trying out a brand-new or less familiar stroke makes the brain learn an entirely new movement pattern. In the water, you are unlikely to twist or hurt a joint, so it's a good low-impact workout. You just need to be a fairly confident swimmer.

Exercise 8: Mix It Up

Step 1

Select one of your daily routines that you can vary safely. Most personal hygiene activities and cleaning activities are fair game, but routines associated with caring for infants and elders are not.

Step 2

Change the sequence of your chosen routine. For example, if you typically shave, brush your teeth and floss, then comb your hair, you might comb your hair, shave and floss, then brush your teeth.

Step 3

Repeat the sequence you chose in Step 2 the following day.

Step 4

Each day, keep repeating your routine in the new sequence until the variation becomes a smooth routine.

Step 5

Change the sequence of your routine again, performing the steps in a new and different order. Repeat the new sequence every day until the variation becomes a smooth routine.

What does this exercise accomplish?

Changing the order in which you perform everyday tasks is a direct way to get the brain to work harder and get smarter. Many daily routines consist of choreographed movements that have been repeated thousands of times. When you repeat the same sequences with no variations over a lifetime, you miss a simple and effective way to train the brain by making new connections.

Exercise 9: Up or Down?

Step 1

Sit comfortably in a chair with your hands resting on your lap.

Step 2

Close your eyes.

Step 3

Have an assistant bend your big (great) toe up or down, then tell him or her which way your toe is bent. The assistant will tell you if you are correct.

Step 4

Repeat Step 3 using the big toe on the opposite foot.

Step 5

If you misidentified which way your toe was bent in Step 3 and/or 4, repeat the steps until you have correctly identified up or down for both big toes. If you still can't tell which direction the toe is pointing after three attempts on each side, you will likely never be able to access this particular sensory information (see box, below).

What does this exercise accomplish?

This is very much a sensory exercise, but it focuses on the kind of sensory information that you need in order to use your muscles correctly. This exercise might seem easy, but people who suffer from diabetes or other conditions that make the feet numb or painful might find it challenging.

Did You Know?

Numb Toes

When you're doing Exercise 9: Up or Down?, remain focused on the sensations you feel. If you discover that you can't sense the position of your toes in this exercise, speak with your doctor right away. Lack of position sense can be a sign of nerve damage.

Exercise 10: Learn to Sign

Step 1

Visit a sign language education website. A good place to start is the American Sign Language University at www.lifeprint.com.

Step 2

Watch a video demonstrating the sign for a common word.

Step 3

Make the sign, following along with the video.

Step 4

Make the sign on your own, without the help of the video.

Step 5

Re-watch the video to see if you are correct.

Step 6

Practice until you can perform the sign from memory.

Step 7

Repeat Steps 1 through 6 to learn two more common signs.

What does this exercise accomplish?

Learning sign language ties together many areas of and pathways in your brain. You have to learn new movements, use visual cues and tie all of this into your understanding of language. This exercise will get several pathways in your brain to light up as you learn this new mode of communication.

Exercise 11: Quick Changes

Step 1

Reach your right hand behind your head and touch your left shoulder once.

Step 2

With your left hand, tap your left knee twice.

Step 3

Stand up if you are sitting down. Touch your left foot to your right knee, then run it down the inside of your lower leg to the ankle.

Step 4

Plant both feet on the floor, then raise your right leg in front of you, bending it at the knee.

Step 5

Plant both feet on the floor, then squat all the way down to the floor.

Step 6

Stand up and do one jumping jack.

Step 7

Stand perfectly straight, as if a string were pulling up the top of your head, and look straight ahead.

Step 8

Tuck your chin in, touching it to your chest.

Step 9

Look up at the ceiling.

Step 10

Return to standing straight, but in a more relaxed stance.

Step 11

Run in place for 15 seconds.

What does this exercise accomplish?

This exercise is simply a way to get your nervous system to coordinate sensory information from your limbs and eyes so that the brain, nervous system and muscles sit up and pay attention. By switching from one motion to the next in rapid succession, your brain must process sensory information and send orders to your muscles fairly quickly. While purposeful meditative exercises such as swimming and tai chi are important in an exercise regimen, quick-fire exercises like this are also important and provide a different experience for your brain.

Exercise 12: Dance, Dance, Dance

Step 1

Visit a website that gives step-by-step instructions for specific dance steps, such as www.arthurmurraycincinnati.com/learn-dances.html.

Step 2

Pick a dance that you don't know. (Make sure it's one you can do without hurting yourself!)

Step 3

Study the written instructions carefully and visualize yourself making these movements.

Step 4

Move through the steps, one by one, until the movement pattern makes sense.

Step 5

Attempt to do the steps slowly in order, all the way through, referring to the instructions when needed

Step 6

Do the steps all the way through, without reading the instructions.

Step 7

Do five repetitions of the full movement pattern as fluidly as possible. Don't rest between repetitions.

What does this exercise accomplish?

By trying a new dance, your brain learns a new motor pattern. Many parts of the brain get involved here: the part that initiates movement, the part that helps refine it and the part that coordinates it. Plus, this exercise might even help your social life!

Exercise 13: Cook Something New

Step 1

Look through a cookbook (such as the recipes in this book) or use a food website or app (such as www.thejoykitchen.com) and find a cooking technique you've never tried. It could be something complicated like boning a turkey or something simple like stuffing grape leaves. Pick a technique that requires manual dexterity and involves a number of steps. Make sure it's doable — you might not want to attempt fancy cutting techniques if you don't have good basic knife skills or a steady grip.

Step 2

Work through the technique, following the instructions. Before you perform each new step (for example, mixing two ingredients together), visualize how you are going to do it.

Step 3

Select other techniques to try. Practice these on the delicious brain-boosting recipes starting on page 199. There are so many options to cook and enjoy.

What does this exercise accomplish?

Performing an unfamiliar physical task — especially one that involves some hand–eye coordination — prompts your brain to recruit the muscles under control of the frontal cortex (following instructions) and the prefrontal cortex (planning ahead). The texture and aroma of the food are also enjoyable and stimulating.

Exercise 14: Try Yoga

Step 1

Learn a bit about yoga postures from an instructional yoga book or video. Or look for yoga routines and instructional videos online (for example, at https://yogainternational.com).

Step 2

Choose a yoga posture that you can do comfortably, one that will not strain your body. It should be appropriate to your fitness and flexibility level.

Step 3

Studying the written or spoken instructions, break down the pose, looking at the specific positions of the hands, feet, trunk, head, etc.

Step 4

Having figured out the correct positions of the various body parts, try everything you've learned together and carefully perform the actual pose.

Caution

Do not cause yourself pain and do not push through this exercise if you don't understand the pose and movement. A one-on-one session with a good yoga teacher, who will explain the pose, help position you and won't push too hard, might be valuable.

What does this exercise accomplish?

Yoga is a very special form of exercise that focuses the mind and the breath. It stimulates the brain, and one 2012 research study found that the gray matter in the brain — where the cells involved in information processing are found — increased in regular practitioners of yoga. By building up this area, you enhance parts of the brain that "map" the body and contain knowledge of other body parts and their locations in space. That mapping may actually increase brain cell growth!

Did You Know?

Yoga Caution

Yoga is typically relaxing, but it can take years of practice to attain a high level of skill. When you are starting out, be careful and avoid stressing your joints or muscles excessively. Taking the time to find a well-informed, qualified yoga instructor is a good investment that will help you enjoy and benefit from this mind–body practice.

Exercise 15: Notice Your Breath

Step 1

Sit down in a comfortable, quiet place and relax.

Step 2

Become aware of your breathing.

Step 3

Place your hand on your abdomen.

Step 4

Slowly breathe down into your belly, inflating your diaphragm (the muscle under your lungs that pushes air out and sucks it in). This will push your hand outward on your belly.

Step 5

Exhale slowly and watch your hand sink back in. With every inhalation and exhalation, visualize your diaphragm working hard.

Step 6

Repeat Steps 2 to 5 for a total of five repetitions.

What does this exercise accomplish?

This exercise helps you focus on the often underused diaphragm muscle. Poor posture and sitting for extended periods force us to breathe shallowly, high in our chests. Deep breathing is a better, healthier way to inhale what you need and exhale what you don't. It also helps activate the core muscles. Breathing deeply with the diaphragm delivers plenty of oxygen to the bloodstream, which is of vital importance to a healthy brain.

Exercise 16: Try Chopsticks

Step 1

Head to a kitchen- or restaurant-supply store and buy some chopsticks.

Step 2

Research how to use chopsticks. There are plenty of online tutorials that can teach you how to grip and manipulate chopsticks successfully. Visit www.wikihow.com/Eat-with-Chopsticks to find helpful step-by-step video demonstrations.

Step 3

Pick up and use your chopsticks in the air, practicing the proper grip and pinching movements.

Step 4

As the motion becomes easier and more natural, practice using your chopsticks to pick up larger pieces of food. Small meatballs, pieces of broccoli or small dumplings can be a good (and delicious) place to start.

Step 5

As you improve, practice using your chopsticks to pick up smaller items, such as small clumps of rice or individual green peas.

What does this exercise accomplish?

Learning to use chopsticks successfully is a continued, purposeful type of training that exercises fine motor skills. It also doesn't hurt to enjoy interesting aromas and tastes while you practice.

Exercise 17: Practice Tai Chi

Step 1

Learn a little about this ancient form of bodywork. Tai chi chuan is an ancient form of physical and breath exercise that also involves meditative practice. It is closely related to traditional Chinese medicine and involves gentle movement patterns that do not stress the joints or the heart. In traditional Chinese medicine, the goal is to balance the energies of the body and bring a person into harmony with both the internal and natural worlds. Check out local resources or online sources such as www.americantaichi.org/about.asp.

Step 2

Find a studio or recreation center in your area that offers beginner tai chi classes.

Step 3

Speak with the instructor about any specific needs you may have, and what the class will involve.

Step 4

Go to classes and practice the movements.

What does this exercise accomplish?

Tai chi is known for increasing feelings of well-being in its practitioners. It is terrific for people of all ages, but seniors especially benefit from it because it promotes better freedom of movement and breathing. Some preliminary scientific research into tai chi indicates that it might improve memory and neuroplasticity (see page 24). This makes sense, because movement stimulates brain growth — and tai chi is all about movement.

Exercise 18: Learn to Sew

Step 1

Find a sewing teacher, such as a knowledgeable relative or an instructor at a fabric shop or craft store. If you can't do this in person, there are some excellent books and videos that can instruct you in the basics.

Step 2

Choose a pattern and assemble the materials you need. The project should be challenging but not too complex. Keep it fun.

Step 3

With your instructor's help, follow the pattern and finish the project.

What does this exercise accomplish?

Sewing is fantastic for building fine motor control and hand–eye coordination. Coordinating what you see and feel requires your brain to fine-tune and manage tiny movements. Threading a needle is particularly challenging for the brain (and hands), because it requires very well-tuned muscle control. Sewing is not a daily activity for most people, as it once was, but there are still plenty of sewers. Besides being a fun hobby, sewing brings generations together and is economical. No more mending fees at the dry cleaner!

Did You Know?

Your Brain on Knitting

One way to strengthen the sensory areas of your brain is to take up knitting as a hobby. Knitting requires sensory information from your hands and eyes but also allows that sensory activity to guide muscle activity in your hands. Plus you get to wear what you make and have the satisfaction of creating something beautiful.

Exercise 19: Try Pilates

Step 1

Research Pilates a bit, either by reading about it or talking with an instructor. The basics: Pilates involves the very deliberate use of body position, speed and force in exercises that strengthen the core of the body, which is centered around the abdominal muscles. This amazing exercise system was created by Joseph Pilates in the early decades of the 20th century. Originally from Germany, Pilates immigrated to the United States and began to train dancers and athletes in his methods. Word of his work quickly spread way beyond his New York City studio, and Pilates classes are now found all over the world.

Step 2

Attend a beginner-level class taught by a certified Pilates instructor (see box, below). You may want to take a group class or have one-on-one private instruction.

What does this exercise accomplish?

Pilates is an incredible strengthening method, but it offers much more than that. It stimulates mental awareness of movement and ensures that you have a strong core that supports other muscles. As we age, we tend to neglect our core muscles by sitting too much at work, at home and in the car, and we lose the capacity to integrate movement the way we did as children. We can also neglect the core by focusing too much on cardio or non-core exercises. Pilates builds the core back up and teaches the body purposeful, refined movement.

Did You Know?

Qualified Instructors

When an unqualified teacher of Pilates, yoga or another mind–body discipline lacks experience or an understanding of human anatomy, injuries can result. Well-qualified teachers have taken the time to study and fine-tune the movements they teach their students. Some may also be certified by a governing body (visit www.pilatesmethodalliance.org for an example). In any case, never let an instructor push you beyond what seems right or comfortable.

Exercise 20: Posture Perfect

Step 1

Stand in front of a full-length mirror. A three-way mirror is best because you can see multiple angles at once (like in the change room of a clothing store).

Step 2

Examine your posture. Do your shoulders slump forward? Is your head thrust forward while your chin points upward? Is your lower back overly arched? Keep in mind that the human body is not linear — it has natural, normal curves, like the stacked S curves of the spine. This means that a military-style, ramrod-straight back is not a sign of good posture.

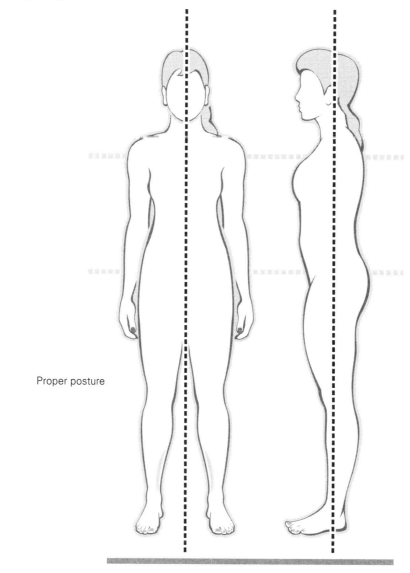

Proper posture

Step 3

Plant your feet firmly on the ground, about one hand's width apart.

Step 4

Place your hands on your sacrum, the triangular bone in your lower back that's located just above the coccyx, or tailbone. It usually starts around the inside corners of the back pockets of your jeans. Feel around the area as you stand straight. Is your sacrum curled in under your body? Is the lower part of the bone tilted toward the front of your body? This can encourage your shoulders to round and undermine good posture.

Step 5

Gently press your sacrum back so that it points more toward the rear of your body. More of the bone's length should press against your hand in this position, and you'll feel the normal curve returning to your lower spine.

Step 6

Now that you have a solid foundation, take a deep breath. Exhale.

Step 7

Square your shoulders. Move them back slightly but not too much.

Step 8

Tuck your chin in slightly, without feeling any tightness around your throat. Nod very slightly.

Step 9

Move your head back a bit so that its weight rests evenly over your shoulders, which are positioned in line with your stable lower back. It might help, at this point, to picture a string at the top of your head pulling up while the ground securely pulls your feet down.

Step 10

Take another deep breath. Exhale.

What does this exercise accomplish?

Gravity, slouching, poorly built chairs, bad mattresses and aging can all make dents in our posture over the years. This exercise helps restore normal structure and function to your body, aligning everything so that the whole body moves more efficiently. This allows your brain to smoothly control movement, and the joints and muscles to work the way they were designed to.

Caution

If you have had surgery or injuries or cannot quite get your posture in order, make sure to review this exercise with your doctor before attempting it. You may want to review your posture with a naturopathic physician, chiropractor or physical therapist as well.

Memory Augmentation Exercises

Memory is essential to our lives, and we are still learning about how it works. But some of the processes of making memories (if not exactly how they are stored) are well understood. Memorization exercises can be beneficial, as can developing better strategies for memorization: giving the brain clues and aids to rely on in memory making and retrieval.

Exercise 1: Pick a Card

Step 1

Open a regular deck of 52 cards and shuffle it.

Step 2

Deal three cards to yourself face down.

Step 3

Pick up each card, look at it and turn it face down again.

Step 4

Wait 10 seconds.

Step 5

Name all three cards out loud.

Step 6

Flip the cards over and see if you were right.

Step 7

Repeat Steps 1 through 6, increasing the waiting time in Step 4 to 20 seconds.

What does this exercise accomplish?

In this activity, you are testing your short-term memory. By waiting for 10 or 20 seconds before naming the cards, you move an image (and the recognition of what it means) from your sensory memory to your working memory.

Exercise 2: Top 5 List

Step 1

Pick a topic that interests you or is important to you, with items you can rank. You might try listing your top 5 favorite actors, your top 5 favorite restaurants or your top 5 inspiring historical figures.

Step 2

Create a Top 5 list for items in your chosen topic.

Step 3

Write down the list and memorize it.

1. ....

2. ....

3. ....

4. ....

5. ....

Step 4

Put the list away and don't look at it for 24 hours.

Step 5

The next day, try to recall your Top 5 list. Check the written list: did you remember every item on it?

What does this exercise accomplish?

This is both an exercise in recall and a tool for developing your memory — especially the initial conversion of memory from short-term to long-term. You can create lots of Top 5 lists that can help you remember important facts. Five is a small number and easy for the memory to manage. To keep building your memory, repeat this exercise daily, making a new list each time. Keep a running list of the topics of your Top 5 lists and see how well you can remember them all.

Exercise 3: Reconstruct the Day

Step 1

At the end of the day, sit down in a quiet place. You should be relaxed but not too tired.

Step 2

Think back over the day's events.

Step 3

Identify the major events and portions of the day. Where did you go? What important things happened? To which events do you have a strong emotional connection? What did you spend a lot of your time doing?

Step 4

Put these events in sequence (ideally in your mind, but you may write a list if that helps).

Step 5

Repeat the list to yourself, saying each event in its correct chronological order. You may do this silently or out loud.

What does this exercise accomplish?

This is a memory workout, but it is also a tool that will help you order items on a list. Mentally putting the day's events in order helps you remember sequences, just as organizing a cupboard helps you remember where to find the items in it. This exercise will help your brain transfer information from short-term memory to long-term memory, which involves many regions of the brain, but particularly the hippocampus (the structure responsible for the creation of long-term memories).

Did You Know?

Short-Term versus Sensory Memory

Short-term memory is actually very short — just a few seconds — but still longer than the imprint on our brain from sensory information, which is called sensory memory (like continuing to see a strong light for a split second after the light is turned off).

Exercise 4: Memorize a New Place

Step 1

Go to an unfamiliar place, such as a neighborhood you've never visited in your town, a neighboring town, a favorite vacation spot or a new mall.

Step 2

Walk around this new place. As you observe it, create a story about the experience. For example, if you've gone to the mall, tell yourself that you're not just on a random walk but rather a quest (to find new shoes, perhaps).

Step 3

Describe to yourself the places you visited and the significant people you met on this outing. Focus on the details that stood out.

Step 4

Retell this story to a friend or family member, including all the salient details you noted.

What does this exercise accomplish?

Using this narrative, or storytelling, technique helps you memorize new experiences and places more effectively. It allows you to place your memories into a framework that can be recalled at another time.

Did You Know?

Drama Helps Memory

People can often recall scenes in a movie that had compelling dramatic arcs. Doing exercises that ask you to create a story around an activity helps you remember details within the context of the story. The brain seems to prefer capturing memorable experiences in this manner.

Exercise 5: Memorize a Task

Step 1

Choose a new task you want to learn how to do. It can be repairing something around the house, doing a craft project or creating something artistic.

Step 2

Learn how to perform the steps needed to do this new task. Follow written instructions, watch a video or have a friend show you the process.

Step 3

Think back through the steps involved in the task, without performing them.

Step 4

Perform the steps and work through the stages of the project until you have finished it. As you work, describe each part of the process to yourself.

Step 5

Describe this new task to a friend or family member, including all the details you noted as you worked through the steps.

What does this exercise accomplish?

This exercise builds on the narrative memory technique you worked on in Exercise 4: Memorize a New Place. The brain builds memories more successfully when information is repeated back to us or when we relay it to another person. This is why students often find they retain material better when they form study groups and "teach" each other the material.

Exercise 6: Shop by Memory

Step 1

Make a list of 20 grocery items you need to buy. Include some items that you do not routinely buy every week, and some that offer a few different choices (such as "fruit — bananas or oranges").

Step 2

Review your list carefully, then put it away so you can't refer to it.

Step 3

Within the following two to six hours, do your shopping without referring to the list.

Step 4

Go home, take out the list and compare it to what you bought. Did you get everything on the list?

What does this exercise accomplish?

This exercise is a way to practice the consolidation of short-term memories into long-term memories. That process can take repetition and time, but we do know that structural changes in the brain can transpire in the first minutes and hours after you hear or learn something new. You can do variations on this exercise to keep it challenging. Try ordering your list by department (such as produce, bakery, dairy, etc.) and memorize what is located in each department. Or wait a full day after putting away your list — the longer lag makes the activity quite a bit tougher.

Exercise 7: Memorize New Countries

Step 1

Get out your world atlas or find some maps on the Internet.

Step 2

Pick 10 countries from an unfamiliar continent (France and Switzerland in Europe probably won't challenge a lot of people).

Step 3

Write down your list of countries and their continent.

1. ....
2. ....
3. ....
4. ....
5. ....
6. ....
7. ....
8. ....
9. ....
10. ....

Step 4

Review the list carefully, at least three times, looking at the names and hearing yourself (out loud or mentally) saying the names of the countries and their continent. Put it away so you can't refer to it, and wait 24 hours.

Step 5

The next day, try to write out your list without referring to it — or to other aids!

Step 6

Take out the original list and compare it to the one you just wrote. How many countries could you remember?

What does this exercise accomplish?

This memory workout exercises learning systems in the brain that take declarative information (such as saying something) and encode them into your long-term memory. To some extent, new synapses (the chemical connections between brain cells) are formed to create the memory.

Exercise 8: Memorize 10 World Capitals

Step 1

Get out (and dust off) your world atlas or find a list of world capital cities on the Internet.

Step 2

Pick 10 countries with capitals that are not familiar to you (Paris, France, probably won't challenge most people).

Step 3

Write down your list of countries and their capitals.

1. ....

2. ....

3. ....

4. ....

5. ....

6. ....

7. ....

8. ....

9. ....

10. ....

Step 4

Review the list carefully, at least three times, looking at the names and hearing yourself (out loud or mentally) saying the names of the cities. Put the list away so you can't refer to it, and wait 24 hours.

Step 5

The next day, try to write out your list without referring to it — or to other aids!

Step 6

Take out the original list and compare it to the one you just wrote. How many capitals did you get right?

What does this exercise accomplish?

Like Exercise 7: Memorize New Countries, this activity requires you to process unfamiliar information and commit it to long-term memory.

Exercise 9: Name Association

Step 1

Try this next time you meet someone new. It should be someone you will encounter again, at a place where you both turn up from time to time. After you hear the person's name for the first time, use it immediately; you might say, "It's nice to meet you, Sue" or "Do you come to this coffee shop often, Brian?"

Step 2

Create an association to help you memorize the name. You can connect the name and face of this new acquaintance with another person you know, or think of a word that rhymes with this person's name. You can also associate the name with the person's background (such as Joanie from the Bronx).

Step 3

The next time you see that person, try to recall the association you created. Greet the person using his or her name. If you have forgotten it, ask again and repeat Steps 1 through 3.

What does this exercise accomplish?

This activity uses a helpful technique to reinforce memory building. By creating mental associations, you help cement a piece of verbal information (the name) into your long-term memory. This creates connections that will help you retrieve it at a later date.

Exercise 10: Create a Mnemonic

Step 1

Think of a list you want to remember. It could be the names of people in a group or the ingredients for a recipe.

Step 2

Write down the names or ingredients and note the first letter of each word.

Step 3

Try to spell a word using these letters, creating a mnemonic. If you can't make a good word with the letters, try substituting another term or nickname for one of the names on your list to help you make an easy-to-remember word.

Step 4

Several times over the next few days, say the mnemonic out loud (either to yourself or to others, if you can find a way to work it into conversation).

Step 5

Write yourself a note on your calendar to check your recall in one week's time.

Step 6

When the week has passed, see if you can use the mnemonic to recall the list of names or ingredients.

What does this exercise accomplish?

Mnemonics help you commit information to your long-term memory. They are useful for people who have trouble retaining lists of new information. When a mnemonic is well rehearsed and interesting enough to stick with you, the brain can usually recall, decode and expand on the word to recreate the list of things you are trying to remember. You are "chunking" information into more manageable pieces and using imagery of some kind (usually a cute or interesting aspect of the mnemonic) to form associations that stick with you.

Did You Know?

Famous Mnemonics

Mnemonics are commonly used memory devices. They involve memorizing a word made up of the first letters of the items on a list; for example, Roy G Biv, which sounds like someone's name, is a handy mnemonic that helps you remember the colors of the rainbow (red, orange, yellow, green, blue, indigo, violet). Another famous mnemonic is HOMES, which helps you remember the names of the Great Lakes (Huron, Ontario, Michigan, Erie, Superior).

Exercise 11: Follow a Mental Map

Step 1

Pick a destination in a less familiar part of town. Choose a place that is not so remote that you could get lost or where it would be stressful to be disoriented (in other words, don't pick a spot in a very busy downtown area). It should not require you to make more than four or five turns to get there, or be very far away.

Step 2

Think through the directions you would have to follow to arrive at that destination.

Step 3

Visualize the street where you start your journey, then the first turn you'll take. What landmarks will you see along the way? Which streets are at the intersection where you will make that first turn?

Step 4

Continue to mentally construct your map this way, turn by turn. Stop after four or five turns — that's far enough.

Step 5

Drive to your destination, following your mental map. Don't get frustrated if you miss the mark. Pull over someplace safe and look at a map or a GPS device. How close were you?

What does this exercise accomplish?

This exercise gives your long-term memory a workout, forcing you to recall information you already know about local geography and to recall your own mental directions. It also makes demands on your visual-spatial intelligence.

Exercise 12: Be Aware

Step 1

Go to a completely new place, such as a recently opened store or restaurant.

Step 2

Observe the details of this environment. Where do people enter and exit from? What does the staff do? Where do they produce and keep their goods? Where do customers go to be served? What does the decor look like? What is the design of the space?

Step 3

Return home. Within an hour of returning, write down all your recollections of this new place.

Step 4

Return to the new place with list in hand. Did you remember the details correctly? How many things do you now notice that you did not before?

What does this exercise accomplish?

When you practice situational awareness, as you did in this exercise, you increase your observational powers and your memory's ability to encode the details of what is happening around you. Practicing this skill in a low-intensity manner can help you notice more and richer details in your surroundings, and better recollect places and events.

Exercise 13: Memorize Addresses

Step 1

Look through your email inbox and your list of contacts.

Step 2

Write out one email address (a personal one if possible). Memorize this address.

Step 3

Every day for the next week, recall the email address you memorized the previous day, then repeat Step 2 with a new address.

Step 4

At the end of the week, recall all seven email addresses you've memorized.

What does this exercise accomplish?

This exercise focuses on your power of recall. Using personal email addresses makes it more challenging, because most business emails often have simple naming conventions, such as first initial plus last name, that don't require you to memorize much. Note: If you do not use email, you can substitute telephone numbers in this exercise.

Exercise 14: Name 10 Foods

Step 1

Using a dictionary (either printed or online), look up the words for 10 different foods in a language you don't speak.

Step 2

Write a list of these words and their translations — original words in one column and translations in the other.

1. ....
2. ....
3. ....
4. ....
5. ....
6. ....
7. ....
8. ....
9. ....
10. ....

Step 3

Read through your list every day for three days. Try to use the words in your daily life — when you cook or eat the foods, or see them in the supermarket, call them by their name in the new language.

Step 4

Refer to your list every few days after the initial three-day period. Each time, cover up the English side and see if you can remember the translation of each food name.

What does this exercise accomplish?

Some memories are made by extending or attaching new meanings to old ones. This exercise does just that. It helps you incorporate new memories into everyday life and attaches a new word to an existing word that already has meaning for you.

Exercise 15: Sum Up a Show

Step 1

Watch a television show that you have not seen before. Try to find a show that will be repeated or that you can replay at another time.

Step 2

After the show has finished, take a break for one hour.

Step 3

Write a synopsis of the plot of the show you watched. Describe the main events in 12 to 15 points. Put away your synopsis and wait for 24 hours.

Step 4

The next day, mentally run through the plot of the show and your synopsis.

Step 5

Take out your written synopsis and read it again. Were your memories accurate?

Step 6

Watch or skim through the show again. Did you leave anything out of your original synopsis?

What does this exercise accomplish?

This activity encourages your brain to recall priority items in a dramatic context. When you assign importance to events or ideas, your brain records them as such. The act of reviewing your written synopsis and comparing it to your memories, then checking it against the actual show, is an excellent way to measure how well — and how accurately — you remember.

Part 3
Brain Hygiene Exercises

••

Sleep and Rest Exercises

Although the brain is never entirely at rest, it does need a period of consolidation and self-repair in order to function. If you cannot sleep, your brain will eventually fail to work properly. According to sleep foundations, the average North American gets about an hour less sleep than is needed for optimal health — much less in some cases. Shift work, late-night use of electronic devices, caffeine and many other things can disturb or postpone our sleep. The brain cannot fully consolidate learning or "reboot" itself without deep sleep.

These exercises, while they may seem to be more about feeling refreshed, go right to the heart of what it means to have a "fit brain."

If you cannot sleep, your brain will eventually fail to work properly.

Did You Know?

Growth Hormone
Growth hormone, an important repair hormone for the body that helps maintain muscle mass, is secreted during the periods of our deepest sleep.

Exercise 1: Begin Your Descent

Step 1

Decide what time you will go to bed, and be prepared to stick to it.

Step 2

Three hours before bedtime, stop consuming drinks and foods that contain caffeine, including cola, coffee, tea and chocolate. If you are sensitive to caffeine, stop six hours or more before bedtime. Any snacks you have at this point should be relatively small and easy to digest.

Step 3

Two hours before bedtime, stop working or watching the news (or anything distressing). Do not have any more snacks after this point.

Step 4

One hour before bedtime, turn off the television and all electronic devices. That means absolutely no web surfing, no social networking, no video game playing and no YouTube watching.

Step 5

In the final hour before bedtime, do relaxing activities. Take a warm bath scented with calming aromatherapy oils or bath salts. Get your oral hygiene routine done and drink just enough water to stay hydrated through the night. Read a pleasing, easy novel or magazine. Avoid distressing novels or page-turners that will keep you up until all hours.

Step 6

Before you go to sleep, reflect on the day. Think about any troubling issues and try to find the causes, especially if you feel you might be at fault. Make a mental (or written) note to adjust your behavior if necessary the next day, even if that includes apologizing to someone. Forgive people who have disturbed you during the day and put them out of your mind.

Step 7

Tell the people you live with that you love them.

Step 8

Conclude the day with any meditations, prayers or affirmations that you typically do.

Step 9

Sleep peacefully.

What does this exercise accomplish?

Sleep deprivation is a known cause of memory loss and cognitive impairment. The techniques used in this exercise increase the likelihood that you will fall asleep on time and experience high-quality sleep.

Create a Sleep Haven

You may prepare your body and mind properly, but if your sleeping quarters are not suitable, you won't be able to get the rest you need to keep your brain healthy. To create the right environment for sleep, follow these steps:

1. Examine your mattress closely. Does it provide adequate support? Is it comfortable?

2. Examine your pillows closely. Do they provide adequate support? Are they comfortable? Would you be better off with a cervical pillow that supports your neck and spine properly?

3. Examine your linens. Are they warm enough? Too warm? Are they scratchy?

4. Assess the air quality of your bedroom. Is there adequate air circulation? Is there too much dust? Is there mold?

5. Examine your bedroom at night with the lights off. Are there artificial light sources outside your windows that intrude into the darkened room? If so, should you put up light-blocking blinds, curtains or drapes?

6. Listen to the noise level in your bedroom at night. Is it quiet? Can you hear noises from inside the house? Can they be diminished? Are there outside noises and can you dampen their impact?

7. Examine the electronic devices in your bedroom. Many common gizmos emit light and make noise, which can disturb sleep. Figure out which ones you can switch off before you go to bed. (The only ones you really can't avoid are your alarm clock and maybe a phone.)

8. Make changes to your bedroom to fix the problems you found in the preceding steps.

Did You Know?

Getting Back to Nature

When city dwellers head out into nature, to a place with no artificial light at night, such as on a camping trip or an ocean cruise, they tend to be surprised by how dark nighttime truly is. They soon learn that their body wants to sync with the natural cycle of light and darkness. Getting back to nature makes it very clear just how overstimulated with light urban folks really are.

Exercise 2: Take a Catnap

Step 1

Find something written that you want to understand, such as a set of instructions. Pick a time when you can take a short nap without inconveniencing yourself or others.

Step 2

Read over the written item for 10 minutes if it's a general explanation of something. For a set of instructions, read them all the way through. Then put the written item down.

Step 3

Set an alarm for 25 minutes and lie down. If you are not able to use your bed, relax on a couch or a very comfortable chair that supports your head and neck and lets you recline and fall asleep.

Step 4

When the alarm goes off, take a few minutes to wake up.

Step 5

Return to what you were reading before your nap. Did this brief rest after a period of study improve your recollection? If not, did your nap at least give you a second wind to continue?

What does this exercise accomplish?

A catnap offers your brain a quick recharge, which can be great for problem solving and dissolving stress. You may need to experiment with this technique; it works for some people, but others actually feel worse after a nap.

Did You Know?

Famous Nappers

Some famous world leaders — such as John F. Kennedy, Eleanor Roosevelt and Winston Churchill — were daily nap devotees. They used short periods of sleep to keep their minds creative and resilient in the face of enormous amounts of stress.

Exercise 3: Take Five

Step 1

Find a time during your busy day when you can withdraw from the hustle and bustle.

Step 2

Isolate yourself in a place free of conversation, noise, television, radio, the Internet and so on.

Step 3

Relax and think about something positive, such as an event you are looking forward to or a good memory. Alternatively, you can do a bit of meditative (but light) reading.

Step 4

Return to your activities.

Step 5

Make this a daily habit. Train yourself to do this when you feel tired, anxious or agitated. Repeat this exercise more than once on particularly busy days.

What does this exercise accomplish?

This technique stops you from staying in overdrive all day long. Our bodies and brains are meant to relax periodically, and we work better when we do. The idea is to pause, unwind, refresh your thinking and return to your active role in life with renewed strength.

Exercise 4: Alternate Nostril Breathing

Step 1

Sit down in a comfortable, quiet place, maintaining good posture.

Step 2

Become aware of your breathing. Is it shallow? Is it rapid? Is it high in your chest or low in your belly?

Step 3

Using your right thumb, close off your right nostril. Inhale slowly through your left nostril.

Step 4

Release your right nostril and, using your left thumb, block off your left nostril. Exhale slowly through your right nostril.

Step 5

Repeat in the opposite order, inhaling through your right nostril (with your left nostril blocked by your left thumb) and exhaling through your left nostril (with your right nostril blocked).

What does this exercise accomplish?

This is a relaxation exercise that derives from meditative practices. The alternate breathing may stimulate the two hemispheres of your brain, with the right nostril stimulating the left hemisphere and the left nostril stimulating the right hemisphere. The science backing up this theory is incomplete, but one thing is for sure: alternate nostril breathing is relaxing.

Sports and Recreation Exercises

If you don't engage in sports or fun activities — or if you have done the same ones for as long as you can remember — it may be time to switch things up. Movement and the mental engagement of new activities can stimulate overall learning in the brain.

Exercise 1: Go Fly a Kite!

Step 1

Go to a hobby store or the recreation section of a department store and buy a kite, or borrow one from a friend.

Step 2

Read the instructions on how to assemble and use the kite. Assemble it.

Step 3

Find a suitable place to fly your kite on a breezy day. Make sure there are no power lines around.

Step 4

Let your kite fly and enjoy the exhilaration.

What does this exercise accomplish?

Kite flying is relaxing, and being surrounded by nature is something our minds and bodies crave. Relearning an activity you did as a child, one that is still fun and enriching for an adult, is a great way to make your brain open to new information and learning — as it was when you were young.

Exercise 2: Take a Stroll

Step 1

Choose a time when you can take a walk and commit to it. Write it down in your calendar.

Step 2

Select a pleasant walking route. This can be through an interesting walkable downtown area where pedestrians are welcome. Try to choose a route where the focus is on walking rather than window-shopping, and where you don't have to cross massive streets that are not pedestrian-friendly. Alternatively, you can try a route through a pretty, safe park or a walkable residential neighborhood.

Step 3

Lace up some good walking shoes. They should offer adequate cushioning and support. Leave the flip-flops at home or by the pool.

Step 4

Take your walk and enjoy seeing the sights, including other people coming and going.

What does this exercise accomplish?

Walking is a good workout. The human body needs to move to stimulate the nervous system, and you can benefit from this type of exercise even if you walk for just 30 minutes three or four times a week.

Did You Know?

Why Walking Works

Walking helps counteract the large amount of time people spend being sedentary in modern society — such as the hours spent sitting in cars, on couches or at desks. Walking also provides sensory input to the brain as you encounter new sights, sounds, smells and the sensation of varying terrain on your trek.

Exercise 3: Try Gardening

Step 1

Find a place to garden. This can be in your yard, on your balcony or at a community garden.

Step 2

Choose what you want to grow. Do you like ornamental plants? Flowers? Vegetables? Herbs?

Step 3

Figure out how much you want to take on. Do you want a small, easy-to-maintain patch or a garden that occupies a large portion of your yard? (Hint: If you've never gardened before, start small.)

Step 4

Buy a book or read gardening websites for advice on plant care.

Step 5

Set up your garden area with the right soil, and remove stones and weeds.

Step 6

Purchase seeds or young plants at a garden center. Speak with the staff about care instructions.

Step 7

Plant your garden. Remember to give plants room to grow and to plant them to the depth they need. This information is usually found on the label of the seed packet or pot.

Step 8

Tend to your garden daily. Water the appropriate amount and inspect your plants daily for insect or fungal damage. Try to deal with those problems in an environmentally friendly way.

What does this exercise accomplish?

A lot is happening in this exercise. The outdoor work — handling the plants, soil and water — and the physical movement (which can be scaled to your ability and agility) are good for both the body and brain. At the same time, you are learning new skills, which also stimulates brain function. The aromas of the soil and the plants stimulate your olfactory (smell) nerves. Your frontal cortex and prefrontal cortex get into the act to help you organize, plan and tend your garden. Getting outside in the sunshine and fresh air, surrounded by nature, has a beneficial effect on body and mind as well.

Exercise 4: Go Biking

Step 1

If you don't already have one, find a bicycle that suits your body and skill level. Many beginners will prefer a modern bike with wider tires that offer good stability.

Step 2

Buy the bike. Read the manual and become familiar with the bike and how to maintain it (count on getting a good tire pump). If you already own a bike, make sure it's in good repair.

Step 3

Invest in a good helmet and other protective gear.

Step 4

Prepare for a ride. Find a safe route on which you don't have to cross multiple lanes or ride in heavy traffic. If there are paved bike trails near you, use them.

Step 5

Stretch and limber up your muscles before you climb on your bike. Focus on the hamstrings (which run along the backs of the thighs down behind the knees) and the quadriceps (which run down the fronts of the thighs). Both work hard when you're pedaling.

Step 6

Enjoy your ride.

What does this exercise accomplish?

Biking is a great cardiovascular workout, and the movement, like walking and other activities, provides important sensory input into your brain. The brain must process incoming sensory information from your joints, muscles and skin as you move and coordinate continued movement. The scenery and the fresh air are pretty spectacular, too. If you learn about bike repair as well, you're mastering another new skill and challenging your learning powers. Or you can skip that step and find a helpful bike repair shop nearby if it's not your thing.

Exercise 5: Go Sailing

Step 1

Find a sailing club or association in your area.

Step 2

Research sailing lessons. Choose a sailing school with certified and experienced instructors to ensure your safety. Sign up for lessons on your preferred craft (see box, below).

Step 3

Obtain all the required safety gear. Sure, you need sunscreen, but a personal flotation device (better known as a life jacket) is the most important investment. Always wear it. If your boat tips and you are thrown overboard, a properly fitted life jacket can save your life and make it easier for others to rescue you.

Step 4

Go sailing. Enjoy the waves, breeze and sun. Make sure to hydrate, wear sunscreen and always have some extra dry clothes and layers with you. Wear your life jacket and use common sense. Always go with experienced sailors, and remember that the skipper is responsible for the boat. If the crew seems reckless or inexperienced, find another boat. If you like competition, a fun option is to help out in a race (ask for a simple job on the boat if you are a beginner). If you simply want a pleasant afternoon, go cruising.

What does this exercise accomplish?

This is another excellent physical exercise that requires you to learn a new skill. Sailing gives your brain the chance to absorb multiple sensory inputs at one time: the motion of the waves, the color of the sky, the feel of the breeze, and the sights and sounds of the activity on the boat. Sailing also requires physical movement and offers a friendly, fun camaraderie with fellow sailors.

Did You Know?

Choosing Sailing Crafts

Make sure that the type of sailboat you learn on suits you physically. Avoid dinghies (small sailboats that can tip easily) if you have arthritis and/or are not a confident swimmer. If you prefer a stabler ride, sign up for keelboat lessons — they take place on larger crafts (generally 24- to 30-foot/7- to 9-meter boats for beginners) that have stabilizing fins underneath.

Social Support and Emotional Health Exercises

Did You Know?

When to Seek Counseling

If you feel that fear is a big problem in your life, see a counselor or psychologist. Counseling is a great way to work through the fears that come up regularly.

People need people. Our emotional health is important to our quality of life but also to the quality of our brains. When we are properly nourished emotionally and socially, our brains are more stimulated and may actually retain more brain cells. We are hard-wired to be with others, and reaching out to friends and family to ask for and offer support can improve our brain fitness and our lives.

Negative emotions, be they morbid recollections of past hurts or negative projections about what life might bring us, can sap our mental energy like nothing else. Getting rid of negativity — a process that can sometimes be helped along by good support from close friends and family — can elevate your brain health as much as it does your sense of well-being.

Exercise 1: Conquer Fear

Step 1

Find a quiet place where you can reflect without interruptions. Turn off all distractions, such as the television and your phone.

Step 2

Think about something that frightens you, such as a financial problem, your family's safety or world events. It can be an irrational or a rational fear. (Note: The fear you examine shouldn't relate to an imminent danger or your intuition about a scary or untrustworthy person — those fears are actually good and necessary for survival.)

Step 3

Mentally separate the fear you've identified from your reactions to it. Tell yourself that your fear can take on a life of its own and that you can live without it.

Step 4

Think about a source of strength in your life, such as a loved one, a divine presence in the universe or nature, or your faith. Concentrate on this positive thought.

Step 5

Say the following affirmation: "I will let go of needless fear. It is not the real me. I am brave. I am strong."

What does this exercise accomplish?

This exercise helps you become aware of subconscious fears that can erode your sense of well-being. Over time, these fears can alter your thinking and create negative thought and behavior patterns. Facing these worries frees up vital mental, physical and emotional resources.

Exercise 2: Banish Resentment

Step 1

Find a quiet, comfortable place where you can reflect without interruptions. Turn off all distractions, such as the television and your phone.

Step 2

Think about something troubling from your past that you can't let go. For example, perhaps someone didn't invite you to an important event or hurt your feelings publicly. Even if it is years later, you may still feel angry about it and you may keep reliving the hurt. The word "resentment" comes from Latin, and means "to feel something over and over." Because you are still holding on to the hurtful emotion, you may still be harboring a grudge against the person who hurt you.

Caution

This common human situation is different from deeper traumas such as abuse, which require healing and insight beyond this exercise. If the source of your anger is a traumatic event, seek the help of a licensed psychotherapist, psychologist or counselor, who can provide guidance and treatment.

Step 3

Think about the person who hurt or offended you. What got under your skin, and why?

Step 4

Think about your involvement in the situation. Did any of your actions or expectations make it worse? Perhaps you were expecting someone to be nice when he or she never is. Perhaps you ended up someplace you should not have been. Perhaps the situation is in no way your fault, but it is good to ask yourself this question.

Step 5

Tell yourself that no matter how wrong the other person was, there must be something missing or wrong in his or her life that provoked this behavior. Wish the person well, and let your resentment go.

Step 6

Immediately turn your attention toward constructive thoughts. Think about someone you love, someone you can help or a happy memory. Do not dwell on the past offense anymore.

Step 7

Don't expect old hurts to disappear easily. Repeat this exercise if the feelings resurface, then move on to better thoughts.

What does this exercise accomplish?

This is an effective technique for letting go of resentment, hatred and anger from the past. These negative emotions can become embedded in the psyche, wasting enormous amounts of energy. If you have anger you can't let go of, see a counselor or psychologist. Some resentment is linked to traumas that require professional attention and a sympathetic ear. Sometimes people think asking for help is a sign of weakness, but it's just the opposite — it is a sign of wisdom.

Exercise 3: Positive Visualization

Step 1

Find a quiet, comfortable place where you can relax without interruptions. Turn off all distractions, such as the television and your phone.

Step 2

Close your eyes.

Step 3

Think of a beautiful place you've visited or a pleasant memory.

Step 4

Recreate the setting in your mind. Focus on the little details that you remember. For example, maybe it's a beautiful Caribbean beach under crystal-clear blue skies, or a wonderful birthday party with the best cake you've ever tasted.

Step 5

Spend a few minutes with this memory, keeping your eyes closed. Try to clearly picture what it looked like and what happened.

What does this exercise accomplish?

This exercise is a type of mental vacation, and it engages memories that tap into the visual processing area of the brain. There are many types of visualization exercises. This simple one aims to help you remember what it's like to feel really good. When you relive these feelings, a number of neurochemical and hormonal changes occur. The brain learns to adopt certain patterns — of anxiety, of gloom or of well-being. This visualization is a way to condition your brain to feel happy.

Exercise 4: Say an Affirmation

Step 1

Find an affirmation — either in inspirational literature or on a website — that you like. For example, an affirmation could be "I am worthy to give and receive love" or "I am able to meet the challenges of today and to help others along the way."

Step 2

Find a quiet, comfortable place where you can meditate for a few minutes, undisturbed, on this affirmation.

Step 3

Repeat the affirmation. Don't force it or try to make yourself feel a certain way. Just repeat the words and let their meaning wash over you. Even if part of your brain tells you not to embrace the affirmation, ignore it and calmly repeat the affirmation.

What does this exercise accomplish?

Affirmations are similar to visualizations. They help condition the brain and, in time, can teach you to adapt to new beliefs and behaviors. Obviously, an affirmation needs to be rooted in the truth. It is most effective when it refers to constructive issues that are within your grasp.

Exercise 5: Practice Gratitude

Step 1

Think about the nature of gratitude. We are grateful for things that are meaningful or valuable to us. These are the good things in our lives, including health, support, family, friends and the natural beauty around us.

Step 2

Think about gratitude as an action. It is the act of making those good things important. We often dwell on and place great importance on the bad things we cannot change. Gratitude is about focusing on the good forces in our lives.

Step 3

Write a list of the good things in your life. Think about the things you want to value.

Step 4

Read over your list and think about what your life would be like without those things. Say "thank you" for each one of them.

What does this exercise accomplish?

Being grateful creates good feelings and thoughts and moves your focus from negative to positive. It also allows you to take better care of the good people and things around you. Gratefulness enhances the "stress letdown response," which means you embrace what is good in your life and release tense feelings. If you can stay in this state a fair amount of the time, you will experience positive effects on your hormonal system and your immune system.

Exercise 6: Make a Call

Step 1

Think of someone with whom you have not connected for a while. Don't start with someone with whom you had a major falling out or a troubled relationship. Just think of someone you wish you spoke to more.

Step 2

Give that person a cheerful or concerned phone call.

Step 3

Agree with that person to keep in touch, and set a time or date to speak again. Better yet, if possible, make a date for a fun breakfast, lunch, dinner or coffee together. If the person you call is far away, just hearing his or her voice is enough.

What does this exercise accomplish?

Maintaining your social connections is extremely important for brain health and function. We too often let these relationships lapse when we are busy. It's good to remember that we can reconnect with great people with just a few pushes of a button.

Did You Know?

Video Conferencing

Two-way video conferencing is now easy with programs such as Skype and FaceTime, which allow you to both see and hear people in other places. All you need is a computer, phone or tablet with a camera, a microphone and speakers. These programs are easy to use and free for casual users.

Exercise 7: Write a Letter

Step 1

Think of someone you have lost touch with. It shouldn't be someone with whom you've had great troubles — just someone you haven't caught up with in a while.

Step 2

Sit down and write the person a letter. An email can work, but the personal touch of a letter is even more valuable.

Step 3

Mention in the letter that you'd like to have a chat sometime. Don't spend the entire letter recounting your news. Ask the person some questions about his or her life, recall some good memories of times you spent together or share some plans for the future.

Step 4

Close the letter by wishing the person well and asking him or her to keep in touch.

What does this exercise accomplish?

Writing a letter is similar to making a phone call: it helps you stay connected with people in your life. Without social input, the brain withers. An old-fashioned handwritten letter is a treat to receive — even for people who typically use email or social networking exclusively.

Exercise 8: Join a Club

Step 1

Find a local club or organization that piques your interest.

Step 2

Find out about the club. Does it cost money to join? Are there any requirements you need to meet in order to join? What are the obligations of the members? What is the club's reputation in the community? Where does it meet and how often? What activities do members participate in?

Step 3

If the club seems right for you, apply for membership.

What does this exercise accomplish?

Social networking was around a long time before websites were invented. People love and need to gather together, and clubs allow them to share information. Some clubs focus on service, which offers an extra benefit: the good feelings you experience when you give to others. Clubs that are built around a shared interest in a specific hobby or topic are wonderful, too. Many of us need to spend less time staring at television, computer, cellphone and tablet screens, and a club offers you a way to do that and spend time with other people while doing interesting things.

Exercise 9: Throw a Dinner Party

Step 1

Create a list of interesting and enjoyable guests.

Step 2

Plan a small, informal gathering at a convenient time.

Step 3

Invite your guests, making sure the invitation asks them to RSVP.

Step 4

Create a menu with a selection of simple foods that people can savor —
small plates or appetizers are fun and interesting to share.

Step 5

If possible, ask an assistant to help you shop for ingredients and prepare.
If cooking is not your thing, you can have the party catered. Remember, the
menu doesn't have to be expensive. Many reasonably priced restaurants
offer catering options, and you can pick up dinner for 8 to 10 people without
a huge bill.

Step 6

Welcome your guests and enjoy their company.

What does this exercise accomplish?

This fun exercise is another way to satisfy the brain's (and the heart's) need
for human interaction. The nice thing about a casual dinner party is that there
is time to talk as you eat. Engaging in interesting conversations, trading
stories and telling jokes are some of the most stimulating activities for your
brain. Your temporal lobe and prefrontal cortex all get in on the act as you
make conversation, learn new things and laugh. Bonding with others and
the feeling of camaraderie have a positive effect on your limbic system, a
driver of emotional responses, such as the affection you feel for a pleasant
group of companions.

Exercise 10: Volunteer

Step 1

Find a volunteer organization, such as a food bank, a drop-in center, a hospital or a long-term care home for seniors.

Step 2

Ask the program manager what the organization needs and what he or she expects of volunteers.

Step 3

Look at your own abilities and talents. Do they fit well with what the institution needs?

Step 4

If your skills are a good match, sign up for some volunteer work.

What does this exercise accomplish?

Volunteering gets you in contact with new people and offers you the chance to learn new skills or put skills you already have to good use. The mental rewards a volunteer gets from helping others are well documented. This is also a chance to focus on the positive changes you can make in a chaotic world. It can help boost the spirits of anyone who is fed up with monotonous daily routines or who is disheartened by too much bad news on television.

Language Acquisition Exercises

From our first days of life through our time as toddlers, our brains were exploding with growth. During this important phase, we acquired a remarkable skill: the use of language. The ability to make sense of sounds and communicate with others is innate, yet it needs to be cultivated and emerges only through interaction with others. While learning even a single language is an amazing accomplishment, studies show that people who learn two or more languages may have a slower cognitive decline later in life.

Further research is needed before it will be clear whether the longevity benefits of multilingualism apply only to those who learned other languages early in life or whether they extend to those who study other languages as adults. Regardless, one of the central themes in this book is that we should activate the learning powers of the brain beyond daily routines that require very little thought or effort. Learning a new language can help us pursue this goal.

> Studies show that people who learn two or more languages may have a slower cognitive decline later in life.

Exercise 1: Learn 10 Words in a Foreign Language

Step 1

Find a foreign-language teaching resource, such as a dictionary or an online resource, for a language you've never studied.

Step 2

Identify 10 words you want to learn how to say in that language.

Step 3

Find the translation and study the pronunciation of each of your 10 words. As you study each word, link it to a mental image, associating it with something that is likely to evoke memories. For instance, if the foreign word is the name of a food, think of a great (or bad!) experience you've had with that food.

Step 4

Practice pronouncing the words and memorize their meanings, spending a few minutes on each word.

continued, next page...

Exercise 1: Learn 10 Words in a Foreign Language (continued)

Step 5

Write down the words and their meanings. Set aside your notes for 24 hours.

1. ....
2. ....
3. ....
4. ....
5. ....
6. ....
7. ....
8. ....
9. ....
10. ....

Step 6

The next day, try to recall and say all 10 words.

Step 7

Compare what you remembered with what you wrote down.

Step 8

If you know someone who speaks your chosen language, try out your 10 words on him or her.

What does this exercise accomplish?

Language acquisition activates pathways in the brain that we use frequently as children but that may lie dormant in adults. By learning these 10 words, you open up those pathways and make new connections in the brain.

Did You Know?

Audio-Visual Aids

Foreign-language DVDs and websites are excellent resources because they contain both audio samples that enable you to hear correct pronunciations and videos that enable you to see someone saying the new words.

Exercise 2: Take a Class

Step 1

Find a foreign-language class in your area. Community centers are a good place to look, and many cities have institutes that specialize in specific languages and the cultures of the people who speak them.

Step 2

Sign up for an introductory class.

Step 3

Attend classes and try to speak as much as possible. Remember, using a language regularly in different situations is the best way to learn.

What does this exercise accomplish?

Learning a new language involves memorizing vocabulary and grammar and learning pronunciation and meanings of phrases. Studying a foreign language, especially in a systematic way in a class, stimulates the learning pathways of your brain.

Exercise 3: Take a Trip

Step 1

Study a foreign language until you have a degree of competence in it. Take classes, in a school or via DVDs or the Internet, and focus on learning how to use that language in daily interactions.

Step 2

Plan a trip to a country where that language is spoken.

Step 3

Ask a travel agent to help you book a trip that will let you speak and interact with people but that is safe and not overwhelming. It is not fun to be in a place where people can't communicate with you or where you feel out of your element. Plus, tourists can be targets in some places. On the other hand, you won't learn much if you're locked away on a tour bus with other English-speakers. Look for a balanced experience.

Step 4

Take your trip, explore and interact with people in their language. Make sure to study cultural norms as well before you jump in. Different cultures have different rules on acceptable levels of eye contact, directness and polite terms of address (such as when to use "sir," "Mr." and "madam").

What does this exercise accomplish?

Traveling is the ultimate way to get out of the repetitive, sedating routines of life. The trick to a successful journey is good planning and awareness. Both minimize any risks while maximizing opportunities for fun and learning.

Exercise 4: Eat Globally

Step 1

Find a restaurant that serves cuisine from another culture. Look for an authentic experience. For example, a takeout Thai place at the food court might make a great snack, but unless you visit at a slow time and the staff are of Thai ancestry or origin, you might not encounter much in the way of Thai culture. A family-run Thai restaurant may provide more authentic sensory stimulation.

Step 2

Find a quiet time to dine at your chosen restaurant, when it is not swamped with customers.

Step 3

Examine the words and dishes on the menu. Ask your server about the meanings of the names.

Step 4

Get to know the owner or the host, and learn how to identify foods by their proper names. Inquiring about the pronunciation of the foods and the history of the dishes can teach you about the culture.

What does this exercise accomplish?

This exercise is a lighter way to study language. Learning about a country's food is a great way to get to know its culture. You learn new words, history and cultural information at the same time. Dining is a rich experience for the senses, and the new words will have staying power in your brain because they are relevant and learned in a pleasant, delicious context.

Exercise 5: Find a Pen Pal

Step 1

Find a pen pal service. Research it thoroughly before you join (unfortunately, there are some that are simply scams to steal money). Ask friends for recommendations and look at online reviews. Alternatively, you may want to contact smaller foreign aid organizations that might be glad to help you form pen pal relationships with the people they sponsor.

Step 2

Once you have a pen pal, write to him or her regularly. Share interesting facts and details about your home and culture.

Step 3

Ask your pen pal to teach you some new words in his or her native language. Start with terms for everyday things and move on to local sayings or issues in your pen pal's life.

What does this exercise accomplish?

Writing to a pen pal is a way to enrich your linguistic knowledge through personal exchanges with another person. Once you've established a relationship, you may want to take a class in your pen pal's language and practice writing to him or her in it.

Part 4
A Healthy Brain in a Healthy Body

Did You Know?

Endorphins

When the body is engaged in intense exercise, powerful pain-suppressing and pleasure-promoting compounds called endorphins are released into your bloodstream. They give us a release from stress and tension. They are one of the components of "runner's high," the rush of exhilaration that exercise can deliver. The best part: you don't have to be a marathon runner or even in peak physical condition to get this type of pleasure from exercise.

Physical Exercise Benefits the Brain

This book focuses on mental exercises you can do to give your brain the workout it needs, but living a healthy physical life plays an important role in supporting those efforts. The brain depends on the rest of the body, so your physical activities influence how your brain works. Depending on what you do (or don't do), you can either build up or undermine brain health.

We need to move. Our bodies are meant to stay active, and the brain responds powerfully to exercise. The brain is such a magnificent, adaptive organ: people who are bedridden or whose bodies are immobilized can still engage in the highest, most complex forms of thought and imagination. But this capacity is enhanced when we move, and if we are able to do so, we should exercise and explore the world freely at every opportunity.

Exercise Enhances Circulation

When you exercise, blood flow to your brain increases. This is a simple outcome of speeding up your circulation. Increased blood flow to the brain leads to feelings of well-being — it's no accident that some people do their best thinking on long walks. The motion, the rhythm and the enhanced circulation in the brain all help inspire their thoughts.

Movement Stimulates Growth

When we move, certain brain-related growth factors are released. These growth factors cause us to sprout new connections in the brain and even grow new brain cells. That means that exercise helps rewire the brain, making you smarter.

It also means that physical activity doesn't just improve the condition of your heart and joints; it also boosts your mental powers. The brain craves the sensory input that exercise provides when you move around in your world. All this makes it even more important to feed the brain more of the essential lifestyle "nutrients" it desires: movement and exercise.

Best Workouts

There are so many sports and recreational activities to choose from. In fact, there is an almost overwhelming amount of choice out there. The key is to find the ones that work for you. That means your body needs to be up to the challenge, and you need to enjoy the activity and have fun doing it. Here are some of the many options.

Aerobic Exercises

These activities get your heart rate up and increase circulation. They are not directly geared toward increasing your physical strength, but they have that effect indirectly. Because these types of exercises raise your heart rate significantly, consult with a physician before you start any of them. This is especially important for people with a history of heart disease or stroke. Some options to try:

- Running
- Cycling
- Exercise classes, such as aerobics or dance-based workouts

Strength Training

These activities are specifically designed to build muscle strength. They also make demands on the heart and increase circulation, but not to the same degree as aerobic activities.

Did You Know?

Watch Your Joints

Many types of high-intensity aerobic exercises — such as running, cycling, high-impact aerobics and so on — can put excessive stress on your joints. The good news is that there are adapted exercises and lower-impact options that don't do the same amount of damage. Never push yourself so hard you injure your joints, and ask trainers or coaches for advice on making exercises work for your particular needs.

Proper form and respect for limits are important to keep in mind when doing these types of training. If you're just starting out, working with a trainer or coach can protect you from injury. Some activities to try:

- Weight lifting
- Isometrics, a muscle contraction technique that builds strength quickly
- Classic strength exercises that use the body's own weight as resistance, such as push-ups, chin-ups, and so on

Swimming

Swimming offers the best of both worlds: it improves aerobic capacity and builds strength. It doesn't require the joints to bear weight, so it is a terrific option for people with arthritis or back pain. Another option is water-based fitness classes, which can be challenging and not quite as gentle on the joints. These classes use aerobic-style motions and allow you to do moderate exercise in a more buoyant environment.

Organized Sports

There are tons of different sports for many different tastes. They may be team-based, such as baseball or soccer; opponent-focused, such as tennis; or individual-oriented, such as golf. No matter which one you prefer, sports blend movement, fun, coordination, visual-spatial intelligence, teamwork and interpersonal interaction. And you can enjoy a variety of levels of exercise (some quite intense), depending on the activities you prefer.

Did You Know?

Tailored Yoga Classes

You can find yoga classes specially designed for people who have had injuries and for the elderly. It never pays to go over your level of tolerance in any type of exercise, and yoga is no exception. Take an adapted class if you need to, so you can stay within your physical limits while still enjoying the benefits this exercise provides.

Mind–Body Exercises

Asia has provided many of the mind–body exercises that are popular today. Both tai chi and qigong were created as components of traditional Chinese medicine. Both promote the flow of energy (which is called qi, or chi) in the body. They are excellent for getting the body to move through full ranges of motion and to stretch the muscles and ligaments around joints.

Yoga is a form of meditation and mind–body exercise from South Asia that is astoundingly popular all over the world. It can be great for centering the breath and increasing flexibility. Many of the poses also really test muscle strength and balance. A good rule is not to overdo it — especially when you're starting out — and to take classes that suit your body (see box, at left).

Return to Nature

Human beings thrive when they are exposed to the outdoors. They naturally crave connections with nature. In our artificially created world of tightly sealed housing, large buildings, cars, 24-hour-a-day lighting and endless glowing screens, we cut ourselves off from the world around us. It's important for your physical and mental well-being to fight that trend and reestablish this natural bond.

FAQ

Q. *How does getting in touch with nature encourage brain health?*

A. Besides being good for you physically, going outside and being active can positively influence the function and health of your brain. Getting in touch with nature can:

- Reduce anxiety
- Improve learning
- Improve cognition
- Increase feelings of well-being
- Improve feelings and attitudes toward others

Easy Ways to Reconnect with Nature

It sounds like a big job, but building connections with the natural world doesn't have to be. There are plenty of simple ways to do this, and you can incorporate many of these activities or strategies into your everyday life. Here are just a few ideas.

- Take a walk in the park.
- Grow more plants in your house.
- Get a pet (and walk with it outdoors whenever possible).
- Plant and tend a garden.
- Hike along a nature trail.
- Walk barefoot on a beach.
- Go boating with friends.
- Visit national parks and monuments erected in beautiful natural settings.

Inflammation and the Brain

Did You Know?

Inflammation

Inflammation is a normal, healthy part of our body's defense mechanism, helping to remodel damaged tissue. However, when it is chronic or out of control, it becomes dangerous.

Unlike muscle tissues, brain cells cannot make energy if they are deprived of oxygen for even a short period of time.

Inflammation is a complex function that has both good and bad aspects. On the positive side, it helps the body fight off infections and respond to injuries. This usually involves special chemicals released by our cells that lead to increased blood flow, redness, swelling and pain, all of which can actually help the body heal and fight off intruders. On the negative side, inflammation can also damage body structures and functions and lead to the development of diseases.

Many brain conditions — including stroke and dementia — have a large inflammatory component. To understand one example of how inflammation ages the brain, let's start with the brain's need for a vast network of healthy blood vessels to supply oxygen. Neurons are very active cells that create their own energy by what is called aerobic metabolism. They take glucose (a sugar) from the bloodstream and break it down into smaller compounds that can be torn apart to release their potential energy. For brain cells, oxygen is a crucial part of the process of energy creation. Unlike muscle tissues, brain cells cannot make energy if they are deprived of oxygen for even a short period of time.

In health and (usually) in youth, the brain is saturated with a seemingly endless branching structure of blood vessels, from large to very small. In atherosclerosis, a common condition that erodes the health of the vascular system, plaque accumulates in arteries of various sizes, but especially those of medium size. Although cholesterol levels are an important predictor of risk for atherosclerosis, it is now understood that inflammation drives this process. The arteries become narrowed with cholesterol deposits and abnormal tissue (similar to scar tissue) as the plaques advance, and they become stiffer. Eventually, when one of the plaques ruptures, a blood clot may form. Sometimes the clot is so large that it blocks the artery.

When a large clot blocks a diseased artery in the brain, it is known as a cerebral vascular event, or infarct (in the heart, it is called a myocardial infarction). In plain English, we call this a stroke (although a stroke can also be caused by a blood vessel bursting). A significant amount of brain tissue can die as a result.

But even when only tiny blood vessels deteriorate because of inflammation, damage to the brain becomes apparent as the brain cells are cut off from healthy circulation. The inflammation might not lead to a catastrophic event such as a stroke, but brain scans will show less gray matter (brain cells) and white matter (the connections or pathways between brain cells and brain regions). The brain may, in fact, actually shrink.

Inflammation thus plays a part in other forms of dementia and neurological aging, although it is not the sole culprit. Regardless, it makes sense to attempt to decrease it. The typical North American diet includes many foods that promote inflammation, such as saturated fats and processed ingredients. Moreover, it is deficient in healthy fats, including omega-3 fatty acids, and plant-based foods, which provide numerous protective anti-inflammatory compounds. Eating a diet of high-fat processed foods, without enough fruits and vegetables, can age the body.

This high-fat, overly processed diet has led to a very high rate of metabolic syndrome, an inflammatory condition characterized by high blood glucose, high blood pressure and (usually) obesity. One of the root causes is that the muscle cells of the body become resistant to the hormone insulin, which plays an important role in moving glucose from the bloodstream into tissue cells. When you eat foods that cause your blood glucose to skyrocket, your body responds by dumping a lot of insulin into your bloodstream. When that occurs day after day, year after year, eventually the body can become less sensitive to insulin: it takes more and more insulin to get blood sugar levels under control. High levels of insulin contribute to obesity and increase some inflammatory activities in the body. (For some people, a preexisting inflammatory state might contribute to their insulin resistance in a vicious cycle.)

When blood glucose levels remain high much of the time, brain cells are damaged. Glucose binds to the proteins in brain cells, distorting their original structure and leading to accelerated aging. The support cells of the nervous system — glial and Schwann cells — are damaged as well. The high blood pressure that goes along with metabolic syndrome can further damage blood vessels in the brain.

Current obesity rates are as follows: 35% of adults and 18% of children in the United States; 25% of adults and 12% of children in Canada. These individuals are not just overweight but are at a high enough weight and body fat content to be at risk for metabolic syndrome and other health risks. The long-term impact of this reality on aging, heart health and brain health has yet to be fully realized.

The good news is that nutrition and dietary changes can help discourage excess inflammation, lower the risk of metabolic syndrome and increase overall health and vitality. In Part 5, you'll learn strategies for making these positive changes to your eating habits.

Nutrition and dietary changes can help discourage excess inflammation, lower the risk of metabolic syndrome and increase overall health and vitality.

Part 5
Brain Food

• •

Foods for a Healthy Brain

Did You Know?

Addressing Metabolic Dysfunctions

When a naturopathic doctor recommends a diet, dysfunctions in the patient's physiology need to be considered before anything else. A patient assessment usually shows what is out of balance or going wrong in the diet, and a naturopathic doctor can outline a modified diet that is therapeutic. For example, a patient with impaired kidney function may need a specific amount of certain high-quality proteins. Treatment may involve dietary restrictions as well as other measures to restore health. Your best bet before you embark on a new diet is to work through any issues with your health-care provider.

Let's start by acknowledging that no one food can meet all the brain's needs. Food doesn't work that way. The human metabolism requires a number of energy sources and special chemical compounds to maintain good health. The brain is no different. It follows the same rules as the rest of the body. Brain cells need to burn energy and repair themselves, and they require vitamins and minerals to perform certain chemical reactions.

No Diet Is Perfect

Nutrition affects every individual differently. We all have slightly different metabolic needs, and there are variations in the quantities of vitamins and minerals we require. Moreover, food sensitivities and allergies cause many people trouble with specific foods. A diet that leaves one person feeling energized can leave another in a higher state of inflammation and feeling sluggish. Remember, foods are not innately good or bad. For example, wheat is fine for some people, but others may not digest or tolerate it — for people with celiac disease, the immune system reacts negatively to the gluten it contains and wheat can make them seriously ill. The key is to eat healthy, whole foods as often as possible, and to respect what works for your body.

Brains Need Glucose

The brain prefers glucose as an energy source. For that reason, you need to consume carbohydrates that slowly and steadily release energy. Simple carbohydrates consist of a single sugar molecule or a pair of sugar molecules. Your cells burn simple carbs quickly, then the energy they provide disappears. Complex carbohydrates, on the other hand, consist of chains of sugar molecules. Cells burn them more slowly, giving you longer-lasting energy.

The Glycemic Index

The glycemic index (GI) is a way of measuring how quickly a specific food sends sugar into the bloodstream after it is eaten. Pure glucose is the simplest form of sugar in the human bloodstream, and it's absorbed very rapidly. Therefore, it has the highest score on the GI index: 100. A high-GI food behaves like glucose, raising the blood sugar level quickly, while a low-GI food behaves in the opposite manner, raising the blood sugar level slowly and steadily.

FAQ

Q. *Are starchy foods made with refined flour as high on the glycemic index as sugar?*

A. Yes. Some starchy foods raise blood sugar almost as fast as pure glucose. Let's take white bread as an example. It turns into glucose almost immediately upon consumption and raises blood sugar quite high at a rapid pace, leading to peaks and valleys in your energy level.

Why Low-GI Foods Are Best

Complex carbohydrates take time to break down in the body, which is why they release their energy slowly and have a lower GI value. Whole grains are a prime example: the carbohydrates they contain are attached to the bran and germ of the kernel (the seed portion of a grain plant). These two parts of the grain are harder for the body to digest, so they don't slam the bloodstream with instantly available glucose.

Foods that contain a larger proportion of fat or protein also rank lower on the GI scale. They release glucose into the bloodstream slowly. When you mix fats or proteins with carbohydrates, they can slow down digestion, which creates a kind of time-released sugar supply for cells.

Brains Need Fat, Too

Another key aspect of brain nutrition is fat consumption. The types of fats we consume matter greatly in the quest to keep brain cells in top condition.

The brain contains a very high percentage of omega-3 fatty acids. It uses them in its cell structure and they form a large component of brain mass. These fatty acids are in the cell membrane (the outer surface), which conducts the electrical

Did You Know?

Weston Price

Weston Price was a dentist who explored the relationship between nutrition and health in the early 20th century. His book *Nutrition and Physical Degeneration: A Comparison of Primitive and Modern Diets and Their Effects*, originally published in 1939, is still relevant today. It shows how intelligent observation and research can guide our food choices.

signals that allow brain cells to communicate. Omega-3 fats can't be made by the body, so it is essential to consume foods that are rich in them. The brain has a powerful need for omega-3 fatty acids, especially when we are young. The brain acquires most of its mass in our first several years of life (although lifelong nutrition is certainly important). Cells require omega-3 fats even before we are born, which is why pure and safe sources of omega-3 fats are important supplements for pregnant women. For more on the fats your brain needs, see page 174.

Antioxidants and Phytochemicals

The brain is susceptible to a variety of factors that cause premature aging, as you learned early on in this book. To protect brain tissue, people need antioxidants and a variety of plant compounds, or phytochemicals, which protect cells from damage. Some of these compounds protect brain cells directly, while others focus more on protecting blood vessels (both large and minute) that the brain needs in order to function. For more on antioxidants, see page 183.

Eating Well Is Simple

Our tendency lately is to make eating so complex and mysterious that we need multiple experts to tell us what to do. But it doesn't have to be difficult. In this section, you'll learn about foods that can, over time and in large quantities, harm the brain. But you'll also learn which foods encourage general health and brain fitness, and discover recipes that use these nutritious foods in delicious, simple ways. These guideposts will help you make healthy choices and not obsess over what's good and what's bad.

Eat Real, Whole Foods

In the wise words of food commentator and author Michael Pollan, "Eat food." In other words, eat real food, not fake food. Natural, whole foods are superior to artificially colored, flavored and texturized pseudo-foods that have had a few nutrients added back into them. Excessive amounts of high-fructose corn syrup in packaged foods, artificial sweeteners and other nutritionally poor ingredients are not components of a brain-boosting diet.

Realistically, most people in North America will consume some processed food. And you can debate for days about what constitutes "processed"; organic pasta sauce in a jar is, to some degree, processed. But a frozen ready-made pasta dish that has upward of 30 ingredients on the label is more processed. Always choose the simpler option.

Keeping a Brain Food Diary

Before you can build a brain-enhancing diet plan, you need to analyze how well you're doing already. You can accomplish this by keeping a brain food diary for four days. Using the diary below as an example, list everything you eat each day. Write down the approximate quantity of each food as well (but don't bother weighing every single thing you eat). Include snacks and beverages.

Four-Day Diet Diary

Day 1
Breakfast:
Morning snack:
Lunch:
Afternoon snack:
Dinner:
Evening snack:
Beverages:

Day 2

Breakfast:

Morning snack:

Lunch:

Afternoon snack:

Dinner:

Evening snack:

Beverages:

Day 3

Breakfast:

Morning snack:

Lunch:

Afternoon snack:

Dinner:

Evening snack:

Beverages:

Day 4

Breakfast:	
Morning snack:	
Lunch:	
Afternoon snack:	
Dinner:	
Evening snack:	
Beverages:	

How Did You Do?

Take a look at your four-day diet diary. Did you discover where you get most of your energy from? Did you try to eat at least five servings of fruits and vegetables a day?

Tally Your Brain Food Score

1. Look at one of the days in your four-day diet diary.
2. Add 1 point for each serving of vegetable or fruit you ate.
3. Add 1 point for each serving of fish, fish oil, flax seeds, flaxseed oil, walnuts or walnut oil you consumed.
4. Subtract 1 point for each deep-fried or sugary item you ate.
5. Subtract 1 point if you had more than two very-high-fat items.
6. Total your score for that day. A positive score of at least 2 or 3 points should be your goal.
7. Repeat Steps 1 through 6 for the other three days in your diary.
8. Total the points for all four days. A positive score of 10 points is good; anything less means there is room for improvement.

Substituting Good Brain Foods for Bad

Did You Know?

Be Consistent

In a healthy diet, there is room for fun foods and even low-nutrient foods on occasion. But the only way to ensure that your diet is nutritionally sound over the long term is to consistently make good choices on a day-to-day basis.

While some foods have both good and bad aspects, many have more of one than the other. To make informed choices, you need to be able to screen for problematic foods that are nutritionally useless or even potentially harmful in large amounts. This requires reading food labels carefully and sticking with foods that are not overly processed. If it takes a long time to read a label, the food item probably contains too many synthetic ingredients.

When preparing your menus or eating out, take a good look at the two lists that follow for sound advice on which foods to avoid and which foods to favor.

Brain-Harming Foods, Drinks and Additives

Alcohol abuse has been proven to lead to brain impairment, in both the short and the long term.

- **Alcohol:** Excessive alcohol can be toxic to brain cells. Even in moderation, alcohol causes sedation (acting like an anesthetic agent and slowing the transmission of signals in the brain). Overconsumption can lead to increased risk of early death. While moderate use of alcohol is okay for most people, some people cannot tolerate a single drop. Alcohol abuse has been proven to lead to brain impairment, in both the short and the long term.

- **Aspartame:** This artificial sweetener contains methanol, a type of alcohol that the body can metabolize into formaldehyde. The amounts are small, but some people can feel their mood and thinking change instantly when they ingest aspartame.

- **Carcinogenic foods:** These are foods that are known or suspected to cause cancer, such as charred or burnt foods. They create oxidative stress in the body and can turn on certain biological processes that might increase your risk of developing cancer.

- **Excessive omega-6 fatty acids:** The body requires an adequate amount of omega-6 fatty acids, which we consume in meats, seed oils such as canola, corn and many other foods. But in the Western diet, our omega-6 intake often far exceeds our omega-3 intake. This can increase inflammation in the body and crowd out the omega-3s we really should be getting (from fatty fish, flax seeds, borage oil and so on).

- **Food colorings and additives:** Some people feel that their attention and concentration are affected by food coloring, while others do not. In children, some hyperactivity is associated with certain food additives, such as tartrazine (yellow dye number 5), blue dyes numbers 1 and 2, and several others.

- **High-sugar foods and highly refined foods:** These give the brain a sugar rush — and then a letdown. A huge letdown. They cause blood sugar levels to skyrocket, then plummet as the body releases insulin. This leads to difficulty concentrating, mood changes, irritability and erratic thinking. Some people may eventually develop metabolic syndrome and/or diabetes after a lifetime of consuming such foods.

- **Trans fats:** These fats are structured differently than natural fats because they are created through an industrial process called hydrogenation, which hardens them into shelf-stable products. They are best avoided or consumed minimally, because they do not behave the same way that healthy fats do in the brain. They also increase your risk for heart disease.

> In the Western diet, our omega-6 intake often far exceeds our omega-3 intake. This can increase inflammation in the body and crowd out the omega-3s we really should be getting

Brain-Strengthening Foods and Nutrients

- **Antioxidants:** There are many food superheroes that contain these important damage-fighting nutrients. Broccoli, for example, has specific antioxidant molecules that, when metabolized, protect the brain. Green tea has a type of molecule that absorbs free radicals (unpaired electrons and chemical compounds that contain them), which can disrupt cells and cellular DNA. Natural honey also has compounds that can take on antioxidant duties in the body.

- **Cinnamon:** This spice tastes wonderful, but it also contains components that help regulate blood sugar.

- **Fruits and vegetables:** In general, fruits and vegetables are rich sources of nutrients. They contain a variety of cancer-preventive molecules, antioxidants and key vitamins.

- **Garlic and onions:** These two aromatics are wonderful for the vascular system. They have mild blood-thinning properties, which is good for circulation — but don't overdo your consumption of garlic and onions if you are already taking blood-thinning medications.

- **Healthy oils:** The body needs fatty acids for energy and structure, and healthy oils such as extra virgin olive oil, safflower oil, sunflower oil, flaxseed oil and walnut oil are good, safe sources. Extra virgin olive oil even has some antioxidant properties.

- **Medicinal mushrooms:** Certain mushroom varieties, such as maitake (hen-of-the-wood), shiitake and reishi (*ling zhi*), stimulate the immune system. They are also delicious in cooking.

- **Omega-3 fatty acids:** These fatty acids are essential for the human body. They occur naturally in fatty fish, fish oil, flax seeds, flaxseed oil and pastured meats. Some foods are fortified with them, including eggs laid by hens fed a diet that includes flax seeds.

- **Pastured meats:** Animals reared this way are raised and finished in pastures rather than feedlots. They forage freely on natural pasture grasses rather than being fed large amounts of corn in order to fatten them up for slaughter. Their grass-based diet means the meat they yield is high in healthy omega-3 fatty acids.

- **Quinoa:** This so-called supergrain, which is actually the seed of an ancient pseudocereal plant, is gluten-free. It has all the positive attributes of whole grains plus an excellent array of vitamins.

- **Sage:** This fragrant, tasty herb has been shown to improve cognition. The essential oils in sage may increase the levels of acetylcholine, a neurotransmitter (a chemical involved in brain signals) that can be low in people with brain-aging diseases such as Alzheimer's disease.

- **Squashes and red bell peppers:** These nutritional powerhouses contain carotenoids, a class of pigments that are excellent sources of vitamin A and act as powerful antioxidants.

- **Turmeric:** This rhizome is dried and ground to make the brilliant yellow powder that's one of the bases of curry powder. It is known for its anti-inflammatory and anti-cancer effects.

- **Whole grains:** These provide a steady source of energy for the brain. Whole grains are packed with B vitamins, which help cells burn carbohydrates in their metabolic "furnaces," the mitochondria. Whole wheat, amaranth, brown rice, oats and barley are just a few delicious examples.

Shopping for Brain Foods

Where should you shop for the best brain-building foods? It doesn't really matter, as long as you get them at a store that carries a wide variety of natural, whole foods, including fresh fruits, vegetables and whole grains. It's helpful if the store offers organic as well as conventionally raised foods, and if it carries meats that have been pasture-raised.

Sure, a higher-end brand-name grocery store that focuses on these ingredients is great. But it can be expensive, and it's not the only option. Food cooperatives deliver local products that emphasize whole foods, and most regular supermarket chains now provide some or many of these choices. Don't forget community-sponsored agriculture (CSA) organizations either. When you buy a share in a CSA, you receive a box full of beautiful local (often organically grown) produce for a set number of weeks through the growing season. It's a delicious, civic-minded choice.

Did You Know?

Stick to the Edges
When you're shopping in a large supermarket, focus on foods sold around the perimeter. Choose your produce first, then meat, then dairy (don't forget the yogurt!). Most of the whole foods are displayed around the edges of the store, while the interior aisles contain all the processed and packaged foods you probably want to avoid.

Top Shopping Tips

- **Read the label:** If a food contains dozens of ingredients (especially ones you can't pronounce), this might be a good reason to avoid it. Skip foods that look like they came from a factory, not a field, or that contain artificial flavorings and colorings.

- **Buy whole foods:** Eat foods in as close to their natural state as possible. Even if you cook them, you'll know that they started out as unadulterated, wholesome ingredients.

- **Eat organic:** When you do this, you know your food has never been contaminated with pesticides, herbicides, antibiotics or other unnecessary substances. Remember, even if it's organic, you still need to wash it well. And make sure to cook meat and eggs to the proper temperature to ensure that any bacteria are killed.

- **Buy local:** Supporting local agriculture and farming ensures a safe and healthy food supply for generations to come. If you can't buy local, avoid foods produced in places that have had quality or safety issues. The United States, Canada, Australia, New Zealand, the United Kingdom and other European Union countries tend to produce safe-to-consume foods. This doesn't mean that products from other countries can't be perfectly fine, or that any food from a "safe" country is always problem-free. Keep in mind that *E. coli* infections caused by lack of sanitation in U.S. meat processing plants have caused serious illnesses (and deaths) in the past. That's why local and ethically raised foods beat factory-farmed options as a general rule.

Brain Food Budget

One handy way to create a balanced brain-boosting diet is to plan it according to your budget. By allocating money this way, you ensure that you include a wide variety of healthy nutrients and stay within your means. Plan to spend:

- 30% on fruits, vegetables and spices
- 20% on meat, eggs and fish
- 20% on whole grains (including bread and pasta) and legumes (beans, lentils, etc.)
- 10% on yogurt, cheese, butter, buttermilk, sour cream and milk
- 10% on healthy oils, such as cold-pressed olive oil, safflower oil or flaxseed oil
- 10% on nuts, nutritious snacks, chocolate, tea, coffee and treats

An Anti-Inflammatory Diet

An athlete who trains very hard but does not adequately nourish his or her body may not be able to achieve his or her goals. The same can be said for our brains — without proper nutrition, they may not benefit as much as they could from purposeful activity and mental exercises. To ensure good brain "fitness," you must consume an array of essential nutrients every day in order for the brain to work properly.

Moreover, there is an important factor that can hasten neurological decline, and it's far too prevalent in our society. That factor is inflammation, and modern diets often promote it. In Part 4 of this book, we explored the connection between inflammation, brain aging and repair, and how inflammation can negatively impact brain health. In this section, we will discover how good nutrition can fight this damaging process.

The Macronutrients You Need

There's one recurring question that just about everyone debates: exactly how much of the big three macronutrients — carbohydrates, proteins and fats — do we need? The answer to this question has changed over the years.

In the media, all these nutrients have taken a turn being the bad guy (see box, page 173). Today, the debate still rages over what percentage of calories in the diet should come from carbohydrates, proteins and fats. What seems to make the biggest difference in promoting health is not finding this magical ratio, but rather the quality of the food we eat.

Carbohydrates

The body needs carbohydrates to provide glucose to the brain so it can function. We can't survive without some carbohydrates in the diet. When you severely limit them, your body stockpiles their energy in the liver, because the brain prefers glucose for energy. In absolute carbohydrate restriction, the brain can use ketones for energy, but this puts a burden on the body.

Forms of Carbohydrates

Carbohydrates are not one single compound but rather a class of them. There are a number of very different types of sugar and starch molecules that count as carbohydrates in the diet:

- Monosaccharides, such as glucose and fructose
- Disaccharides, such as sucrose and lactose
- Polysaccharides, such as starch (which the body digests) and dietary fiber (which the body does not digest)

Simple versus Complex Carbohydrates

In general, naturopathic physicians and other nutrition-oriented practitioners recommend that you get the majority of your carbohydrate calories from complex carbohydrate sources. This provides a steady stream of energy for the brain and is the least likely to stress your insulin system.

Simple carbohydrates, such as high-fructose corn syrup (which contains both glucose and fructose), are generally easy for the body to digest and absorb (with some exceptions). The glucose they contain usually enters the bloodstream very quickly, resulting in a rapid rise in the blood sugar level. This energy spike induces the pancreas to send out a burst of the hormone insulin to help that sugar enter muscle or fat cells. Over time, this can cause insulin resistance (see box, page 174).

Complex carbohydrates, such as whole grains, are generally digested more slowly and do not provoke insulin secretion to as great a degree as simple carbohydrates. Complex carbs come in many forms. Naturopathic physicians tend to encourage patients to choose whole, or unrefined, grains, such as brown rice and whole-grain flour, instead of their white, or refined, counterparts. Whole grains contain polyphenolic molecules and lignans, which may have an inflammation-reducing effect; certainly the slower digestion of whole grains and the fact that they don't trigger large surges of insulin are helpful in keeping inflammation in check.

Food "Villains"

The diet industry goes through cycles. Typically, about every five years, a certain type of food, nutrient or component is singled out as *the* thing to avoid. A current example is gluten, a component of wheat protein (and some other grains). These food villains provide an interesting snapshot of the psychology of food. They live at the intersection of science, clinical reasoning, common wisdom and marketing hyperbole.

Fat is a good historical example. When links were discovered between saturated fat intake and heart disease and cancer, they were taken out of context. That caused many people to adhere to very-low-fat diets, even though they did not need to. They substituted protein or carbohydrates, which created new problems (see Carbohydrates, page 172). While some people do need to reduce their overall fat intake to protect their cardiovascular health, this does not apply to everyone. And while too much saturated fat might promote some forms of cancer and increase the risk of heart disease, that is no reason to go completely fat-free! Fatty acids are vital for metabolism and energy production. Essential fatty acids, such as omega-3s and omega-6s, are important components of the diet and should not be avoided.

When fat was the villain in the 1980s, carbs were kind — everyone was encouraged to eat plenty of grains in place of fat. Then, in the 1990s and 2000s, it became apparent that high carb intake was making obesity rates skyrocket (with sugar and refined grains like white bread being the major culprits). And so protein ruled, and carbs became the new food villain.

Cutting back on simple carbs and starchy foods does offer some short-term benefits. When consumed in excess, and combined with physical inactivity, they promote inflammation and can cause insulin resistance (see box, page 174). When people reduce their sugar intake, they start seeing beneficial changes to their blood sugar — not surprising when you consider the glucose content of an extra-large sugary soda or a couple of glazed donuts for breakfast.

But excessive protein consumption has its problems, too. When you eliminate most carbohydrate-rich foods from the diet and eat lots of meat, dairy and fats, you are enjoying foods that are lower on the GI scale (see page 161), which can help keep your blood sugar in check. But they can stress the metabolic pathways of some individuals — among other issues, very high protein consumption creates a lot of ammonia that the body needs to detoxify. The bottom line: no food is perfect, and variety is the key to good health.

Naturopathic practitioners in the early 20th century observed that patients who relied heavily on refined carbohydrates (such as sugar and white flour) were less healthy. It turned out that the very nutrients needed to metabolize these substances were missing or reduced in refined foods. As they are metabolized, these foods use up more B-complex vitamins and trace minerals than they contribute. If you consume a varied diet

Did You Know?

Insulin Resistance

Chronic high insulin levels are thought to be linked to the gradual development of obesity. Over time, muscle tissues are too well supplied with glucose, so they stop paying attention to those bursts of insulin. Unfortunately, this leads to more aggressive insulin release from the pancreas, which is trying to cope with the overabundance of glucose in the blood. This condition is called insulin resistance, and in some people it can lead to diabetes.

FAQ

Q. *What are whole grains?*

A. Whole grains contain all the components of the kernel: the bran, the germ and the endosperm. When grains are refined, the nutritious bran and germ are stripped away, along with the nutrients, fiber and antioxidants they contain. While some refined flours are fortified, or enriched, with nutrients — such as thiamine (vitamin B_1), riboflavin (vitamin B_2) and niacin (vitamin B_3) — they are still missing many important nutrients that were removed during processing.

that contains a variety of whole foods, your body can tolerate a certain amount of these highly refined foods. However, large quantities of simple carbs simply elbow out more nutritious alternatives.

Protein

Amino acids are the building blocks of proteins. The body digests these compounds from the foods we eat, then our cells assemble the amino acids into a variety of proteins that run our organs and enable important functions, such as immune system responses and nerve transmission. Brain cells must make special proteins called neurotransmitters, which carry a signal from one cell in the brain, spinal cord or nerve to another cell.

Once cells have used their quota of protein, any excess is broken down and turned into energy. The body is constantly losing protein, thanks to skin cell turnover, the renewal of mucosal surfaces and digestive secretions. And certain life events, such as pregnancy, growth spurts in kids and injury repair, cause the body to require increased levels of proteins.

All this means that the diet should always contain adequate sources of protein. Protein should not be our main source of energy, but having enough of it helps keep us from overindulging in carbohydrates.

Fat

Fat is essential for the construction of cell membranes and is the richest source of energy the body can take in. Some fats support healing processes, while others contribute to disease processes.

There are a variety of different types of fat, which are just different forms of fatty acids. Some consist of long chains of fatty acids (with 16, 18 or more carbon units) and others consist of short chains of fatty acids (such as the butyric acid found in butter, which contains only three carbon units).

The body stores these fatty acids to use as fuel. They are sometimes present in food in the form of triglycerides, which are made up of three fatty acids stuck to a backbone molecule called glycerol. A triglyceride is how the body puts fat in the bank — it waits patiently until it needs to be released to meet the body's energy needs.

Saturated versus Unsaturated Fats

Saturated fat contains carbon bonds that are fully saturated with hydrogen, which is why they are often solid at room temperature. This type of fat can be harmful to the body when consumed in large quantities. Animal-derived foods, such as meat and dairy products, are high in saturated fat. In general, naturopathic physicians follow the recommendations of the major nutritional authorities and advise patients to restrict the amount of saturated fat in their diets. Some saturated fats (such as those from meat) contain high amounts of arachidonic acid. Although arachidonic acid is an essential fatty acid, it is instrumental in the inflammatory process, so it should be consumed only in moderation.

On the other side of the coin are unsaturated fats: monounsaturated fats and polyunsaturated fats, which are liquid at room temperature. Both appear to decrease blood cholesterol, lowering the risk for vascular (blood vessel) disease.

> Saturated fat can be harmful to the body when consumed in large quantities.

FAQ

Q. *So is fat good or bad for you?*

A. Fat is essential for life, and healthy fats are very good for you. What's bad for you is overconsumption of high-fat foods and those that contain unhealthy fat (such as trans fats), which can lead to obesity, elevated cholesterol, atherosclerosis, heart disease, stroke, gallstones and many other health problems. And it doesn't take much fat to deliver quite a lot of calories. For example, even after cooking, extra-lean ground beef gets more than half its calories from fat. Another example of a fat-dense food is cheese: more than 70% of its energy content comes from fat. You can handle reasonable portions of this in your diet, but it's wise not to overindulge. And remember that the quality of the fat you eat is as important as the quantity.

Cooking with Healthy Oils

Polyunsaturated fatty acids are damaged by heat. Therefore, it is best to avoid cooking at high temperatures with polyunsaturated oils, especially more delicate oils such as flaxseed oil. When flaxseed oil is heated, it becomes bitter and rancid. (Interestingly, the fatty acids in flax seeds can survive higher temperatures, such as when the seeds are baked in muffins or bread. It's only when the oil is extracted that the fatty acids become vulnerable.) Olive oil — a monounsaturated oil — is better for cooking, but still should not be heated to the point that it smokes.

Monounsaturated fats contain one unsaturated carbon-to-carbon bond; polyunsaturated fats have several double bonds between carbon atoms. Because of their double bonds, polyunsaturated fats are more susceptible than monounsaturated fats to being attacked by oxygen, which reacts very easily with other chemical compounds (browning apple slices and rusty nails are examples of oxidation). However, polyunsaturated fats are less likely than saturated fats to cause the buildup of fatty plaques in the arteries, which can contribute to the incidence of heart attack and stroke.

Monounsaturated fats are found in avocados and avocado oil, canola oil, peanuts and peanut oil, and olives and olive oil. Polyunsaturated fatty acids, which include the essential fatty acids discussed below, are found in nuts and nut oils, seeds and seed oils, canola oil, safflower oil, corn and corn oil, soybeans and soy oil, and fish and fish oil.

Essential Fatty Acids

Did You Know?

Prostaglandins

Prostaglandins were first discovered in the prostate glands of sheep. That is how they got their name.

Some polyunsaturated fats are called essential fatty acids (EFAs) because they cannot be synthesized from other fatty acids in the body, and must be consumed in food. They play a critical role in the creation of prostaglandins, the chemical messengers that exert control over inflammatory activity, blood vessel tone (how tense or relaxed the blood vessels are) and clotting. Prostaglandins influence the function of specific body tissues and play a large role in controlling inflammation throughout the body.

Essential fatty acids come in two types: omega-3 and omega-6. "Omega" refers to a structural detail of these fatty acids — namely, where one of the double bonds in the molecule is located. "Omega-3" means the double bond starts at the third carbon atom from the end of the carbon chain (the carbon atoms are the backbone of the fatty acid). An omega-6 fatty acid has the first double bond at the sixth carbon atom from the end. This detail makes a difference in how the body uses it. Some types of both omega-3 and omega-6 fatty acids are considered essential and help form both prostaglandins and other similar molecules.

- **Omega-3 fatty acids** help reduce inflammation and also aid platelet aggregation, or the formation of clots. Essential omega-3 fatty acids include alpha-linolenic acid (ALA), found in walnuts, flax seeds and hemp seeds, and docosahexaenoic acid (DHA) and eicosapentaenoic acid (EPA), both of which are found in fatty fish, such as salmon, herring and sardines.

- **Omega-6 fatty acids** are important for energy production. The omega-6 called linoleic acid (found in many sources, including corn, soy, sunflower and evening primrose oils) can be turned into special molecules that act as switches for inflammation, blood clotting and other actions that are important for healing wounds and improving our general response to injury. On the negative side, an omega-6 called arachidonic acid (AA) — which the body can make from linoleic acid and is also found in animal fats — tends to lead to inflammation when overconsumed and when our diet lacks sufficient intake of omega-3 fats. Our body uses arachidonic acid to make chemical messengers that trigger more inflammation.

We need both omega-3s and omega-6s, but there is a catch: the modern diet is way out of balance when it comes to the proportions of these fats. Many herbivorous animals consume more omega-3s than 6s. Humans, when raised on a natural hunter-gatherer diet, consume large amounts of omega-3 fatty acids. Unfortunately, modern humans who follow a Western diet often consume much higher amounts of omega-6s than omega-3s. This imbalance is likely to promote inflammation and cause disease. A healthy ratio of omega-6 fatty acids to omega-3 fatty acids is somewhere between 10:1 and 6:1. The lower ratio is desirable for people who suffer from inflammatory diseases and who want to reduce inflammation.

Trans Fatty Acids

Trans fatty acids start out with the same chemical formula as normal fatty acids, but through a manufacturing process called hydrogenation, the orientation of their hydrogen atoms (around a carbon-to-carbon double bond) is altered. In plain English, this means that trans fats are produced from the same chemical elements as normal fat, but they are stuck together in a slightly different way.

Trans fats occur in small amounts in nature. But most are created through the hydrogenation of oils; these fatty acids are present in many types of margarine, vegetable shortenings and deep-fryer oils. In the case of margarine and shortening, the aim of the hydrogenation process is to make a product that is more stable at room temperature; with deep-fryer oils, the hydrogenated product is more resistant to heat.

Did You Know?

Choose Cold-Pressed

Many natural vegetable oils contain essential fatty acids, provided that they have not been overly processed. It is best to choose cold-pressed oils that have not been refined.

Did You Know?

Mercury Caution

Certain predatory fish, such as tuna and swordfish, can accumulate the toxic metal mercury in their bodies as they feast on fish lower on the food chain. These types of fish should be eaten in moderation, no more than once a week, and not at all during pregnancy. Some fish oil supplements are purified, filtered and guaranteed to be mercury-free, but be a wise consumer: not all fish oil supplements are equal. Check to see what certifications — such as U.S. Pharmacopeial Convention (USP) — the manufacturer has.

Did You Know?

Palm Oil: Not Always Eco-Friendly

There is a current craze for substituting palm oil for trans fats. One factor you should keep in mind is that many palm-growing operations around the world are built on land where rainforests — sometimes very ancient rainforests — have been cut down. Look for sustainable, eco-friendly fats as you move away from synthetic fats.

Did You Know?

Keep Oil in the Dark

Cold-pressed oils, especially those that contain a lot of polyunsaturated fat, should always be protected from light, which can lead to rancidity. Keep them in the refrigerator and take them out only when you need them. You might find that letting them warm to room temperature for a few minutes before preparing food makes them easier to pour.

The chemical change that trans fats undergo has a big impact on what those fats do inside the body once consumed. And trans fats can be dangerous. They promote inflammation, become incorporated into brain structures, and have been linked to increased risk of cardiovascular disease. They replace fats present in normal cell membranes, affecting the fluidity of the membrane and reactions inside the cells. Brain cells depend on healthy cell membranes to conduct electrical signals.

The good news is that food is increasingly being processed using alternative oils and being prepared commercially without the use of trans fats. But it still pays to read the labels on prepared foods. Be aware that if the amount of trans fats is less than 0.5 gram (for example, 0.4 gram), the manufacturer is allowed to list the content as 0 gram, so look to see if "hydrogenated fats" appears anywhere in the ingredient list.

Natural Fats Are Best

Fats that have not been chemically modified are the healthiest ones to include in your diet. But many readily available oils and fats are not processed in ways that preserve their nutrients and protect you from disease. Old-school is best when it comes to fat: if you could produce it yourself, it will be friendlier to your body than a fat that requires a team of chemical engineers to bring it to the supermarket shelf.

Even though it's well known that vegetable oils that are high in polyunsaturated fats, such as sunflower seed oil, are susceptible to oxidation, these oils are often stripped of their antioxidants (such as beta-carotene and vitamin E) during processing. As mentioned earlier, they don't make great cooking oils. Heating these oils, whether during extraction or in cooking, can lead to the formation of trans fats and epoxides. Epoxides are oxygen-damaged fatty acids that generate free radicals in the body, which can encourage disease processes.

Cold-pressed oils are the best choice, because neither heat nor chemical solvents are used to extract the oil. Olive oil is high in monounsaturated fat; look for cold-pressed extra virgin versions, which come from the first pressing. Flaxseed oil, a source of both linoleic acid (an omega-6 fatty acid) and alpha-linolenic acid (an omega-3 fatty acid), should never be used for cooking — heat makes it rancid and unfit for consumption.

Dietary Fiber

Dietary fiber is another nutritional necessity. Fiber is an indigestible form of carbohydrate that humans cannot enzymatically break down. It adds bulk to stool and makes it easier for the colon to function. You'll find dietary fiber in whole grains, fruits and vegetables.

Insoluble versus Soluble Fiber

You probably already know that fiber is your body's friend. And the more of it you take in, the better.

Dietary fiber is divided into two basic types: soluble and insoluble. Insoluble fiber includes cellulose and hemicellulose, two components of plant cell walls. This type of fiber helps stool pass more easily through the intestines. You get insoluble fiber in bran, whole-grain flours (such as whole wheat), cabbage, peas, beans and root vegetables.

Soluble fiber is composed of nonstructural polysaccharides and includes pectins, gums and mucilages. All these impressive compounds have something in common: they can absorb water and form gels. This bulks up stool, which is vital for the gut to function properly. Pectins are found in apples, citrus fruits, carrots, sweet potatoes and bananas. Gums and mucilages are found in oatmeal, dried beans and other legumes.

FAQ

Q. *Does soluble fiber reduce cholesterol?*

A. Yes, it does. Soluble fiber binds with cholesterol in the gut, removing it from the body and lowering blood cholesterol levels. It also slows down gastric emptying, a fancy term for how fast food passes through the stomach. This is beneficial for people with impaired glucose tolerance (such as those who have diabetes), because it makes the absorption of glucose into the bloodstream more gradual.

More Fiber Benefits

Fiber can also benefit the colon in another way. Bacteria in the colon ferment fiber, breaking down links in the cellulose chains. The end products of this bacterial fiber feast are short-chain fatty acids, such as butyrate and acetate. These molecules are an important energy source for the colonic mucosal cells. When you increase your fiber intake, your gut enjoys this secondary benefit.

When to Increase Fiber Intake

There are many good reasons to increase your fiber intake. When you eat foods that are high in fiber, you can reduce your food intake and achieve or maintain a healthy weight. (Obesity is rare in populations where the diet is high in fiber.) This may be because fiber is relatively low in calories or because it increases the feeling of fullness when you eat. One caution: fiber can bind with and remove certain essential minerals in the gut, such as zinc. However, if you eat a varied diet that contains lots of mineral-rich foods, this is not a significant concern.

Modern North Americans take in much less fiber than their ancestors, thanks in part to a shift from whole grains to refined grains. But it's an easy-to-remedy situation, because you can get all the fiber you need from eating a whole-food diet that includes plenty of whole grains, fruits and vegetables. Naturopathic physicians sometimes recommend fiber supplements, such as those that contain ground psyllium. These can be helpful — but, again, food is the best source.

Fiber Fights Disease

Epidemiological studies have shown that fiber protects against diverticular disease and colon cancer. In diverticulitis, small pouches called diverticula develop along the intestinal walls as a result of chronic constipation and straining during defecation. The pressure causes them to bulge, and they can become inflamed and infected. Fiber decreases the pressure on them and can help prevent illness. Colon cancer can occur when carcinogens stay in prolonged contact with the bowel. By increasing your fiber intake, you prevent constipation and thereby reduce the amount of time that toxins stay in the gut.

When to Reduce Fiber Intake

In some people, fiber needs to be reduced. This is the case in Crohn's disease, which can narrow segments of the intestine. The pulpy undigested fiber can become trapped in these narrow passages, leading to bowel obstruction. Any disease that involves partial obstruction of the gastrointestinal tract may require you to lower your fiber intake (and especially avoid whole seeds or large flakes of bran). Like most things, fiber is not a one-size-fits-all solution.

Fruits and Vegetables

Fruits and vegetables are very low in fat and high in dietary fiber, so they are emphasized in most naturopathic approaches to nutrition. In addition, they provide micronutrients such as vitamins and minerals, which the body needs in order to digest and absorb macronutrients.

The form and amount of fruits and vegetables you eat can be adjusted to suit your needs. People with intestinal yeast overgrowth (such as *Candida* in the bowel) or poorly controlled diabetes shouldn't eat an excessive amount of fruit, because it contains too much sugar for them. Vegetables are easier to digest when cooked, which may be desirable for some people, while others will benefit from the bowel-cleansing effects of raw vegetables. Experiment and see what works for your body.

Water

People often need encouragement to increase their water intake. Most of us simply don't drink enough, and many circumstances can cause us to need more than we realize. Plus, the feeling of thirst does not always occur at the moment when we need water most. You shouldn't assume that you've met your body's water needs just because you don't feel thirsty.

Higher fiber intake, especially in supplement form, requires higher water intake. High levels of exercise or perspiration can lead to dehydration; increased water intake is necessary to replenish water lost to sweat. The use of laxatives or diuretics, including coffee, can also increase your water needs.

FAQ

Q. How much water should I drink per day?

A. Consume at least 8 cups (2 L) of water daily — 12 cups (3 L) is even better. More than that is not necessary, and excessive amounts can actually be harmful. (Note: If you are a high-performance athlete, live in a very hot climate or are new to a hot climate, your water needs may be higher. Discuss this with a physician.)

Most people don't drink enough water simply because they haven't developed the habit of doing so. If you keep a source of drinking water handy throughout the day, you will have no difficulty meeting your needs.

So what should you drink? Filtered or spring water is ideal. Distilled water is good for a clothes iron but not for people, because it is devoid of minerals. Drinking distilled water for prolonged periods can create a mineral imbalance in the body.

Vitamins

Diets that are low in whole foods and high in processed foods can be deficient in certain vitamins. Although some processed grains are "enriched" to add back some of the vitamins that were lost in processing, in general, starchy or essentially synthetic foods (think packaged pastry or cheese-flavored cornmeal puffs) are calorie-rich and vitamin-poor.

The nutritional choices recommended in this book cover a wide variety of foods, many of them unprocessed or minimally processed, which is the key to ensuring good vitamin intake. Supplementation with a multivitamin or specific vitamins can help, but food sources of vitamins are the best choice.

Minerals

When people consume a diet full of highly processed foods, they can lack key minerals — particularly iron, calcium, magnesium and zinc. For example, many women in North America have calcium and iron intakes that fall below the recommended dietary allowance (RDA). This leaves them susceptible to osteoporosis and microcytic anemia.

In addition, food in some areas is grown in mineral-depleted soil; this is especially true in fields that have been over-cultivated. This can lead to suboptimal mineral content in the foods grown in the soil. In some cases, eating these foods can cause outright deficiencies of minerals that the body requires in smaller quantities, such as selenium and chromium.

To avoid mineral depletion in the diet, naturopathic doctors often recommend that you eat organic foods. Organic agriculture uses methods that conserve nutrients and support the soil, ensuring that the minerals in it are maintained or replenished. In addition, the topsoil (where the real growing occurs) is much thinner than it used to be in some North American farmlands, and good organic practices help conserve this important growing medium.

Soil is an organic, living matrix of plant matter and microorganisms. While foods grown with the use of chemical fertilizers, pesticides, herbicides and fungicides can be nutritious, organically produced foods are not as hard on the earth and can be more nutritionally complete. Crops will grow when they are fed (literally) tons of fertilizer. But these fertilizers are just nitrogen, phosphorus and potassium — they lack the other trace minerals the soil (and our bodies) requires.

Why Sustainable Foods Matter

Over-cultivation degrades the amount of nutrients in the topsoil, so intensive agricultural operations must compensate by using massive amounts of fertilizers. The manufacturing and application of fertilizers rely heavily on fossil fuels, and these fertilizers end up polluting lakes, rivers, wells and even oceans. Our modern food supply is also heavily dependent on factory-farming technology and efficient transportation systems and ignores natural crop cycles — all of which is ecologically shortsighted.

Increasingly, foods are transported long distances to meet consumer demands for exotic or off-season ingredients. In grocery stores, we now find heavily fertilized, oversize fruits and vegetables flown in from far-flung places year-round. Exotic foods transported long distances lose much of their nutrient content, making them less nutritious than similar locally grown, organic options.

Foods produced using sustainable agricultural practices and sold locally not only enrich the diet but also help support local farming communities. The choices you make as a consumer directly influence the food supply. Choosing local leads to more sustainable choices, now and for future generations.

Antioxidant Power

Antioxidants are key protective substances in the body. They neutralize free radicals (also called reactive oxygen species) and protect all cell components, including DNA and cell membranes, from damage. Oxidative stress caused by free radicals can promote heart disease and cancer, so antioxidants play a vital role in their prevention.

Our cells manufacture some very powerful antioxidants of their own, but we can enhance their action by consuming dietary antioxidants, which are plentiful in fruits and vegetables. When one of our self-made antioxidants is "spent" absorbing a free radical, the body uses helpful dietary antioxidants, such as vitamin C, to "recycle" it so that it can be used again.

A diet can meet the recommended daily intake for all nutrients but still lack some of the great plant-derived antioxidants, which is one reason nutrition experts are increasingly emphasizing that we should eat lots of fruits and vegetables.

Oxidative stress caused by free radicals can promote heart disease and cancer, so antioxidants play a vital role in their prevention.

Fermented Foods

Those of us who don't eat fermented foods are missing out on a terrific supply of gut-friendly bacteria.

Many cultures include some kind of fermented food in their diet, and those of us who don't eat fermented foods are missing out on a terrific supply of gut-friendly bacteria. There are trillions of bacteria in our guts, and they can influence our genes and possibly our risk for some diseases — Parkinson's disease may be one of them.

The research in this area is still new and untested, but it's clear that we should be eating these beneficial organisms. They help maintain a healthy bacterial and viral balance in the gut, and by keeping the "bad guys" in check, they reduce or prevent the inflammation that arises from having our immune system activated by intestinal bacteria that could threaten the body.

Here are some fermented foods to try:

- **Active-culture yogurt** contains live *Lactobacillus acidophilus* and other bacteria naturally found in a healthy human digestive tract. They coexist with other types of microflora and keep aggressive bacteria in check. They also produce important nutrients, such as vitamin K, in the gut. Yogurt also supplies some protein.

- **Kimchi** is the generic name for Korean pickled vegetables. The best-known types in North America are made from cabbage and radishes, hot chile peppers, garlic and salt. They provide healthy bacteria to the gut, and cabbage-based kimchi is a source of vitamin C, too.

- **Miso** is a familiar Japanese seasoning paste made from fermented ground soybeans, salt and barley or rice. It offers lots of healthy bacteria, protein and savory flavor.

- **Sauerkraut** is a German dish made by salting and fermenting sliced cabbage. It has a pungent smell but a wonderful, slightly sweet and tangy taste. It is packed with fiber and healthy probiotic bacteria.

- **Tempeh** is a pressed patty of fermented soybeans. It can be sliced and used as a protein source in stir-fries and many other dishes. It has a nutty flavor and is a complete source of vegetarian protein.

The Mechanics of Digestion

Food must be well digested for the body to absorb nutrients properly. Many people are too busy multitasking to even chew their food properly, which automatically reduces the percentage of digestible nutrients in that food. Digestive enzymes must be able to penetrate food particles; if they are too large, the enzymes can't do their job as efficiently. Likewise, eating under emotional pressure or in a hurry can lead to impaired digestive function. Stress hormones automatically decrease gastrointestinal tract function, diverting blood to the peripheral muscles.

The major consequence of poor digestion and nutrient malabsorption is that the body is deprived of the things it needs to work well. For example, malabsorption of fat leads to deficiencies in fat-soluble vitamins. Malabsorption of protein can lead to muscle wasting and immune system dysfunction. The key is to maximize your digestive powers for each type of macronutrient you consume.

Many people are too busy multitasking to even chew their food properly, which automatically reduces the percentage of digestible nutrients in that food.

Digestive Aids

You can take digestive enzyme supplements if you don't have a sufficient natural supply. Proteases, lipases and amylases (enzymes that break down protein, fat and starch, respectively) all come in pill form. Hydrochloric acid can also be given as a supplement to help the stomach do its job; however, this therapy is not recommended for people who have inflamed or ulcerated gastric mucosa (the mucous membranes that line the stomach).

Macronutrients and Digestion

- **Fat is the hardest substance to digest.** Bile acts as a kind of detergent on ingested food, causing the fat in it to micellize, or form small groups (micelles) of fat molecules. Enzymes then break down these smaller particles so the body can absorb them. People who have had their gallbladders removed do not have the reserve of bile they need to emulsify fats.

- **Stomach acid activates protein digestion.** The hydrochloric acid in the stomach hydrolyzes proteins and begins to break them down. Many patients over the age of 60 don't make enough stomach acid. Others reduce their stomach acid by taking medications for heartburn or indigestion.

- **Carbohydrate digestion begins right away.** Salivary amylase, an enzyme in the mouth, starts to break down carbs immediately. Digestion continues in the small intestine with pancreatic amylase, another enzyme. Disaccharidase, an enzyme present on the intestinal surface, splits the disaccharides sucrose, lactose and maltose into simpler monosaccharides for digestion. Another important carb-digesting enzyme is lactase, which breaks down lactose, a type of sugar present in dairy products. Patients who lack this enzyme have lactose intolerance.

Lactase supplements (for digesting lactose) are a common sight in pharmacies. So are amylase supplements, which break down the starch in legumes. When this starch is not digested properly, it can ferment in the colon, causing flatulence.

Choosing Digestible Foods

Undigested food can become a burden to the body. It allows some kinds of bacteria to grow out of control, and the byproducts of bacterial digestion can be reabsorbed and strain the liver, which must detoxify them.

A food is nutritious only if your body can digest it and absorb its nutrients properly. Undigested food can become a burden to the body. It allows some kinds of bacteria to grow out of control, and the byproducts of bacterial digestion can be reabsorbed and strain the liver, which must detoxify them.

Foods that are excessively high in fat can impair digestion. Foods that are high in proteins, such as wheat gluten, can also pose a digestive problem for some people. And while a person's health status is often the culprit in these scenarios, some foods are better than others in this regard. For example, some people rely on protein snack bars to get through the day. Some of these bars have a super-sticky texture, making them difficult for the stomach to dissolve. The bars are also heat-treated to increase their shelf life, which denatures their proteins and makes them even less bioavailable.

Maximizing Nutrient Values

Although storage, cooking and other processing can decrease it, the nutrient value of a food can be assessed easily from a medical point of view. Detailed tables of food nutrient values have been compiled for years, and much of that information is available online. With just a few clicks of a mouse or a couple of swipes on your tablet, you can discover the nutritional differences between a boiled potato and a fried one, or the iron content of a 3-oz (90 g) hamburger versus a 3-oz (90 g) piece of steak.

A food's nutrient value can be determined by its level of a single nutrient, or by a combination of them. A food can be considered nutritious even if it is high in only a few nutrients. For example, fruits contain high levels of vitamin C and some beneficial plant molecules, such as fiber, but they are not good sources of protein. Are they still nutritious foods? Definitely! Likewise, chicken breast is a good source of protein, but it is not high in vitamins A or C. But it is still considered nutritious.

FAQ

Q. *How do I get all the nutrients I need?*

A. Eating a variety of foods is the best way to ensure that you consume a wide array of valuable nutrients. By eating many different foods that contain different amounts of macro- and micro-nutrients, you achieve a balance — foods that are higher in certain nutrients will make up for others that are lower in them, and vice versa. Make sure you eat a diet that contains a mix of protein, fat and carbohydrates. If you eat lots of different whole foods and don't turn any one food or category of nutrients into a villain (see page 173), your body will get the nutrition it needs.

Combining Foods

Eating high-nutrient-value foods in specific combinations makes sense. Naturopathic practitioners always try to keep this principle in mind when planning a patient's diet. Some foods are more nutrient dense, meaning they are rich in several different nutrients, while others are superstars for just one important nutrient.

When you combine foods, you combine their strengths and their different components. For example, when you eat legumes with grains (such as pita and hummus made from chickpeas, or soybeans and rice), you consume the complete spectrum of essential amino acids. You wouldn't get that balance from just one of those items. Another example: whole grains are not high in vitamin C, but vegetables, such as bell peppers, and many fruits are; combine them and you get a good selection of the nutrients your body needs.

Avoiding Displacement

A human being can ingest and digest only so much per day. If you eat mostly foods packed with simple sugars, starches or trans fats — and those with low levels of micronutrients, high-quality essential fats or healthy proteins — they displace more nutritious foods. Likewise, someone who eats too much of a single food or food group might not include enough foods that contain different essential nutrients.

Here's an example: children who fill up on dairy products won't have room for fruits and vegetables, which contain adequate zinc, vitamin C and fiber for their growing bodies. A more extreme example is children who eat excessive amounts of processed and deep-fried foods — such as frozen pizza pockets, toaster pastries, chicken nuggets breaded in cornmeal and so on. These foods crowd out vegetables, fruits, nuts, seeds, better protein sources and high-fiber foods. The more low-nutrient-value foods people eat, the fewer opportunities they have to get all of the nutrients they need.

Preventing Toxicity

All foods have the potential to contain toxic substances that your body must break down and eliminate. You can't control every single factor when it comes to choosing foods. But you can do your research and choose foods that are free of external toxins. In case you are exposed, you can also add detoxifying foods to your diet. Examples include cruciferous vegetables (such as cauliflower and Brussels sprouts), green tea, turmeric and rosemary.

Modern conventional agriculture makes extensive use of pesticides and herbicides to reduce crop damage. These chemicals place heavy demands on the body's detoxification systems. Both plastics used for storage (see page 189) and environmental contaminants, such as pesticides, can dysregulate the body's hormonal system.

Did You Know?

Statistics versus You

Remember that your body is unique. Your nutrient needs are different from everyone else's. In some instances, your body may demand more of a certain nutrient than the statistical average for the entire population. Check with your health-care providers about what your needs might be. Support and celebrate your uniqueness.

Another issue to consider is the origin of your food. In this global age, foods from all over the world end up at your local supermarket. Pesticide usage laws are more liberal in some countries, and the use of banned pesticides continues in some places as well. Environmental degradation and heavy-metal contamination of foods can also be inadvertent sources of toxicity. A recent example is farm-raised seafood exported by China to other countries that had high heavy metal and antibiotic content that are not allowed in other countries.

Pesticide usage laws are more liberal in some countries, and the use of banned pesticides continues in some places as well.

Food Allergies and Intolerances

Many diseases are the result of systemic inflammatory responses to food allergies or intolerances. For example, naturopathic physicians often find that children with chronic otitis media (infection of the middle ear) had dairy, grains and meats introduced into their diets before the age of 6 months. These children are more prone to developing immunologic sensitivity to foods. And this predisposition extends beyond the foods they ate during their early development. These children seem more allergy-prone in later life, too. The too-early introduction of certain foods seems to set them up for a lifetime of food sensitivity.

FAQ

Q. *Should I avoid foods wrapped or stored in plastic?*

A. When you store or cook food in plastic, you may be getting more than you bargained for. Plastics can release harmful substances into food; both the type of plastic and the storage time can influence this. Canned foods are an excellent example of this: many are lined with a plastic coating that can leach chemicals into the food and increase the level of bisphenol A (an endocrine disruptor) in the blood.

The field of immunology began to make advances in the early 1960s. Each cohort of children born since that era has had a progressively higher incidence of allergic diseases.

The field of immunology began to make advances in the early 1960s. Each cohort of children born since that era has had a progressively higher incidence of allergic diseases, especially atopic asthma and atopic dermatitis. Current rates of these maladies are three times higher than they were in 1960. This tendency has become common in the developed Western countries, in particular in higher socioeconomic subgroups. And it has had an enormous impact on health care: asthma treatment alone is a multibillion-dollar industry.

FAQ

Q. *How can I find out if I have specific food allergies or intolerances?*

A. Each person has a unique food-tolerance profile, and some people have immune reactions to specific foods. Blood tests, such as the enzyme-linked immunosorbent assay (ELISA) test, can help detect levels of the antibodies immunoglobulin E (IgE) and immunoglobulin G (IgG) in relation to different foods. This can tell you what to avoid or limit in your diet.

Common Food Intolerances

- Dairy products (lactose)
- Grain products (gluten)
- Corn products
- Meat products
- Citrus
- Soy

Part 6
Brain Food Menu Plans and Recipes

....

Guide to Using the Menu Plans

The two-week menu plans on pages 192–195 provide multiple servings of brain-supportive foods and minimize foods that might have an adverse effect on the brain and body over time. Whole foods, ample plant foods and whole grains are emphasized and processed foods minimized.

The meal plans are intended to be guidelines, not prescriptions. Feel free to substitute healthy foods and recipes — from this book or from your personal collection — that better suit your tastes. Once you have adapted the menu plans to your liking, look up the recipes you intend to prepare over the following week. Create a shopping list based on the recipes and meal plans.

As much as possible, try to eat your meals with other people, as human interaction stimulates the brain. If you don't have housemates to eat with, invite friends over. Or create a rotating supper or lunch club. Make mealtime stimulating instead of just a way to get calories.

As much as possible, try to eat your meals with other people, as human interaction stimulates the brain.

Two-Week Menu Plans

Menu Plan Week 1

	Monday	Tuesday	Wednesday	
Breakfast	Power Granola* ¾ cup (175 mL) low-fat organic milk or fortified almond or rice milk ⅓ cup (75 mL) organic applesauce	Spiced Fruit and Grain Cereal* ⅓ cup (75 mL) blueberries ½ cup (125 mL) unsweetened plain yogurt	Power Granola* 1 banana ½ cup (125 mL) unsweetened plain yogurt ¾ cup (175 mL) low-fat organic milk or fortified almond or rice milk	
Morning snack	Cranberry Walnut Muffin*	Cinnamon Apple Chips*	Cranberry Walnut Muffin*	
Lunch	Quinoa Salad*	Couscous Salad with Basil and Pine Nuts*	Broccoli and Quinoa Enchiladas*	
Afternoon snack	Trail Mix*	3 tbsp (45 mL) roasted almonds	Trail Mix*	
Dinner	Chicken Paprika with Noodles* Roasted Butternut Squash Chowder with Sage Butter*	Shrimp Risotto with Artichoke Hearts and Parmesan*	Shepherd's Pie with Creamy Corn Filling* Everyday Salad*	
Evening snack	1 orange	Cherry Juice*	1 pear	

* The recipe is in this book; unless otherwise indicated, the amount is 1 serving.

Thursday	Friday	Saturday	Sunday
Spiced Fruit and Grain Cereal* ½ cup (125 mL) hulled strawberries ½ cup (125 mL) unsweetened plain yogurt ¾ cup (175 mL) grape juice (purple, unclarified)	Power Granola* ¾ cup (175 mL) low-fat organic milk or fortified almond or rice milk ¾ cup (175 mL) grape juice (purple, unclarified)	Walnut Flax Waffles* ⅓ cup (75 mL) blueberries ½ cup (125 mL) unsweetened plain yogurt ¾ cup (175 mL) grape juice (purple, unclarified)	Sage and Savory Mushroom Frittata* ¾ cup (175 mL) low-fat organic milk or fortified almond or rice milk
Cinnamon Apple Chips*	Cranberry Walnut Muffin*	Super Antioxidant Smoothie*	C-Blitz*
Curried Chicken Salad Wraps*	Salmon Chowder*	Creamy Mushroom Walnut Toasts*	Saffron Paella Soup*
3 tbsp (45 mL) roasted almonds	8 to 10 carrot sticks 2 oz (60 g) low-fat cheese	8 to 10 carrot sticks 2 oz (60 g) low-fat cheese	Slippery Beet*
Vegetable Cheese Loaf with Lemon Tomato Sauce*	Pasta with Shrimp and Peas* Roasted Bell Peppers*	Saucy Swiss Steak* New Orleans Braised Onions* Spinach Salad with Oranges and Mushrooms*	Turkey Cutlets in Gingery Lemon Gravy with Cranberry Rice* Insalata Caprese*
⅓ cup (75 mL) blueberries	⅓ cup (75 mL) blueberries	Chocolate Chile Cupcake*	1 slice Cinnamon Cake with Whipped Mocha Frosting*

Menu Plan Week 2

	Monday	Tuesday	Wednesday
Breakfast	Hot Breakfast Cereal Mix* ½ cup (125 mL) unsweetened plain yogurt ¾ cup (175 mL) grape juice (purple, unclarified)	Avocado and Egg Breakfast Wrap* ½ cup (125 mL) unsweetened plain yogurt ¾ cup (175 mL) low-fat organic milk or fortified almond or rice milk	Hot Breakfast Cereal Mix* ½ cup (125 mL) unsweetened plain yogurt ¾ cup (175 mL) grape juice (purple, unclarified)
Morning snack	Date and Walnut Muffin*	Cinnamon Apple Chips*	2 oz (60 g) low-fat cheese ½ cup (125 mL) sliced peaches
Lunch	Cream of Broccoli Soup*	Tabbouleh*	Three-Bean Chili*
Afternoon snack	3 tbsp (45 mL) cashew butter 6 rice crackers	Chunky Guacamole* 10 corn tortilla chips	3 tbsp (45 mL) cashew butter 6 rice crackers
Dinner	Peppery Meatloaf with Quinoa* Everyday Salad*	Three-Spice Chicken with Potatoes* Roasted Beet and Beet Greens Salad*	Pad Thai* Simple Stir-Fried Kale*
Evening snack	Cherry Juice*	1 apple	C-Blitz*

* The recipe is in this book; unless otherwise indicated, the amount is 1 serving.

Thursday	Friday	Saturday	Sunday
Cranberry Quinoa Porridge* 1 pat butter ¾ cup (175 mL) low-fat organic milk or fortified almond or rice milk	Cranberry Quinoa Porridge* 1 pat butter ¾ cup (175 mL) grape juice (purple, unclarified)	Home-Style Pancakes* ½ cup (125 mL) unsweetened plain yogurt ¾ cup (175 mL) grape juice (purple, unclarified)	Tomato and Asiago Cheese Strata* ⅓ cup (75 mL) organic applesauce ¾ cup (175 mL) freshly squeezed orange juice
Date and Walnut Muffin*	2 oz (60 g) low-fat cheese ½ cup (125 mL) sliced peaches	Super Antioxidant Smoothie*	C-Blitz*
Lunch Box Peachy Sweet Potato and Couscous*	Minestrone*	Open-Face Salmon Salad Sandwich with Apple and Ginger*	Tuna Salad Melt*
Chunky Guacamole* 10 corn tortilla chips	3 tbsp (45 mL) cashew butter 6 rice crackers	Cell Support Juice*	Dandelion Slam Dunk*
Barbecued Lemongrass Pork* Broccoli Carrot Slaw with Cranberries and Sunflower Seeds*	Beef with Broccoli* Cranberry Mandarin Coleslaw with Walnuts and Raisins*	Lamb Tagine with Chickpeas and Apricots* Moroccan Pumpkin Soup* Sweet Cinnamon Waldorf Salad*	Rosemary Chicken Breasts with Sweet Potatoes and Onions* Roasted Peppers Antipasto*
1 peach	1 apple	Dark Chocolate Mousse*	1 slice Perfect Chocolate Bundt*

Cooking Brain Food Recipes

Cooking is a mental, physical and sensory experience, so the act of cooking is good brain exercise — better than microwaving a frozen meal or ordering takeout.

Cooking is a mental, physical and sensory experience, so the act of cooking is good brain exercise — better than microwaving a frozen meal or ordering takeout. Brain foods (especially the recipes in this book) are delicious, so the rewards are doubled — you boost your mental powers and enjoy the sensory pleasures of eating tasty meals. Try to cook daily, even if all you feel like making is a simple recipe or two. For some dishes, such as casseroles, whole roasted chicken or soups, cooking double batches is easy, practical and great for leftovers on days when you don't feel like cooking.

The recipes in this book yield wonderful results. They not only ensure that you'll enjoy eating well, but you'll also learn some new techniques in the process. As you perfect new skills and get to know what foods you like, you might eventually try your hand at creating your own healthy recipes. Above all, enjoy the cooking process and the good health it brings.

Top 12 Cooking Tips

1 Use stainless steel or enamel cookware. Nonstick surfaces can release unwanted chemicals into your food. The exception is cast iron, which can develop a natural nonstick coating if the pan is seasoned properly with regular cooking oil.

2 Don't burn your food. Consuming charred or burnt food creates free-radical stress in the body and may activate enzymes that can increase your risk for cancer.

3 Don't boil vegetables unless you are making soup and plan to include the broth they create. Steaming is a better choice for preserving vitamins and minerals.

4 Rinse whole grains before you cook them and discard the rinse water. It may contain phytates, naturally occurring compounds that bind with and leach necessary minerals from the diet.

5 Use fresh ingredients and avoid overly salted, phony-tasting "starters" as the base of your recipes.

6 Don't cook or store foods in plastic. It can release endocrine-disrupting compounds into foods, especially those that contain fat. Use ceramic or glass containers to store leftovers.

7 If you use the microwave to reheat dishes, use glass or unglazed ceramic cookware. Remember, the microwave is best for reheating, not cooking from scratch. (Please don't destroy good vegetables by microwaving them!)

8 Don't overheat oils. When an oil reaches its smoke point, it's a sign that the fatty acids that comprise the oil are becoming oxidized — or, to put it another way, rancid.

9 Don't cook with polyunsaturated oils, such as safflower, corn or canola. They are highly susceptible to damage from heat, light and oxygen. For cooking, use olive oil or butter and cook them at as low a temperature as is practical.

10 Avoid aluminum cookware. When acidic foods, such as tomato sauce, are cooked in aluminum, the metal leaches out and becomes part of the dish. Aluminum can cause oxidative stress in brain tissue. Although normal dietary amounts of aluminum are tolerable, why add to the burden on the brain?

11 Thaw, cook and store foods at the right temperature. That's a good rule for all foods, and especially for meats and dairy products. Avoid leaving food out for long periods of time, and follow established safety guidelines to prevent cross-contamination. There is excellent information at www.foodsafety.gov and www.hc-sc.gc.ca/fn-an/securit/kitchen-cuisine/index-eng.php.

12 Don't overheat foods. Delicate nutrients, such as omega-3 fatty acids and antioxidants, can be damaged by heat.

Aluminum can cause oxidative stress in brain tissue. Although normal dietary amounts of aluminum are tolerable, why add to the burden on the brain?

About the Nutrient Analyses

The nutrient analysis done on the recipes in this book was derived from the Food Processor SQL Nutrition Analysis software, version 10.9, ESHA Research (2011). Where necessary, data was supplemented using the USDA National Nutrient Database for Standard Reference, Release #26 (2014), retrieved January 2014 from the USDA Agricultural Research Service website: www.nal.usda.gov/fnic/foodcomp/search.

Recipes were evaluated as follows:

- The larger number of servings was used where a range is given.
- Where alternatives are given, the first ingredient and amount listed were used.
- Optional ingredients and ingredients that are not quantified were not included.
- Calculations were based on imperial measures and weights.
- Nutrient values were rounded to the nearest whole number for calories, fat, carbohydrate, protein, vitamin C, vitamin D, vitamin E, niacin, folate and selenium.
- Nutrient values were rounded to one decimal point for vitamin B_6, vitamin B_{12} and zinc.
- The smaller quantity of an ingredient was used where a range is provided.
- Reduced-sodium broth, 1% milk, light mayonnaise and light sour cream were used where these ingredients are listed as broth, milk, mayonnaise and sour cream.
- Calculations involving meat and poultry used lean portions.
- Canola oil was used where the type of fat was not specified.
- Recipes were analyzed prior to cooking.

It is important to note that the cooking method used to prepare the recipe may alter the nutrient content per serving, as may ingredient substitutions and differences among brand-name products.

Breakfast

Power Granola

This recipe provides a steady source of energy at the beginning of the day, or as a snack. Whole grains are an excellent way to sustain an even blood sugar level, and this is a delicious and convenient way to get some whole grains first thing in the morning.

Makes about 3½ cups (875 mL)

Tip

Look for packages of ready-ground flax seeds, which may be labeled "flaxseed meal," or use a spice or coffee grinder to grind whole flax seeds to a very fine meal.

- **Preheat oven to 300°F (150°C)**
- **Large rimmed baking sheet, lined with parchment paper**

2 cups	large-flake (old-fashioned) rolled oats	500 mL
½ cup	chopped pecans	125 mL
⅓ cup	ground flax seeds (flaxseed meal)	75 mL
2 tsp	ground cinnamon	10 mL
½ cup	unsweetened apple juice	125 mL
½ cup	brown rice syrup or liquid honey	125 mL
1 tbsp	vegetable oil	15 mL
2 tsp	vanilla extract	10 mL
½ cup	dried blueberries, cranberries or cherries	125 mL

1. In a large bowl, whisk together oats, pecans, flax seeds and cinnamon.

2. In a medium bowl, whisk together apple juice, brown rice syrup, oil and vanilla until well blended.

3. Add the apple juice mixture to the oats mixture and stir until well coated. Spread mixture in a single layer on prepared baking sheet.

4. Bake in preheated oven for 20 to 25 minutes or until oats are golden brown. Let cool completely on pan.

5. Transfer granola to an airtight container and stir in blueberries. Store at room temperature for up to 2 weeks.

> ▶ **Health Tip**
>
> Berries are a great source of antioxidants — some of the best nature provides — flaxseeds and walnuts provide brain-boosting omega-3 fats, and cinnamon helps regulate blood sugar. This recipe is a winner.

Nutrients per ¼ cup (60 mL)	
Calories	204
Fat	7 g
Carbohydrate	31 g
Protein	5 g
Vitamin C	0 mg
Vitamin D	0 IU
Vitamin E	0 mg
Niacin	0 mg
Folate	16 mcg
Vitamin B$_6$	0.1 mg
Vitamin B$_{12}$	0.0 mcg
Zinc	0.2 mg
Selenium	1 mcg

Toasted Oat Muesli with Dried Fruit and Pecans

This convenient breakfast cereal delivers slow-burning energy so you won't feel faint or famished an hour later.

Makes about 6 cups (1.5 L)

Tip

Some bran cereals are high in sugar, and although some sugar content is acceptable, make sure to read the ingredients list on the bran cereal you choose for this recipe — no high-fructose corn syrup allowed!

- **Preheat oven to 350°F (180°C)**
- **Large rimmed baking sheet, lined with parchment paper**

3 cups	large-flake (old-fashioned) rolled oats	750 mL
1/2 cup	chopped pecans	125 mL
1 cup	bran cereal (such as All-Bran)	250 mL
1 1/2 cups	chopped mixed dried fruit	375 mL
1/2 cup	ground flax seeds (flaxseed meal)	125 mL

Suggested Accompaniments

Skim milk, non-dairy milk or nonfat plain yogurt (regular or Greek)

Liquid honey or agave nectar

1. Spread oats and pecans in a single layer on prepared baking sheet. Bake in preheated oven for 7 to 8 minutes or until golden and fragrant. Let cool completely on pan.

2. In an airtight container, combine oat mixture, bran cereal, dried fruit and flax seeds. Store in the refrigerator for up to 1 month.

3. Serve with any of the suggested accompaniments, as desired.

> ▶ **Health Tip**
>
> Grinding flax seeds into flaxmeal releases their many benefits: high fiber, lignans (which can reduce cholesterol), omega-3 fats and more. This recipe does toast the muesli but does not overheat it, so the value of the flaxmeal and its compounds is preserved.

Nutrients per 1/4 cup (60 mL)	
Calories	107
Fat	3 g
Carbohydrate	18 g
Protein	3 g
Vitamin C	1 mg
Vitamin D	3 IU
Vitamin E	0 mg
Niacin	1 mg
Folate	34 mcg
Vitamin B$_6$	0.3 mg
Vitamin B$_{12}$	0.5 mcg
Zinc	0.4 mg
Selenium	0 mcg

Spiced Fruit and Grain Cereal

Centuries ago, wars were fought over spices, and when you taste this recipe, you'll be reminded why. Spices give us great flavor, but also digestive support and health benefits.

Tip

Toast walnut halves in a dry skillet over low heat, stirring constantly, for 3 to 4 minutes or until fragrant. Transfer the toasted nuts to a plate and let cool before chopping.

½ cup	quinoa, rinsed	125 mL
⅛ tsp	fine sea salt	0.5 mL
1 cup	water	250 mL
¾ cup	milk or plain non-dairy milk (such as soy, almond, rice or hemp)	175 mL
½ cup	large-flake (old-fashioned) rolled oats	125 mL
3 tbsp	chopped dried figs or dried apricots	45 mL
2 tbsp	ground flax seeds (flaxseed meal)	30 mL
¼ tsp	ground ginger	1 mL
¼ tsp	ground cloves	1 mL
2 tbsp	chopped toasted walnuts	30 mL
2 tbsp	liquid honey	30 mL

1. In a medium saucepan, combine quinoa, salt, water and milk. Bring to a boil over medium-high heat. Reduce heat to low, cover and simmer for 10 minutes.

2. Stir in oats, figs, flax seeds, ginger and cloves. Cover and simmer for 5 to 8 minutes or until most of the liquid is absorbed and quinoa and oats are cooked through. Stir in walnuts and drizzle with honey.

> ▶ **Health Tip**
>
> Ginger contains compounds that are anti-inflammatory and improve digestion and stomach health, cloves are a source of antioxidants, and walnuts are a brain-supportive food.

Nutrients per serving	
Calories	536
Fat	14 g
Carbohydrate	89 g
Protein	19 g
Vitamin C	1 mg
Vitamin D	44 IU
Vitamin E	0 mg
Niacin	1 mg
Folate	37 mcg
Vitamin B_6	0.2 mg
Vitamin B_{12}	0.4 mcg
Zinc	2.6 mg
Selenium	7 mcg

Hot Breakfast Cereal Mix

The taste, texture and simplicity of rolled oats, the fiber of bran and protein from soy make this cereal a great way to stay on an even keel — and you can make your own additions at the breakfast table too!

Tips

For a wholesome breakfast, serve with nuts, fruit and milk or soy beverage on the side.

Enjoy this with a cup of ginger tea. Simply fill a microwave-safe mug with water and add 2 thin slices of peeled gingerroot. Microwave on High for 2 minutes. Remove the ginger and stir in 1 tsp (5 mL) liquid honey, if desired.

2 tbsp	large-flake (old-fashioned) rolled oats	30 mL
2 tbsp	wheat bran	30 mL
1 tbsp	wheat germ	15 mL
1 tbsp	soy beverage powder	15 mL

1. In a small, microwave-safe cup, stir together oats, bran, wheat germ and soy beverage powder. Stir in $\frac{1}{2}$ cup (125 mL) water. Microwave on High for 1 to $1\frac{1}{2}$ minutes or until oats are tender.

Variations

Add nuts and/or fresh or dried fruits of your choice.

Stir in fortified soy beverage or low-fat milk.

Sweeten with brown sugar or maple syrup.

> ▶ **Health Tip**
>
> Wheat germ is an excellent natural source of Vitamin E — a great antioxidant with uses throughout the body and of particular interest to people at risk for dementia.

This recipe courtesy of David Shaikh.

Nutrients per serving	
Calories	137
Fat	2 g
Carbohydrate	21 g
Protein	11 g
Vitamin C	0 mg
Vitamin D	0 IU
Vitamin E	1 mg
Niacin	2 mg
Folate	37 mcg
Vitamin B_6	0.2 mg
Vitamin B_{12}	0 mcg
Zinc	2.2 mg
Selenium	11 mcg

Hot Multigrain Cereal

Hot cereal is a terrific way to begin the day, and happily you can use your slow cooker to ensure that all family members get off to a nutritious start. Cook the cereal overnight and leave the slow cooker on Warm in the morning. Everyone can help themselves according to their schedules.

Makes 6 servings

Tip

When making whole-grain cereals in the slow cooker, be aware that stirring encourages creaminess. Obviously, for convenience, you don't need to wake up during the night to stir the cereal. However, if you have time, let the cereal sit on Warm for at least 15 minutes before serving, and stir it several times.

- **Small to medium (1½- to 3½-quart) slow cooker, lightly greased**

1 cup	multigrain cereal (or half multigrain cereal and half rolled or steel-cut oats)	250 mL
¼ tsp	salt	1 mL
4 cups	water	1 L
2	all-purpose apples, peeled and thickly sliced	2
¼ to ⅓ cup	raisins (optional)	60 to 75 mL
	Milk or non-dairy alternative	

1. In prepared stoneware, combine cereal, salt, water and apples. Stir well. Place a clean tea towel, folded in half (so you have two layers), over top of stoneware to absorb moisture. Cover and cook on Low for 8 hours or overnight or on High for 4 hours. Stir well and set to Warm.

2. Just before serving, place raisins, if using, in a microwave-safe bowl and cover with water. Microwave for 20 seconds to soften. Add to hot cereal. Stir well and serve with milk or non-dairy alternative.

> ▶ **Health Tip**
>
> Multigrain cereal takes longer to break down in the gut and does not flood the bloodstream with glucose, the way some starchy or processed cereals can.

Nutrients per serving	
Calories	88
Fat	1 g
Carbohydrate	20 g
Protein	3 g
Vitamin C	3 mg
Vitamin D	7 IU
Vitamin E	0 mg
Niacin	1 mg
Folate	14 mcg
Vitamin B$_6$	0.1 mg
Vitamin B$_{12}$	0.1 mcg
Zinc	0.7 mg
Selenium	7 mcg

Cranberry Quinoa Porridge

Forget about boring, lumpy porridges — this dish will give you a great start to the day with the energy and protein boost of quinoa and some nutritious natural sweetness from cranberries and honey or maple syrup.

Tip

Unless you have a stove with a true simmer, after reducing the heat to low, place a heat diffuser under the pot to prevent the mixture from boiling. This device also helps ensure that the grains will cook evenly and prevents hot spots, which might cause scorching, from forming. Heat diffusers are available at kitchen supply and hardware stores and are made to work on gas or electric stoves.

3 cups	water	750 mL
1 cup	quinoa, rinsed	250 mL
½ cup	dried cranberries	125 mL
	Maple syrup or honey	
	Milk or non-dairy alternative (optional)	

1. In a saucepan over medium heat, bring water to a boil. Stir in quinoa and cranberries and return to a boil. Reduce heat to low. Cover and simmer until quinoa is cooked (look for a white line around the seeds), about 15 minutes. Remove from heat and let stand, covered, about 5 minutes. Serve with maple syrup and milk or non-dairy alternative (if using).

Variations

Substitute dried cherries or blueberries or raisins for the cranberries.

Use red quinoa for a change.

▶ **Health Tip**

Quinoa contains all the essential amino acids and is a good protein source.

Nutrients per serving	
Calories	135
Fat	2 g
Carbohydrate	27 g
Protein	4 g
Vitamin C	0 mg
Vitamin D	0 IU
Vitamin E	2 mg
Niacin	1 mg
Folate	52 mcg
Vitamin B_6	0.1 mg
Vitamin B_{12}	0 mcg
Zinc	0.9 mg
Selenium	3 mcg

Breakfast Rice

Simple yet delicious, this tasty combination couldn't be easier to make. Also, because rice is a gluten-free grain, it makes a perfect breakfast for people who cannot tolerate that ingredient.

Tip

Made with this quantity of liquid, the rice will be a bit crunchy around the edges. If you prefer a softer version or will be cooking it longer than 8 hours, add ½ cup (125 mL) water or rice milk to the recipe.

Variation

Use half rice and half wheat, spelt or Kamut berries.

- **Small to medium (1½ to 3½ quart) slow cooker, lightly greased**

1 cup	brown rice	250 mL
4 cups	vanilla-flavored enriched rice milk	1 L
½ cup	dried cherries or cranberries	125 mL

1. In prepared slow cooker stoneware, combine rice, rice milk and cherries. Stir well. Place a clean tea towel, folded in half (so you have two layers), over top of stoneware to absorb moisture. Cover and cook on Low for up to 8 hours or overnight or on High for 4 hours. Stir well and serve.

> ▶ **Health Tip**
>
> Rice is a simple and easy-to-digest source of energy.

Nutrients per serving	
Calories	236
Fat	2 g
Carbohydrate	51 g
Protein	3 g
Vitamin C	0 mg
Vitamin D	67 IU
Vitamin E	1 mg
Niacin	2 mg
Folate	6 mcg
Vitamin B$_6$	0.2 mg
Vitamin B$_{12}$	1.0 mcg
Zinc	0.6 mg
Selenium	7 mcg

Power Pitas with Eggs and Vegetables

This dish is an easy-to-prepare breakfast that goes beyond the cereal and toast regimen. It will satisfy but leaves the grease and fat behind.

Makes 2 servings

Tip

If using salsa, select a brand that has a short list of easily identifiable ingredients, for the best flavor and nutrition.

3	large egg whites	3
1	large egg	1
½ cup	drained silken tofu, crumbled	125 mL
1 tsp	extra virgin olive oil	5 mL
½ cup	chopped fresh or thawed frozen broccoli florets	125 mL
½ cup	chopped red bell pepper	125 mL
2	6-inch (15 cm) whole wheat pitas, warmed	2
¼ cup	reduced-sodium salsa (optional)	60 mL

1. In a small bowl, beat egg whites and egg until blended. Stir in tofu.

2. In a small skillet, heat oil over medium-high heat. Add broccoli and red pepper; cook, stirring, for 4 to 5 minutes or until softened. Reduce heat to medium. Pour egg mixture over vegetables and cook, stirring gently with a spatula, for 2 to 4 minutes or until eggs are set.

3. Spoon egg mixture onto warm pitas and top with salsa, if desired. Fold in half and serve right away or wrap in foil to eat on the go.

> ▶ **Health Tip**
>
> Eggs are a fantastic high-value protein, and the addition of tofu offers beneficial soy isoflavones. Broccoli and red peppers ensure that this dish counts as a serving of vegetables — ones that have excellent detoxification and antioxidant properties.

Nutrients per serving	
Calories	306
Fat	8 g
Carbohydrate	41 g
Protein	20 g
Vitamin C	67 mg
Vitamin D	21 IU
Vitamin E	2 mg
Niacin	3 mg
Folate	67 mcg
Vitamin B_6	0.4 mg
Vitamin B_{12}	0.3 mcg
Zinc	1.8 mg
Selenium	46 mcg

Avocado and Egg Breakfast Wraps

Avocado is a versatile food that has grown in popularity. This dish combines it with the savory taste of goat cheese in what could be described as a spinach omelet in a pita.

Makes 2 servings

Tip

Hass avocados (sometimes called Haas avocados) are dark-skinned avocados with nutty, buttery flesh and a longer shelf life than other varieties, making them the most popular avocado in North America. To determine whether a Hass avocado is ripe, look for a purple-black skin and gently press the top — a ripe one will give slightly.

2	large eggs	2
2	large egg whites	2
Pinch	fine sea salt	Pinch
1/4 tsp	freshly ground black pepper	1 mL
1 tsp	extra virgin olive oil	5 mL
3 cups	loosely packed spinach, chopped	750 mL
2 tsp	water	10 mL
2	6-inch (15 cm) whole wheat tortillas, warmed	2
2 tbsp	crumbled soft goat cheese	30 mL
1/2	small ripe Hass avocado, sliced	1/2

1. In a small bowl, beat eggs, egg whites, salt and pepper until blended.

2. In a small skillet, heat oil over medium-high heat. Add spinach and water; cook, stirring, until leaves are wilted. Reduce heat to medium. Pour egg mixture over spinach. Cook, stirring gently with a spatula, for 2 to 4 minutes or until eggs are set.

3. Place half the egg mixture in the center of each warm tortilla and sprinkle each with 1 tbsp (15 mL) goat cheese. Top with avocado and fold or roll up.

> ▶ **Health Tip**
>
> Avocado is rich in healthy fats and increases absorption of carotenoids, the great antioxidant molecules in spinach that give it its green color.

Nutrients per serving	
Calories	315
Fat	20 g
Carbohydrate	22 g
Protein	14 g
Vitamin C	18 mg
Vitamin D	43 IU
Vitamin E	3 mg
Niacin	2 mg
Folate	157 mcg
Vitamin B_6	0.4 mg
Vitamin B_{12}	0.5 mcg
Zinc	1.5 mg
Selenium	23 mcg

Sage and Savory Mushroom Frittata

There is no lack of flavor in this dish, with shallots, mushrooms and sage livening up a protein-packed tofu-based frittata.

Tip

You can substitute 1 tsp (5 mL) dried sage for 1 tbsp (15 mL) fresh sage.

- **Preheat oven to 350°F (180°C)**
- **Cast-iron or other ovenproof skillet**
- **Food processor**

2 tbsp	olive oil	30 mL
1 lb	mushrooms, sliced	500 g
1/4 cup	sliced shallots (about 2 large)	60 mL
1 tbsp	vegan hard margarine	15 mL
1 tbsp	chopped fresh sage leaves (see tip, at left)	15 mL
1 lb	firm tofu, drained and crumbled	500 g
1	package (12.3 oz/350 g) firm silken tofu	1
1/4 cup	plain soy milk	60 mL
2 tbsp	nutritional yeast	30 mL
1 tbsp	cornstarch	15 mL
3/4 tsp	ground turmeric	3 mL
3/4 tsp	salt	3 mL
1/2 tsp	freshly ground black pepper	2 mL

1. Place skillet over medium-high heat and let pan get hot. Add oil and tip pan to coat. Add mushrooms and shallots. Reduce heat to medium and cook, stirring, until softened and lightly browned, 6 to 8 minutes. Add margarine, sage and firm tofu and cook, stirring, for 2 to 3 minutes to let flavors combine. Remove from heat and gently distribute mixture evenly in pan.

2. In food processor, combine silken tofu, soy milk, nutritional yeast, cornstarch, turmeric, salt and pepper and process until smooth. Pour mixture evenly over vegetable mixture in pan, gently lifting and stirring to combine ingredients.

3. Bake in preheated oven until top is firm and golden, 25 to 30 minutes. Let frittata cool slightly, cut into wedges and serve.

> ▶ **Health Tip**
>
> Sage is a brain-boosting food that has been shown to improve cognition.

Nutrients per 1 of 8 servings

Calories	192
Fat	11 g
Carbohydrate	11 g
Protein	15 g
Vitamin C	1 mg
Vitamin D	14 IU
Vitamin E	1 mg
Niacin	9 mg
Folate	92 mcg
Vitamin B$_6$	0.2 mg
Vitamin B$_{12}$	0.1 mcg
Zinc	1.7 mg
Selenium	12 mcg

French-Herbed Strata

A strata is a layered dish using bread as the backbone, and *vive les herbes* — this flavorful dish will nourish and satisfy.

Tip

Leeks are grown in sand and are sometimes difficult to clean. A good method of cleaning is to vertically slice through the white and light green leaves, leaving most of the dark green leaves intact. Grasp the leek by the dark green leaves, fan out the bottom white and light green portions, exposing much of the inside of the leek, and run under cold water.

Nutrients per 1 of 10 servings	
Calories	215
Fat	4 g
Carbohydrate	34 g
Protein	10 g
Vitamin C	5 mg
Vitamin D	11 IU
Vitamin E	1 mg
Niacin	3 mg
Folate	42 mcg
Vitamin B$_6$	0.1 mg
Vitamin B$_{12}$	0.2 mcg
Zinc	1.0 mg
Selenium	15 mcg

- **10-cup (2.5 L) baking dish, lightly oiled**
- **Food processor**

1 tbsp	olive oil	15 mL
2	large leeks, thoroughly washed (see tip, at left) and sliced	2
8 oz	thin asparagus, ends trimmed, cut into 3-inch (7.5 cm) pieces	250 g
3	cloves garlic, chopped	3
1 tbsp	freshly squeezed lemon juice	15 mL
1 tsp	salt, divided	5 mL
1/2 tsp	freshly ground black pepper	2 mL
1/2	loaf (1 lb/500 g) day-old vegan French bread, cut into 2-inch (5 cm) pieces	1/2
1	package (12.3 oz/350 g) firm silken tofu	1
4 oz	medium regular tofu	125 g
1 cup	plain non-dairy milk	250 mL
1/4 cup	dry white wine	60 mL
2 tbsp	cornstarch	30 mL
2 tsp	Dijon mustard	10 mL
1 tsp	onion powder	5 mL
1/4 tsp	ground turmeric	1 mL
1 tbsp	fresh tarragon leaves	15 mL
1 tsp	herbes de Provence	5 mL

1. Place a large skillet over medium heat and let pan get hot. Add oil and tip pan to coat. Add leeks and cook, stirring occasionally, for 3 to 4 minutes. Add asparagus, garlic, lemon juice, 1/2 tsp (2 mL) of the salt and pepper and cook until asparagus turns bright green, 2 to 3 minutes. Remove from heat, stir in bread and transfer to prepared baking dish.

Tip

Choose your favorite non-dairy milk, such as soy, almond, rice or hemp.

2. In food processor, combine silken and regular tofu, milk, wine, cornstarch, mustard, onion powder, $1/2$ tsp (2 mL) salt and turmeric and process until very smooth. Add tarragon and herbes de Provence and process until blended. Pour mixture over vegetables and bread. Cover strata and refrigerate for at least 2 hours or up to overnight, for bread to absorb custard.

3. Preheat oven to 350°F (180°C).

4. Remove strata from refrigerator and allow it to warm to room temperature. Uncover and bake in preheated oven until slightly puffed and firm, 45 minutes to 1 hour. Let stand for 6 to 8 minutes before cutting to serve.

> ▶ **Health Tip**
>
> Tarragon has a very high antioxidant value.

Tomato and Asiago Cheese Strata

This is a more traditional strata with eggs and cheese. This dish is rich but not greasy and has a Mediterranean aspect due to garlic, onions, olive oil and plum tomatoes.

Makes 4 to 6 servings

Tip

If the bread is fresh, place on a baking sheet and toast in 350°F (180°C) oven for 8 to 10 minutes or until crisp around the edges.

Variation

Instead of fresh basil, substitute 2 tbsp (30 mL) parsley and add 1 tsp (5 mL) dried basil to onions when cooking.

- **Preheat oven to 350°F (180°C)**
- **8-inch (20 cm) square baking dish, well greased**

2 tbsp	olive oil	30 mL
1 cup	chopped Spanish onion	250 mL
2	cloves garlic, finely chopped	2
2 cups	chopped seeded plum (Roma) tomatoes (about 5 or 6)	500 mL
½ tsp	salt	2 mL
¼ tsp	freshly ground black pepper	1 mL
2 tbsp	chopped fresh basil	30 mL
6 cups	cubed stale Italian or French bread (see tip, at left)	1.5 L
1½ cups	shredded Asiago or fontina cheese	375 mL
4	large eggs	4
1 cup	ready-to-use vegetable or chicken broth	250 mL

1. In a large nonstick skillet, heat oil over medium-high heat. Cook onion and garlic, stirring, for 2 minutes. Stir in tomatoes, salt and pepper; cook, stirring often, for 5 minutes or until tomatoes are sauce-like. Stir in basil.

2. Layer half of the bread cubes in prepared baking dish. Top with half of the tomato mixture and sprinkle with half of the cheese. Layer with remaining bread and tomato mixture.

3. In a bowl, beat eggs with broth; pour over bread mixture. Sprinkle with remaining cheese. Let stand for 10 minutes for bread to absorb egg mixture. (This can be made a day ahead; cover and refrigerate.)

4. Bake in preheated oven for 35 to 40 minutes (5 to 10 minutes longer if refrigerated), until top is golden and center is set when tested with a knife. Serve warm or at room temperature.

▶ Health Tip

Tomatoes are a great source of lycopene, a potent antioxidant and cell protector (cancer prevention antioxidant) molecule.

Nutrients per 1 of 6 servings	
Calories	403
Fat	18 g
Carbohydrate	42 g
Protein	20 g
Vitamin C	11 mg
Vitamin D	34 IU
Vitamin E	2 mg
Niacin	4 mg
Folate	49 mcg
Vitamin B$_6$	0.2 mg
Vitamin B$_{12}$	0.8 mcg
Zinc	2.2 mg
Selenium	32 mcg

Home-Style Pancakes

This dish is a whole-grain dream, and about as far away from white flour, high-glycemic-index pancakes as you can get. The flavors here come from vanilla and the natural nutty flavor of the grains.

Tip

Choose your favorite gluten-free non-dairy milk, such as soy, rice, almond or potato-based milk, or, if you can tolerate lactose, use regular 1% milk.

½ cup	sorghum flour	125 mL
½ cup	brown rice flour	125 mL
2 tbsp	psyllium husks	30 mL
1 tsp	gluten-free baking powder	5 mL
¼ tsp	baking soda	1 mL
¼ tsp	salt	1 mL
1	large egg	1
1 cup	fortified gluten-free non-dairy milk or lactose-free 1% milk	250 mL
1 tbsp	liquid honey, pure maple syrup or agave nectar	15 mL
2 tsp	grapeseed oil	10 mL
1 tsp	vanilla extract	5 mL
	Butter or grapeseed oil	

1. In a large bowl, combine sorghum flour, brown rice flour, psyllium, baking powder, baking soda and salt.

2. In another bowl, beat egg, milk, honey, oil and vanilla. Pour into flour mixture and whisk for about 1 minute or until smooth.

3. On a griddle or in a nonstick skillet, melt 1 tsp (5 mL) butter over medium heat. For each pancake, pour in ¼ cup (60 mL) batter. Cook for 1 to 2 minutes or until bubbles start to form and edges are firm. Flip over and cook other side for 1 to 2 minutes or until bottom is golden. Transfer to a plate and keep warm. Repeat with the remaining batter, greasing griddle and adjusting heat between batches as needed.

> ▶ **Health Tip**
>
> This dish is an excellent source of dietary fiber. Not only does that help regulate the GI tract, but sources of fiber like whole grains and psyllium help bind some toxins in the gut and whisk them out of the body before they can be reabsorbed.

Nutrients per pancake	
Calories	139
Fat	3 g
Carbohydrate	24 g
Protein	4 g
Vitamin C	0 mg
Vitamin D	21 IU
Vitamin E	1 mg
Niacin	1 mg
Folate	8 mcg
Vitamin B$_6$	0.1 mg
Vitamin B$_{12}$	0.4 mcg
Zinc	0.5 mg
Selenium	3 mcg

Potato Pancakes with Cinnamon Apples and Yogurt Cheese

Make a series of individual pancakes with this recipe or one giant pancake, cutting it into wedges to serve. Serve with back (Canadian) bacon or farmer's sausage, or omit the apple topping and serve it with poached or fried eggs on top.

Makes 4 servings

Tips

Tossing the apples in lemon juice immediately after they have been sliced prevents browning.

You can make this dish with floury, all-purpose or even waxy potatoes, but with waxy potatoes you have to work a little harder to keep the shreds together.

Nutrients per serving	
Calories	499
Fat	29 g
Carbohydrate	52 g
Protein	12 g
Vitamin C	33 mg
Vitamin D	36 IU
Vitamin E	3 mg
Niacin	2 mg
Folate	60 mcg
Vitamin B$_6$	0.4 mg
Vitamin B$_{12}$	0.7 mcg
Zinc	1.5 mg
Selenium	11 mcg

Topping

1 tbsp	butter	15 mL
1 tbsp	olive oil	15 mL
3	apples (Cortland, Crispin or Spartan), peeled, cored, sliced and tossed with 2 tbsp (30 mL) lemon juice	3
½ tsp	ground cinnamon	2 mL
½ tsp	ground nutmeg	2 mL
Pinch	ground allspice	Pinch
1 tbsp	packed brown sugar	15 mL

Pancakes

1 lb	floury potatoes, peeled	500 g
1	small onion	1
3	large eggs, lightly beaten	3
2 to 3 tbsp	all-purpose flour	30 to 45 mL
	Salt and freshly ground black pepper	
3 tbsp	butter (approx.), divided	45 mL
3 tbsp	olive oil (approx.), divided	45 mL
1 cup	plain Greek yogurt	250 mL

1. *Topping:* In a skillet, heat butter and oil over medium heat. Add apples, cinnamon, nutmeg and allspice and cook, stirring, for 10 minutes. Stir in brown sugar and cook for 15 minutes or until apples are glazed (do not overcook; you do not want the apples to become totally soft). Remove from heat and keep warm.

Tips

If you don't work fairly quickly when shredding the potatoes, they may discolor. Transferring them to a bowl of cold water as you work will prevent this, but you will have to work extra diligently to extract the water.

Be careful with the amount of flour — using too much will make the pancakes leaden.

Variation

In season, substitute fresh peaches for the apples. Blanch in boiling water and peel before using in recipes.

2. *Pancakes:* Meanwhile, coarsely shred potatoes (use a food processor fitted with shredding blade or a box grater). Using a slotted spoon, transfer to a clean tea towel, leaving liquid behind. Gather towel around potatoes and, holding it over the sink, squeeze to wring out as much moisture as possible. Over a small bowl, shred onion. Set aside.

3. In a bowl, beat eggs. Lightly stir together potatoes, onion and 2 tbsp (30 mL) flour (if mixture looks too wet, add a little more flour). Season to taste with salt and pepper.

4. Preheat oven to 140°F (60°C). In a large, heavy skillet, heat 1 tbsp (15 mL) butter and 1 tbsp (15 mL) oil over medium-high heat until hot. In batches, drop potato mixture by spoonfuls into pan and, using a metal spatula, gently flatten to about $1/4$ inch (0.5 cm) thick. Cook for about 3 minutes per side or until browned. As completed, transfer to preheated oven to keep warm. Repeat until all the batter has been cooked, adding more butter and oil as necessary and ensuring it is hot before adding next batch.

5. Divide pancakes among four warmed individual serving plates. Top each evenly with apple mixture and a quarter of the yogurt.

> ▶ **Health Tip**
>
> Cinnamon has been shown to encourage the body to make better use of insulin.

Walnut Flax Waffles

This is a hearty waffle that has the flavors of maple syrup and vanilla (very comforting) and the crunch of walnuts.

Makes 8 waffles

Tip

Look for packages of ready-ground flax seeds, which may be labeled "flaxseed meal," or use a spice or coffee grinder to grind whole flax seeds to a very fine meal.

- **Preheat waffle maker to medium-high**
- **Blender**

1 1/2 cups	plain almond milk	375 mL
2 tbsp	vegetable oil	30 mL
1 tbsp	pure maple syrup	15 mL
2 tsp	vanilla extract	10 mL
1 1/2 tsp	cider vinegar	7 mL
3 tbsp	ground flax seeds (flaxseed meal)	45 mL
1 cup	whole wheat flour	250 mL
1 1/2 tsp	baking powder	7 mL
1/2 tsp	baking soda	2 mL
1/8 tsp	fine sea salt	0.5 mL
1/2 cup	chopped toasted walnuts	125 mL
	Nonstick cooking spray	

1. In blender, combine almond milk, oil, maple syrup, vanilla and vinegar. Let stand for 10 minutes. Add flax seeds and blend for 1 minute or until slightly frothy.

2. In a large bowl, whisk together flour, baking powder, baking soda and salt. Add almond milk mixture and stir until just blended. Gently stir in walnuts.

3. Spray preheated waffle maker with cooking spray. For each waffle, pour about 1/3 cup (75 mL) batter into waffle maker. Cook according to manufacturer's instructions until golden brown.

▶ **Health Tip**

Walnuts are a good source of omega-3 fats and one of our top brain-boosting foods. Flax meal, which can be purchased vacuum-packed and kept in the fridge, is yet another good omega-3 source.

Nutrients per waffle

Calories	165
Fat	10 g
Carbohydrate	16 g
Protein	5 g
Vitamin C	0 mg
Vitamin D	19 IU
Vitamin E	1 mg
Niacin	1 mg
Folate	11 mcg
Vitamin B_6	0.1 mg
Vitamin B_{12}	0.0 mcg
Zinc	0.8 mg
Selenium	11 mcg

Snacks and Appetizers

Trail Mix

You don't need to be hiking to enjoy this trail mix — it's an excellent high-energy snack where every bite counts nutritionally.

Makes 3½ cups (875 mL)

Tip

Start with this basic recipe and sub in other ingredients depending on what strikes your fancy and what you have on hand. Good additions include raisins, shredded coconut, hazelnuts and even chunks of dark chocolate. Be creative — trail mix can be a little different every time you make it!

½ cup	dried apricots, cut into quarters	125 mL
½ cup	dried cranberries	125 mL
½ cup	dried goji berries (optional)	125 mL
½ cup	whole almonds	125 mL
½ cup	chopped walnuts	125 mL
½ cup	unsalted sunflower seeds	125 mL
½ cup	raw green pumpkin seeds (pepitas)	125 mL

1. In a large bowl, combine apricots, cranberries, goji berries (if using), almonds, walnuts, sunflower seeds and pumpkin seeds.

2. Store in an airtight container at room temperature for up to 1 month.

> ▶ **Health Tip**
>
> Every ingredient in this trail mix is a concentrated source of antioxidants or healthy fats. This high-energy pick-me-up will leave your body better nourished and get you through your afternoon.

Nutrients per ¼ cup (60 mL)	
Calories	144
Fat	11 g
Carbohydrate	10 g
Protein	5 g
Vitamin C	0 mg
Vitamin D	0 IU
Vitamin E	3 mg
Niacin	1 mg
Folate	15 mcg
Vitamin B_6	0.1 mg
Vitamin B_{12}	0 mcg
Zinc	0.6 mg
Selenium	5 mcg

Cranberry Walnut Muffins

The cranberry is praised for its sauce at the Thanksgiving table, but the ruby fruit is just as delicious when baked into muffins.

Makes 12 muffins

Tips

Look for packages of ready-ground flax seeds, which may be labeled "flaxseed meal," or use a spice or coffee grinder to grind whole flax seeds to a very fine meal.

Toast walnut halves in a dry skillet over low heat, stirring constantly, for 3 to 4 minutes or until fragrant. Transfer the toasted nuts to a plate and let cool before chopping.

- **Preheat oven to 350°F (180°C)**
- **12-cup muffin pan, greased**

1¼ cups	whole wheat pastry flour	300 mL
¼ cup	wheat germ	60 mL
1½ tsp	baking powder	7 mL
1 tsp	ground cinnamon	5 mL
½ tsp	salt	2 mL
¼ tsp	baking soda	1 mL
2	large eggs	2
¼ cup	ground flax seeds (flaxseed meal)	60 mL
½ cup	agave nectar	125 mL
⅓ cup	low-fat (1%) plain yogurt	75 mL
¼ cup	vegetable oil	60 mL
1 tsp	vanilla extract	5 mL
1 cup	fresh cranberries, coarsely chopped	250 mL
1 cup	chopped toasted walnuts	250 mL

1. In a large bowl, whisk together flour, wheat germ, baking powder, cinnamon, salt and baking soda.

2. In a medium bowl, whisk together eggs, flax seeds, agave nectar, yogurt, oil and vanilla, until well blended.

3. Add the egg mixture to the flour mixture and stir until just blended. Gently fold in cranberries and walnuts.

4. Divide batter equally among prepared muffin cups.

5. Bake in preheated oven for 20 to 25 minutes or until tops are golden and a toothpick inserted in the center comes out clean. Let cool in pan on a wire rack for 5 minutes, then transfer to the rack to cool.

> ▶ **Health Tip**
>
> Cranberries are loaded with disease-fighting antioxidants and are a good source of vitamin C, fiber, manganese and potassium.

Nutrients per muffin	
Calories	235
Fat	13 g
Carbohydrate	25 g
Protein	6 g
Vitamin C	2 mg
Vitamin D	7 IU
Vitamin E	1 mg
Niacin	0 mg
Folate	21 mcg
Vitamin B$_6$	0.1 mg
Vitamin B$_{12}$	0.1 mcg
Zinc	0.9 mg
Selenium	7 mcg

Date and Walnut Muffins

This gluten-free muffin provides a great energy boost and healthy snacks for a few days or for one hungry family.

Makes 12 muffins

- **Preheat oven to 350°F (180°C)**
- **12-cup muffin pan, lined with paper liners**

¾ cup	chopped dates	175 mL
⅔ cup	boiling water	150 mL
1½ cups	Brown Rice Flour Blend (see recipe, opposite)	375 mL
1 tsp	xanthan gum	5 mL
¾ tsp	gluten-free baking powder	3 mL
¾ tsp	baking soda	3 mL
¾ tsp	ground cinnamon	3 mL
½ tsp	salt	2 mL
¾ cup	packed dark brown sugar	175 mL
6 tbsp	unsalted butter, softened	90 mL
2	large eggs	2
1 tsp	vanilla extract	5 mL
¾ cup	chopped toasted walnuts	175 mL

1. In a small bowl, combine dates and boiling water. Let stand for 10 minutes (do not drain).

2. In a medium bowl, whisk together flour blend, xanthan gum, baking powder, baking soda, cinnamon and salt.

3. In a large bowl, using an electric mixer on medium speed, beat brown sugar and butter until light and fluffy. Beat in eggs, one at a time, until well blended. Beat in vanilla until blended. Beat in date mixture.

4. Add the flour mixture to the egg mixture and, using a wooden spoon, stir until just blended. Gently fold in walnuts.

5. Divide batter equally among prepared muffin cups.

6. Bake in preheated oven for 16 to 20 minutes or until a toothpick inserted in the center comes out clean. Let cool in pan on a wire rack for 5 minutes, then transfer to the rack to cool.

Nutrients per muffin	
Calories	263
Fat	12 g
Carbohydrate	38 g
Protein	4 g
Vitamin C	0 mg
Vitamin D	11 IU
Vitamin E	1 mg
Niacin	1 mg
Folate	11 mcg
Vitamin B6	0.2 mg
Vitamin B12	0.1 mcg
Zinc	0.7 mg
Selenium	4 mcg

> ▶ **Health Tip**
>
> Walnuts have lots of vitamin E in a rather unusual form, gamma-tocopherol, which has cardiovascular benefits.

Tips

You can also make this blend in smaller amounts by using the basic proportions: 2 parts finely ground brown rice flour, $\frac{2}{3}$ part potato starch and $\frac{1}{3}$ part tapioca starch.

You can double, triple or quadruple the recipe to have it on hand.

Brown Rice Flour Blend

If you are going to do some gluten-free baking, this is a key component for some of the recipes in this book. You can also purchase blends at many supermarkets and certainly at gluten-free shops or health food stores.

2 cups	finely ground brown rice flour	500 mL
$\frac{2}{3}$ cup	potato starch	150 mL
$\frac{1}{3}$ cup	tapioca starch	75 mL

1. In a bowl, whisk together brown rice flour, potato starch and tapioca starch.

2. Store in an airtight container in the refrigerator for up to 4 months, or in the freezer for up to 1 year. Let warm to room temperature before using.

> ▶ **Health Tip**
>
> Flour made from a whole grain, like brown rice flour, still contains most of its original vitamins and minerals.

Nutrients per 2 tbsp (30 mL)	
Calories	68
Fat	0 g
Carbohydrate	15 g
Protein	1 g
Vitamin C	0 mg
Vitamin D	0 IU
Vitamin E	0 mg
Niacin	1 mg
Folate	3 mcg
Vitamin B$_6$	0.1 mg
Vitamin B$_{12}$	0.0 mcg
Zinc	0.3 mg
Selenium	0 mcg

Cinnamon Apple Chips

Combining the tart and sweet flavor of apples with the natural sweetness of stevia and cinnamon, this is an enjoyable but low-glycemic-index treat.

Makes 8 servings

Tip

Be sure to transfer the chips from the parchment paper to a wire rack while still warm, or they will stick.

Variation

Pear Chips: Use 4 medium Bosc pears, halved and cored, in place of the apples.

- **Preheat oven to 325°F (160°C)**
- **2 rimmed baking sheets, lined with parchment paper**

4	large tart-sweet apples (such as Braeburn, Gala or Pippin), halved and cored	4
4 tsp	stevia powder	20 mL
1/2 tsp	ground cinnamon	2 mL
	Nonstick cooking spray (preferably olive oil)	

1. Using a very sharp knife or a mandoline, cut apples into $\frac{1}{8}$-inch (3 mm) thick slices.

2. In a small bowl, combine stevia and cinnamon.

3. Arrange apple slices in a single layer on prepared baking sheets. Spray with cooking spray and sprinkle with stevia mixture.

4. Bake in preheated oven for 35 to 40 minutes or until edges are browned and slices are dry and crispy. Transfer chips to a wire rack and let cool completely (they will crisp more as they cool). Store in an airtight container at room temperature for up to 1 week.

> ▶ **Health Tip**
>
> Recent studies indicate that eating as little as 1/2 tsp (2 mL) of ground cinnamon per day can boost cognitive function and memory.

Nutrients per serving	
Calories	59
Fat	0 g
Carbohydrate	16 g
Protein	0 g
Vitamin C	5 mg
Vitamin D	0 IU
Vitamin E	0 mg
Niacin	0 mg
Folate	3 mcg
Vitamin B$_6$	0.1 mg
Vitamin B$_{12}$	0.0 mcg
Zinc	0.1 mg
Selenium	0 mcg

Cashew Butter

Easy and delicious, this nut butter is great for breakfast on toasted whole wheat bread. It is also a very good substitute for tahini, a sesame paste, because it is milder than peanut butter, which is often used to replace tahini.

Makes 2½ cups (625 mL)

Tip

Brown rice syrup has a light, mild flavor and a similar appearance to honey, though it is less sweet.

- **Blender or food processor**

½ cup	unsweetened apple juice	125 mL
2 cups	lightly salted roasted cashews	500 mL
2 tbsp	brown rice syrup	30 mL
2 tbsp	freshly squeezed lemon juice	30 mL

1. In blender, combine apple juice, cashews, rice syrup and lemon juice. Blend until smooth.

2. Transfer to a clean container with lid. Store spread, tightly covered, in the refrigerator for up to 1 week.

Nutrients per 1 tbsp (15 mL)	
Calories	42
Fat	3 g
Carbohydrate	3 g
Protein	1 g
Vitamin C	0 mg
Vitamin D	0 IU
Vitamin E	0 mg
Niacin	0 mg
Folate	5 mcg
Vitamin B$_6$	0.0 mg
Vitamin B$_{12}$	0.0 mcg
Zinc	0.4 mg
Selenium	1 mcg

Red Pepper Hummus

This hummus gives all sandwiches a wonderful kick. It also works great as an appetizer, served with pita triangles and crudités.

Makes 1½ cups (375 mL)

Tips

Tahini is made of ground sesame seeds. Look for it in the international section of grocery stores. If you can't find tahini, try smooth peanut butter instead.

Substitute cannellini or other white beans for the chickpeas.

- **Food processor**

1	can (14 to 19 oz/398 to 540 mL) chickpeas, drained and rinsed	1
⅓ cup	drained roasted red peppers	75 mL
2	cloves garlic, coarsely chopped	2
¼ cup	tahini (see tip, at left)	60 mL
2 tbsp	minced fresh flat-leaf (Italian) parsley	30 mL
2 tbsp	freshly squeezed lemon juice	30 mL
1½ tsp	ground cumin	7 mL
¼ tsp	kosher salt	1 mL
¼ tsp	cayenne pepper	1 mL

1. In food processor, combine chickpeas, roasted peppers, garlic, tahini, parsley, lemon juice, cumin, salt and cayenne; purée until smooth. Use immediately or cover and refrigerate for up to 2 days.

> ▶ **Health Tip**
>
> The fiber from chickpeas is good for gastrointestinal health.

Nutrients per 2 tbsp (30 mL)	
Calories	67
Fat	3 g
Carbohydrate	9 g
Protein	3 g
Vitamin C	9 mg
Vitamin D	0 IU
Vitamin E	0 mg
Niacin	0 mg
Folate	27 mcg
Vitamin B$_6$	0.2 mg
Vitamin B$_{12}$	0.0 mcg
Zinc	0.6 mg
Selenium	3 mcg

Chunky Guacamole

This rich and creamy guacamole has a full-bodied flavor that will add life to whatever it accompanies. Serve with tortilla chips, crackers or fresh vegetables.

Tips

Use 1 tbsp (15 mL) finely chopped pickled jalapeño peppers if fresh are not available. The added vinegar in the peppers will alter the flavor slightly, so taste before adding the full tablespoon (15 mL) of pickled peppers.

If you prefer a smoother consistency, make the guacamole in a food processor.

2	avocados, peeled, pitted and quartered	2
2	cloves garlic, minced (about 2 tsp/10 mL)	2
1	small tomato, seeded and finely diced	1
1½ tsp	freshly squeezed lime juice	7 mL
1	jalapeño pepper, seeded and finely chopped (optional)	1
½ tsp	hot pepper sauce (or to taste)	2 mL
	Salt and freshly ground black pepper	

1. In a bowl, using a fork or potato masher, mash avocados until the desired consistency is reached. Add garlic, tomato, lime juice, jalapeño pepper (if using) and hot pepper sauce. Mix well and season with salt and freshly ground black pepper to taste. Serve immediately or cover and chill. Guacamole is best eaten within a day.

**Nutrients
per 2 tbsp (30 mL)**

Calories	84
Fat	7 g
Carbohydrate	5 g
Protein	1 g
Vitamin C	7 mg
Vitamin D	0 IU
Vitamin E	1 mg
Niacin	1 mg
Folate	43 mcg
Vitamin B$_6$	0.2 mg
Vitamin B$_{12}$	0.0 mcg
Zinc	0.4 mg
Selenium	0 mcg

Creamy Mushroom Walnut Toasts

This dish will satisfy and impress guests as an appetizer — or just liven up a Sunday afternoon.

Tip

To make crostini: Cut 1 thin baguette into ⅓ inch (8 mm) thick slices. Arrange on a baking sheet; brush lightly with 2 tbsp (30 mL) olive oil or melted butter. Bake in 375°F (190°C) oven for 5 minutes or until edges are lightly toasted.

- **Preheat oven to 375°F (190°C)**
- **Food processor**

1 lb	mushrooms (an assortment of white, oyster and portobello), coarsely chopped	500 g
2 tbsp	butter	30 mL
⅓ cup	finely chopped green onions	75 mL
2	cloves garlic, minced	2
½ tsp	dried thyme	2 mL
4 oz	cream cheese or goat cheese, cut into pieces	125 g
⅓ cup	freshly grated Parmesan cheese (plus extra for topping)	75 mL
⅓ cup	finely chopped walnuts	75 mL
2 tbsp	finely chopped fresh parsley	30 mL
	Salt and freshly ground black pepper	
40	crostini (see tip, at left)	40

1. In food processor, finely chop mushrooms in batches, using on-off turns.

2. In a large skillet, heat butter over medium-high heat. Add mushrooms, green onions, garlic and thyme; cook for 5 to 7 minutes or until mushrooms are softened. Cook 1 to 2 minutes more, if necessary, until all moisture has evaporated. (Mixture should be dry and almost crumbly.) Remove from heat.

3. Add cream cheese, stirring until smooth. Add Parmesan cheese, walnuts and parsley. Season with salt and pepper to taste. Transfer to a bowl; cover and let cool.

Nutrients per appetizer	
Calories	39
Fat	2 g
Carbohydrate	3 g
Protein	1 g
Vitamin C	1 mg
Vitamin D	2 IU
Vitamin E	0 mg
Niacin	1 mg
Folate	7 mcg
Vitamin B$_6$	0.0 mg
Vitamin B$_{12}$	0.0 mcg
Zinc	0.2 mg
Selenium	1 mcg

Tips

Spread toasts with mushroom mixture just before baking to prevent them from turning soggy.

The mushroom-walnut filling can be frozen for up to 1 month.

4. Spread crostini with a generous teaspoonful (5 to 7 mL) of mushroom mixture. Arrange on a baking sheet. Sprinkle tops with additional Parmesan cheese. Bake in preheated oven for 8 to 10 minutes or until edges are toasted.

> ▶ **Health Tip**
>
> Walnuts are a good source of the mineral manganese (not magnesium — manganese), which is important for joint health and is part of a very important antioxidant system that protects the cells in our body.

Roasted Peppers Antipasto

Go Mediterranean with this appetizer that brings out the wonderful sweetness of bell peppers.

Tips

To save time and trouble, core and cut peppers in half before roasting or grilling. This tends to dehydrate and shrink the flesh a little, making it fragile, but it's a heck of a lot easier.

For parties, try serving these peppers with black olives, sun-dried tomatoes, capers, sliced ripe tomatoes, mozzarella or bocconcini cheese, artichoke hearts and marinated mushrooms to create a real Italian appetizer extravaganza.

Nutrients per serving	
Calories	231
Fat	20 g
Carbohydrate	7 g
Protein	6 g
Vitamin C	115 mg
Vitamin D	3 IU
Vitamin E	3 mg
Niacin	1 mg
Folate	44 mcg
Vitamin B_6	0.3 mg
Vitamin B_{12}	0.3 mcg
Zinc	0.8 mg
Selenium	3 mcg

- **Preheat oven to 400°F (200°C)**

3	bell peppers, preferably different colors (e.g., green, red and yellow)	3
1 tsp	vegetable oil	5 mL
1 tbsp	balsamic vinegar	15 mL
1/4 cup	extra virgin olive oil	60 mL
	Salt and freshly ground black pepper	
2 oz	Parmesan cheese, shaved	60 g
1/4 cup	thinly sliced red onion	60 mL
	Few sprigs of fresh basil and/or parsley, chopped	

1. Cut peppers in half lengthwise, then core and deseed them. Brush their skins with the vegetable oil, and arrange the peppers (without crowding) in an oven pan, skin side up. Roast in preheated oven for 20 to 25 minutes, just until the skin has crinkled but before it has blackened. (If you wait until the skin turns black, the flesh of these halved peppers will totally disintegrate.) Remove peppers from oven and let cool for 5 to 10 minutes.

2. Using a spatula, pry the cooled peppers from the pan and transfer them to a work surface. Remove the skins (they should come off easily and more or less in one piece). Cut each into 5 or 6 strips and transfer to a plate.

3. Moisten the pepper strips with vinegar, then douse them with olive oil. Season to taste with salt and pepper. Decorate with Parmesan shavings, onion and basil and/or parsley just prior to serving. The oiled peppers can wait (and improve) for up to 1 hour.

> ▶ **Health Tip**
>
> Balsamic vinegar concentrates some of the powerful antioxidant molecules from grapes, known collectively as polyphenols.

Soups

Gingered Beet and Quinoa Soup

This extremely nutritious soup provides a very satisfying meatless meal but complements a main dish too.

Makes 6 servings

Tips

If you prefer a silken texture, you can purée the finished soup. Working in batches, transfer soup to a food processor or blender (or use an immersion blender in the pot) and purée until smooth. Return soup to pot (if necessary) and heat over low heat, uncovered, for 4 to 5 minutes or until warm.

Store the cooled soup in an airtight container in the refrigerator for up to 2 days or in the freezer for up to 6 months.

4 cups	diced peeled beets	1 L
6 cups	ready-to-use reduced-sodium vegetable or chicken broth, divided	1.5 L
1 tbsp	extra virgin olive oil	15 mL
2 cups	chopped onions	500 mL
1½ tbsp	ground ginger	22 mL
⅔ cup	quinoa, rinsed	150 mL
	Fine sea salt and freshly ground black pepper	
½ cup	plain Greek yogurt	125 mL
⅓ cup	packed fresh mint leaves, chopped	75 mL

1. In a microwave-safe bowl, combine beets and 2 cups (500 mL) of the broth. Cover loosely and microwave on High for 15 minutes or until beets are tender. Set aside.

2. Meanwhile, in a large pot, heat oil over medium-high heat. Add onions and cook, stirring, for 6 to 8 minutes or until softened. Add ginger and cook, stirring, for 30 seconds.

3. Stir in beet mixture, quinoa and the remaining broth; bring to a boil. Reduce heat to low, cover and simmer for 15 to 20 minutes or until quinoa is tender. Season to taste with salt and pepper. Serve dolloped with yogurt and sprinkled with mint.

> ▶ **Health Tip**
>
> Beets give us a great taste but also a health-promoting substance — pigments collectively called betalains that support detoxification in the body and may also reduce the chemical changes to the LDL particle (cholesterol) that can make it more reactive to the body.

Nutrients per serving	
Calories	188
Fat	4 g
Carbohydrate	33 g
Protein	7 g
Vitamin C	9 mg
Vitamin D	0 IU
Vitamin E	1 mg
Niacin	1 mg
Folate	137 mcg
Vitamin B_6	0.2 mg
Vitamin B_{12}	0.0 mcg
Zinc	1.1 mg
Selenium	3 mcg

Cream of Broccoli Soup

This flavorful soup derives protein and fats from cashews and offers a non-meat and non-dairy savory soup option.

Makes 6 servings

Variations

Add ⅛ tsp (0.5 mL) ground nutmeg or allspice or more to taste.

Refrigerate and serve soup chilled.

- **Food processor**

1 cup	raw cashews	250 mL
1 lb	broccoli	500 g
2 tsp	olive oil	10 mL
½	onion, chopped	½
5 cups	ready-to-use vegetable broth	1.25 L
1	russet (Idaho) potato, peeled and cut into 1-inch (2.5 cm) cubes	1
¼ tsp	freshly ground black pepper	1 mL
½ tsp	salt	2 mL

1. Place cashews in a bowl and add water to cover by 3 inches (7.5 cm). Cover bowl and let soak for at least 2 hours.

2. Cut broccoli into 2-inch (5 cm) florets. Peel stalk and cut in half lengthwise and then crosswise into 1-inch (2.5 cm) pieces. You should have about 8 cups (2 L) total. Set aside.

3. Place cashews and 2 tbsp (30 mL) of the soaking water into food processor and process to a semi-smooth paste. Leave in processor and set aside.

4. Place a large saucepan over medium heat and let pan get hot. Add oil and tip pan to coat. Add onion and cook, stirring occasionally, until softened, 3 to 4 minutes. Add vegetable broth and potato, increase heat to high and bring to a boil. Reduce heat and simmer until slightly softened, 5 to 6 minutes. Add broccoli and black pepper, increase heat to high and bring to a boil. Reduce heat and simmer until potato and broccoli are tender, 6 to 8 minutes.

5. Let cool slightly. Working in batches, ladle soup into food processor with cashews and blend until smooth. Return to pan. Stir in salt. Taste and adjust seasonings and heat over low heat, stirring often, until soup is heated through. Serve hot.

Nutrients per serving	
Calories	206
Fat	12 g
Carbohydrate	21 g
Protein	7 g
Vitamin C	73 mg
Vitamin D	0 IU
Vitamin E	1 mg
Niacin	1 mg
Folate	78 mcg
Vitamin B$_6$	0.3 mg
Vitamin B$_{12}$	0.0 mcg
Zinc	1.7 mg
Selenium	5 mcg

> ▶ **Health Tip**
>
> A class of plant compounds called glycosinolates helps give broccoli its powerful role in supporting detoxification and helping the body eliminate some toxins that can promote the aging processes in the brain.

Tomato Basil Soup

This is an easy-to-prepare version of a classic, ideal for busy cooks.

Tip

To keep basil fresh, like other fresh herbs (including parsley), wrap it in several layers of paper towel and place in a plastic bag; store in the warmest part of your fridge — in the butter keeper, for example, or the door.

- **Food processor**

2 tsp	olive oil	10 mL
$\frac{1}{2}$	onion, chopped	$\frac{1}{2}$
1	can (28 oz/796 mL) whole tomatoes, with juice	1
2 cups	ready-to-use vegetable broth	500 mL
2 cups	tomato marinara sauce	500 mL
$\frac{1}{2}$ tsp	salt	2 mL
$\frac{1}{2}$ tsp	freshly ground black pepper	2 mL
$\frac{1}{2}$ cup	packed fresh basil leaves, divided	125 mL
$\frac{1}{4}$ cup	toasted pine nuts	60 mL

1. Place a medium saucepan over medium heat and let pan get hot. Add oil and tip pan to coat. Add onion and cook, stirring occasionally, until softened but not browned, 3 to 4 minutes. Add tomatoes, vegetable broth, marinara sauce, salt and pepper. Reduce heat to low and simmer, stirring occasionally and breaking up tomatoes with the back of a spoon, about 10 minutes. Stir in $\frac{1}{4}$ cup (60 mL) of the basil. Let cool.

2. Transfer soup to food processor and blend until smooth, 20 to 30 seconds. Return soup to saucepan, taste and adjust seasonings. Turn heat to low and simmer until soup is hot throughout. Chiffonade remaining basil leaves. Serve soup hot, topped with a scattering of basil and a sprinkle of pine nuts.

> ▶ **Health Tip**
>
> Basil contains the brain-protective flavonoids orientin and vicenin, which are just some of the amazing compounds in this commonly used herb.

Nutrients per serving	
Calories	151
Fat	9 g
Carbohydrate	18 g
Protein	5 g
Vitamin C	29 mg
Vitamin D	0 IU
Vitamin E	4 mg
Niacin	3 mg
Folate	38 mcg
Vitamin B$_6$	0.4 mg
Vitamin B$_{12}$	0.0 mcg
Zinc	1.1 mg
Selenium	1 mcg

Minestrone

This rich minestrone provides a high level of protein and a wide variety of veggies and spices — a meal in itself.

Tip

A 19-oz (540 mL) can of beans will yield about 2 cups (500 mL) once the beans are drained and rinsed. If you have smaller or larger cans, you can use the volume called for or just add the amount from your can.

Variations

Substitute cooked beef for the chicken.

Add 1 cup (250 mL) cooked gluten-free pasta to the finished minestrone.

1 tbsp	grapeseed oil	15 mL
1	clove garlic, minced	1
1/2 cup	chopped onion	125 mL
1 tbsp	chopped fresh parsley	15 mL
1	potato (unpeeled), chopped	1
1	tomato, chopped	1
2 cups	rinsed drained canned romano beans	500 mL
1 cup	cubed cooked chicken	250 mL
1/2 cup	peas	125 mL
1/2 cup	broccoli florets	125 mL
1/2 cup	chopped celery	125 mL
1/4 cup	chopped dry-packed sun-dried tomatoes	60 mL
	Salt and freshly ground black pepper	

1. In a large saucepan, heat oil over medium heat. Sauté garlic, onion and parsley for 3 to 4 minutes or until onion is softened.

2. Stir in potato, chopped tomato, beans, chicken, peas, broccoli, celery, sun-dried tomatoes and 8 cups (2 L) water; bring to a boil over medium-high heat. Cover, leaving lid ajar, reduce heat to low and simmer, stirring occasionally, for 30 minutes or until vegetables are tender (or for up to $1\frac{1}{2}$ hours if you prefer a very soft texture). Season to taste with salt and pepper.

> ▶ **Health Tip**
>
> Broccoli is a good source of vitamin C and vitamin K.

Nutrients per 1 of 8 servings	
Calories	137
Fat	3 g
Carbohydrate	18 g
Protein	11 g
Vitamin C	16 mg
Vitamin D	1 IU
Vitamin E	1 mg
Niacin	3 mg
Folate	71 mcg
Vitamin B_6	0.3 mg
Vitamin B_{12}	0.1 mcg
Zinc	1.0 mg
Selenium	7 mcg

Moroccan Pumpkin Soup

Pumpkin is a wildly popular flavor these days, but almost always in conjunction with aromatic spices. This dish delivers on that count and more!

Tips

Any small, thick-skinned cooking pumpkin or a butternut squash will work in this recipe.

Pressed curry powder is available in cubes and can usually be found in gourmet or natural food stores.

- **Blender**

1 tsp	whole cumin seeds	5 mL
1 tsp	whole coriander seeds	5 mL
½ tsp	whole fennel seeds	2 mL
3 tbsp	olive oil, divided	45 mL
2	red onions, chopped	2
1 tbsp	blackstrap molasses	15 mL
1	leek, white and green parts, sliced	1
1 tbsp	organic cane sugar	15 mL
1	sweet or pie pumpkin (2 lbs/1 kg), peeled and cut into 1-inch (2.5 cm) cubes	1
2	apples, chopped	2
1 tbsp	curry powder or cube (see tip, at left)	15 mL
1 tsp	ground turmeric	5 mL
½ tsp	ground cinnamon	2 mL
4 cups	ready-to-use vegetable broth or water	1 L
1 cup	rice milk	250 mL
½ cup	cashews	125 mL

1. In a large saucepan, toast cumin, coriander and fennel seeds over high heat until the seeds begin to pop and their fragrance is released, about 2 minutes. Do not allow to smoke or burn. Add 2 tbsp (30 mL) of the oil to pan and heat. Stir in red onions. Reduce heat to medium and cook, stirring frequently, for 10 minutes or until onions are soft and caramelized. Transfer ¾ cup (175 mL) to a bowl and add molasses. Stir and set aside.

Nutrients per serving	
Calories	277
Fat	13 g
Carbohydrate	40 g
Protein	5 g
Vitamin C	22 mg
Vitamin D	17 IU
Vitamin E	3 mg
Niacin	2 mg
Folate	55 mcg
Vitamin B$_6$	0.3 mg
Vitamin B$_{12}$	0.3 mcg
Zinc	1.4 mg
Selenium	4 mcg

Leeks are grown in sand and are sometimes difficult to clean. A good method of cleaning is to vertically slice through the white and light green leaves, leaving most of the dark green leaves intact. Grasp the leek by the dark green leaves, fan out the bottom white and light green portions, exposing much of the inside of the leek, and run under cold water.

2. Add remaining oil to onions in pan and heat over high heat. Stir in leek. Reduce heat to medium and cook, stirring frequently, for 6 minutes or until soft. One at a time, add sugar, pumpkin, apples, curry powder, turmeric and cinnamon, stirring after each addition. Cook, stirring, for 1 minute. Add vegetable broth and bring to a gentle boil over high heat. Cover, reduce heat to medium-low and gently boil for 40 minutes or until vegetables are tender when pierced with the tip of a knife.

3. In blender, combine rice milk and cashews. Blend until smooth. Ladle 2 cups (500 mL) of the soup mixture into blender. Blend with nut mixture until smooth. Stir into soup and heat through. Ladle soup into bowls and float 2 tbsp (30 mL) of the reserved red onion on top of each.

> ▶ **Health Tip**
>
> Cumin, coriander and fennel are potent digestive tonics. Blackstrap molasses is a great source of iron, calcium, manganese and other nutrients.

Curry-Roasted Squash and Apple Soup

This spicy and warming soup tastes great and will stimulate your digestion with its array of active spices and flavors.

Tip

To peel butternut squash, cut it in half crosswise to create two flat surfaces. Place each half on its flat surface and use a sharp knife to remove the tough peel.

Variation

Replace squash with 2 large sweet potatoes, peeled and cut into ½-inch (1 cm) pieces.

Nutrients per serving	
Calories	161
Fat	7 g
Carbohydrate	25 g
Protein	2 g
Vitamin C	33 mg
Vitamin D	0 IU
Vitamin E	3 mg
Niacin	2 mg
Folate	43 mcg
Vitamin B₆	0.3 mg
Vitamin B₁₂	0.0 mcg
Zinc	0.3 mg
Selenium	1 mcg

- **Preheat oven to 450°F (230°C)**
- **Rimmed baking sheet, ungreased**
- **Immersion blender or upright blender**

2 tsp	salt	10 mL
1 tsp	ground coriander	5 mL
1 tsp	ground cumin	5 mL
½ tsp	ground turmeric	2 mL
¼ tsp	ground cinnamon	1 mL
¼ tsp	freshly ground black pepper	1 mL
¼ cup	vegetable oil	60 mL
2 tbsp	cider vinegar or white wine vinegar	30 mL
4	cloves garlic	4
2	tart apples, peeled and chopped	2
1	butternut squash, peeled and cut into ½-inch (1 cm) pieces (about 8 cups/2 L)	1
1	large onion, chopped	1
6 cups	water (approx.)	1.5 L
½ tsp	garam masala, divided	2 mL
	Salt and freshly ground black pepper	

1. In a small bowl, combine salt, coriander, cumin, turmeric, cinnamon, pepper, oil and vinegar.

2. On baking sheet, combine garlic, apples, squash and onion. Drizzle with spice mixture and toss to coat evenly. Roast in preheated oven, stirring twice, for about 45 minutes or until softened and golden brown.

3. Transfer roasted vegetables to a large pot. Add water and bring to a boil over medium-high heat. Reduce heat and simmer, stirring occasionally, until vegetables are very soft and liquid is reduced by about one-third, about 30 minutes. Remove from heat.

Tip

The soup can be made ahead, cooled, covered and refrigerated for up to 2 days or frozen for up to 2 months (thaw overnight in the refrigerator). Reheat over medium heat until steaming and season to taste before serving.

4. Using immersion blender in pot or transferring soup in batches to an upright blender, purée until very smooth. Return to pot, if necessary.

5. Reheat over medium heat until steaming, stirring often. Thin with a little water, if necessary, to desired consistency. Stir in half the garam masala and season to taste with salt and pepper. Ladle into warmed bowls and serve sprinkled with remaining garam masala.

> **▶ Health Tip**
>
> Coriander and cinnamon are promising agents for regulating blood sugar.

Roasted Butternut Squash Chowder with Sage Butter

This is a deeply flavored dish that contains white wine as well as garlic and onions, with a flavorful topping.

Makes 6 servings

Tip

You can use 1½ cups (375 mL) table (18%) cream instead of the half-and-half and whipping creams.

- **Preheat oven to 400°F (200°C)**
- **Rimmed baking sheet, lined with parchment paper**

1	butternut squash (3½ to 4 lbs/ 1.75 to 2 kg), halved lengthwise and seeded	1
¼ cup	olive oil, divided	60 mL
10	fresh sage leaves, thinly sliced	10
1	large onion, finely chopped	1
1	clove garlic, minced	1
1 cup	dry white wine	250 mL
2	large potatoes, peeled and cut into ½-inch (1 cm) dice	2
6 cups	ready-to-use vegetable or chicken broth (or a blend of the two)	1.5 L
1 tsp	salt	5 mL
1 tsp	freshly squeezed lemon juice	5 mL
Pinch	cayenne pepper	Pinch
Pinch	ground nutmeg	Pinch
	Freshly ground black pepper	
1 cup	half-and-half (10%) cream	250 mL
½ cup	heavy or whipping (35%) cream	125 mL
¼ cup	unsalted butter	60 mL
12	whole fresh sage leaves	12

1. Rub the cut side of one of the squash halves with 1 tbsp (15 mL) of the oil and place cut side down on prepared baking sheet. Roast in preheated oven until a knife pierces easily into the thick part of the neck, about 40 minutes. Let cool on pan.

2. Meanwhile, peel and cut the remaining squash half into ½-inch (1 cm) dice; set aside.

Tip

The taste of freshly grated nutmeg is so much better than the preground variety. Whole nutmeg can be found in the spice section of your supermarket or bulk food store. Use a rasp grater (such as a Microplane) to grate nutmeg.

3. In a large pot, heat the remaining oil over medium-high heat. Add sliced sage leaves and sauté until fragrant, about 1 minute. Add onion and sauté until softened, about 4 minutes. Add garlic and sauté until fragrant, about 1 minute. Add wine and cook until reduced by half, about 5 minutes. Add diced squash, potatoes, broth and salt; bring to a boil. Reduce heat and simmer until vegetables are tender, about 20 minutes.

4. Scoop roasted squash from its shell, mash it and add it to the soup. Season with lemon juice, cayenne, nutmeg and black pepper to taste. Stir in half-and-half cream and whipping cream; reheat over medium heat until steaming, stirring often. Taste and adjust seasoning with cayenne, nutmeg, salt and black pepper, if necessary.

5. In a skillet, melt butter over medium heat until sizzling. Add whole sage leaves and sauté until crispy and browned, about 2 minutes. Transfer sage to a plate lined with paper towels. Remove pan from heat.

6. Ladle chowder into heated bowls and top each with a drizzle of sage butter and 2 fried sage leaves.

> **▶ Health Tip**
>
> Sage has been found by researchers to be both a potent antioxidant and a memory booster.

Lentil Soup with Rice

If you can find them, use the small brown Italian lentils from Umbria or the dark green Puy lentils — they don't break up during cooking, and they will nicely absorb any aromatics cooked with them, yet retain their attractive shape. Health-food markets are good sources for a wide range of quality pulses, including organic varieties.

Makes 6 servings

1 tbsp	butter	15 mL
1 tbsp	olive oil	15 mL
2	cloves garlic, finely chopped	2
1	small onion, finely chopped	1
1	stalk celery, finely chopped	1
1	small carrot, finely chopped	1
4 oz	pancetta, finely chopped	125 g
2 tbsp	finely chopped fresh marjoram	30 mL
1½ cups	dried lentils, rinsed and drained	375 mL
1½ cups	canned tomatoes, with juice, finely chopped	375 mL
6 cups	ready-to-use beef broth	1.5 L
½ cup	Arborio rice	125 mL
	Salt and freshly ground black pepper	
½ cup	grated Parmigiano-Reggiano cheese	125 mL
2 tbsp	chopped celery leaves	30 mL

1. In a saucepan, melt butter with olive oil over medium heat. Add garlic, onion, celery, carrot, pancetta and marjoram; sauté for 5 minutes or until vegetables have softened.

2. Stir in lentils and tomatoes; cook for 3 minutes. Add broth and bring to a boil. Reduce heat to low, cover and simmer for 30 minutes or until lentils are almost tender.

3. Stir in rice, cover and simmer, stirring occasionally, for 20 minutes or until rice and lentils are tender. Season to taste with salt and pepper.

4. Serve sprinkled with Parmigiano-Reggiano and celery leaves.

> ▶ **Health Tip**
>
> Lentils are nutritionally loaded. Many people do not know that they contain folate.

Nutrients per serving	
Calories	395
Fat	10 g
Carbohydrate	53 g
Protein	27 g
Vitamin C	9 mg
Vitamin D	3 IU
Vitamin E	1 mg
Niacin	4 mg
Folate	158 mcg
Vitamin B$_6$	0.5 mg
Vitamin B$_{12}$	0.2 mcg
Zinc	3.0 mg
Selenium	11 mcg

Salmon Chowder

This hearty soup creates a fantastic stock from the salmon, broth, milk and herbs.

Tips

Hot-smoked salmon is smoked at a much higher temperature than cold-smoked salmon. This gives it a fuller, smokier flavor and a firmer texture.

If you can't find hot-smoked salmon, add hot pepper flakes to taste along with regular smoked salmon. You can also use smoked whitefish or trout.

▶ Health Tip

Salmon is a source of omega-3 fats in a form that the body can very readily use.

Nutrients per serving

Calories	172
Fat	3 g
Carbohydrate	26 g
Protein	12 g
Vitamin C	30 mg
Vitamin D	202 IU
Vitamin E	1 mg
Niacin	4 mg
Folate	44 mcg
Vitamin B$_6$	0.3 mg
Vitamin B$_{12}$	1.3 mcg
Zinc	0.9 mg
Selenium	11 mcg

- **Preheat barbecue grill or broiler**

1	small onion, cut into $1/4$-inch (0.5 cm) thick slices	1
1	potato, cut into $1/4$-inch (0.5 cm) thick slices	1
1	large carrot, cut lengthwise into $1/4$-inch (0.5 cm) thick slices	1
$1/4$	stalk celery	$1/4$
1	green bell pepper, quartered and seeded	1
2 cups	ready-to-use fish or chicken broth	500 mL
$1/2$ tsp	crumbled dried thyme	2 mL
$1/4$ tsp	crumbled dried basil	1 mL
2 cups	1% milk, divided	500 mL
$1/4$ cup	all-purpose flour	60 mL
4 oz	unsalted hot-smoked salmon or smoked whitefish	125 g
$3/4$ cup	frozen corn kernels	175 mL
Pinch	salt	Pinch
	Freshly ground black pepper	

1. Place onion, potato, carrot, celery and green pepper on barbecue or under broiler; cook, turning occasionally, until distinct grill marks are visible and pepper skin is blackened. Place vegetables in a plastic bag; seal and let stand for 20 minutes.

2. Peel skin off pepper; dice pepper. Dice remaining roasted vegetables and place in a large saucepan. Add 1 cup (250 mL) broth, thyme and basil; bring to a boil. Add remaining broth and $1\frac{1}{2}$ cups (375 mL) milk; bring just to a simmer. Stir flour with remaining milk until smooth; gradually stir into soup. Simmer over low heat for 5 minutes.

3. Remove skin and any bones from fish; cut into $1/4$-inch (0.5 cm) cubes. Add to soup along with corn; cook for 10 minutes. Season with salt, and pepper to taste. Serve hot.

This recipe courtesy of chef Dean Mitchell and dietitian Suzanne Journault-Hemstock.

Shrimp and Corn Bisque

You don't have to live by the sea or a fisherman's wharf to enjoy this soup, but do have fresh or frozen shrimp on hand — you'll still feel like you do when you taste this rich, nutritious dish.

Tip

Small amounts of cayenne and nutmeg add immeasurably to the flavor of soups without announcing their presence.

5 tbsp	unsalted butter, divided	75 mL
2	onions, finely chopped, divided	2
2	stalks celery, diced, divided	2
1	carrot, diced	1
2 lbs	medium shrimp, peeled, deveined and halved lengthwise, shells reserved	1 kg
1	clove garlic, minced	1
6	whole black peppercorns	6
1	bay leaf	1
½ tsp	dried thyme	2 mL
4	ears corn, kernels removed and reserved and cobs cut into quarters	4
8 cups	ready-to-use shellfish, chicken or vegetable broth	2 L
3 tbsp	all-purpose flour	45 mL
½ tsp	salt	2 mL
1 cup	heavy or whipping (35%) cream	250 mL
Pinch	ground nutmeg	Pinch
Pinch	cayenne pepper	Pinch
	Freshly ground black pepper	
3 tbsp	minced fresh chives	45 mL

1. In a large pot, melt 2 tbsp (30 mL) of the butter over medium heat. Add half the onions, half the celery and the carrot; sauté until softened, about 6 minutes. Add shrimp shells, garlic, peppercorns, bay leaf and thyme; sauté until shells turn pink and garlic is fragrant, about 4 minutes. Add corn cobs and broth; bring to a boil. Reduce heat and simmer for 30 minutes.

2. Meanwhile, in a saucepan, melt remaining butter over medium heat. Add remaining onion and celery; sauté until softened, about 6 minutes. Add flour and salt; sauté for 2 minutes. Gradually whisk in cream and cook, stirring, until slightly thickened, about 3 minutes. Remove from heat and set aside.

Nutrients per serving	
Calories	472
Fat	29 g
Carbohydrate	26 g
Protein	31 g
Vitamin C	8 mg
Vitamin D	21 IU
Vitamin E	3 mg
Niacin	9 mg
Folate	66 mcg
Vitamin B$_6$	0.4 mg
Vitamin B$_{12}$	2.1 mcg
Zinc	2.4 mg
Selenium	46 mcg

Is cutting onions
bringing you to tears?
Try placing them in the
freezer for 10 minutes
before chopping.

3. Strain the broth and discard all solids; return broth to the pot and bring to a simmer over medium heat. Add corn kernels and simmer until almost tender, about 5 minutes. Add shrimp and simmer until pink and opaque, about 2 minutes. Add cream mixture and bring to a simmer, stirring often. Stir in nutmeg and cayenne. Season with salt and black pepper to taste.

4. Ladle into heated bowls and garnish with chives.

▶ **Health Tip**

Use shrimp that are ocean-caught (wild) or organically (certified) farm-raised, as some farm-raised shrimp are from contaminated sources — often extremely toxic ponds that are laced with antibiotics.

Saffron Paella Soup

We often think of soup as a starter dish, but this is a meal of a soup. Paella is a traditional dish in Mediterranean cuisine, and this recipe brings out the best of that tradition.

Tip

Have the fishmonger tap each mussel individually to make sure it is alive, and check again just before cooking. Live mussels will close when tapped. Any mussels that do not open while cooking were dead before they were cooked and should be discarded.

¼ cup	olive oil, divided	60 mL
1	large onion, chopped, divided	1
1 lb	chicken thighs	500 g
3	cloves garlic, minced	3
8 cups	ready-to-use chicken broth, divided	2 L
1	can (14 oz/398 mL) diced tomatoes, with juice	1
½ cup	long-grain white rice	125 mL
¼ tsp	salt	1 mL
¼ tsp	saffron threads	1 mL
1	red bell pepper, diced	1
1 lb	smoked Spanish chorizo or andouille sausage, diced	500 g
12	mussels, scrubbed and debearded (see tips)	12
1 cup	frozen peas, thawed	250 mL
1 lb	large shrimp, peeled and deveined	500 g
¼ cup	minced fresh flat-leaf (Italian) parsley	60 mL
	Garlic-seasoned croutons	

1. In a large pot, heat 3 tbsp (45 mL) of the oil over medium-high heat. Add half the onion and sauté until starting to soften, about 2 minutes. Add chicken, skin side down, and cook until browned, about 4 minutes. (Be careful not to let the onion burn.) Turn chicken over and brown the other side. Add garlic and sauté for 2 minutes. Add 5 cups (1.25 L) of the broth and tomatoes; bring to a boil. Reduce heat and simmer until juices run clear when chicken is pierced, about 30 minutes. Remove from heat.

2. Using tongs, transfer chicken to a large plate and let cool slightly. Remove skin and bones and discard. Shred the meat into bite-size pieces and set aside. Set cooking liquid aside.

Nutrients per serving	
Calories	642
Fat	36 g
Carbohydrate	30 g
Protein	50 g
Vitamin C	44 mg
Vitamin D	5 IU
Vitamin E	4 mg
Niacin	15 mg
Folate	109 mcg
Vitamin B$_6$	0.7 mg
Vitamin B$_{12}$	6.7 mcg
Zinc	5.7 mg
Selenium	61 mcg

To scrub and debeard mussels, hold each mussel under cool running water and scrub the shell with a stiff-bristled brush. Next, grab the fibers of the "beard" with your fingers and pull them out, tugging toward the hinged point of the shell.

3. In a saucepan, bring the remaining broth to a simmer over medium heat. Add rice, salt and saffron; cover, reduce heat and simmer until rice is almost tender, about 15 minutes. Remove from heat and let stand, covered, until ready to use.

4. In another large pot, heat the remaining oil over medium heat. Add the remaining onion, red pepper and sausage; sauté until vegetables are softened, about 6 minutes. Add reserved cooking liquid and bring to a simmer. Add reserved chicken and rice, mussels and peas; return to a simmer. Cover, reduce heat to low and simmer gently for 5 minutes. Add shrimp, cover and simmer gently until mussels have opened and shrimp are pink and opaque, 2 to 3 minutes. Discard any mussels that do not open.

5. Ladle into heated bowls, making sure each bowl contains a few shrimp and 2 mussels. Garnish with parsley and croutons.

▶ Health Tip

This dish is a source of omega-3 fatty acids, which are essential for brain health. Because of toxin, parasite and antibiotic concerns, avoid farm-raised seafood unless it is truly organic and sustainable.

Stuffed Cabbage Soup

Stuffed cabbage rolls — or pigs in a blanket, as they call them in West Virginia — also make an excellent soup!

Tip

Napa cabbage is also sometimes called Chinese cabbage. The long leaves are easy to roll up, but if you're a purist, go ahead and use regular round cabbage leaves for these tasty meat-filled bundles.

1½ cups	water	375 mL
¾ cup	long-grain white rice	175 mL
1 tbsp	salt, divided	15 mL
3 tbsp	olive oil, divided	45 mL
3 cups	chopped onion, divided	750 mL
3	cloves garlic, minced, divided	3
8 oz	lean ground beef	250 g
8 oz	regular or lean ground pork	250 g
8 oz	lean ground veal	250 g
1	large egg	1
½ cup	chopped fresh parsley, divided	125 mL
2 tsp	paprika	10 mL
½ tsp	freshly ground black pepper	2 mL
8	large napa cabbage leaves	8
3 cups	chopped napa cabbage	750 mL
2	carrots, sliced	2
1	stalk celery, sliced	1
1	can (28 oz/796 mL) crushed tomatoes	1
1 cup	dry white wine	250 mL
8 cups	ready-to-use beef broth	2 L
1 tbsp	white wine vinegar	15 mL
1 tbsp	packed brown sugar	15 mL

1. In a small saucepan, bring water to a boil over medium heat. Add rice and a pinch of salt; cover, reduce heat to low and simmer gently until water is almost absorbed, about 15 minutes. Remove from heat and let stand until water is absorbed and rice is tender, 2 or 3 minutes. Uncover, fluff with a fork and let cool.

2. In a skillet, heat 1 tbsp (15 mL) oil over medium heat. Add 1 cup (250 mL) onion and one-third of the garlic; sauté until starting to soften, about 3 minutes. Transfer to a large bowl and add ¾ cup (175 mL) rice, beef, pork, veal, egg, half the parsley, paprika, 2 tsp (10 mL) salt and pepper. Use your hands to mix the filling together. Set aside.

Nutrients per serving	
Calories	376
Fat	11 g
Carbohydrate	38 g
Protein	28 g
Vitamin C	42 mg
Vitamin D	7 IU
Vitamin E	2 mg
Niacin	11 mg
Folate	114 mcg
Vitamin B$_6$	0.9 mg
Vitamin B$_{12}$	1.3 mcg
Zinc	4.1 mg
Selenium	26 mcg

3. Bring a large pot of salted water to a boil over medium heat. Add the whole cabbage leaves and cook until tender, 2 to 3 minutes. Drain and refresh under cold running water. Blot dry.

4. Place about $1/3$ cup (75 mL) of the filling in the center of each cabbage leaf and, starting at the thick end, fold the sides in and roll up the cabbage to enclose the filling.

5. In a large pot, heat the remaining oil over medium heat. Add the remaining onion and sauté until starting to soften, about 2 minutes. Add chopped cabbage, carrots, celery and the remaining garlic; sauté until vegetables are almost softened, about 5 minutes.

6. Add tomatoes and wine; bring to a boil. Cook until sauce has thickened, about 5 minutes. Add broth, vinegar, brown sugar and the remaining salt, bring to a boil. Carefully add cabbage rolls and bring back to a boil. Cover, reduce heat to low and simmer gently until cabbage rolls are cooked through, about 30 minutes. Add the remaining rice to thicken the soup, if desired. Taste and adjust seasoning with salt and pepper, if necessary.

7. Place cabbage rolls in heated bowls and top with soup. Garnish with the remaining parsley.

> ▶ **Health Tip**
>
> Cabbage is a natural source of the amino acid glutamine, which is a source of energy for the small intestine.

Navy Bean and Ham Soup

You'll return to this soup time and time again when you're looking for the simple flavors of ham and beans.

Tip

Here's how to quick-soak dried beans: In a colander, rinse beans under cold water and discard any discolored ones. In a saucepan, combine beans with enough cold water to cover them by 2 inches (5 cm). Bring to a boil over medium heat and boil for 2 minutes. Remove from heat and let soak, covered, for 1 hour.

8 cups	cold water	2 L
2 cups	dried navy beans, soaked overnight or quick-soaked (see tip, at left) and drained	500 mL
2	large smoked ham hocks (about 1¾ lbs/875 g total)	2
1	onion, coarsely chopped	1
1	carrot, coarsely chopped	1
1	clove garlic, coarsely chopped	1
2	sprigs fresh thyme	2
1	bay leaf	1
	Salt and freshly ground black pepper	
2 tbsp	chopped fresh parsley	30 mL

1. In a large pot, bring water, beans, ham hocks, onion, carrot, garlic, thyme and bay leaf to a boil over medium heat. Reduce heat and simmer until beans are tender, about 1½ hours.

2. Discard thyme sprigs and bay leaf.

3. Remove ham hocks from the soup and let cool slightly. Pick the meat from the bones and shred into bite-size pieces. Discard bones, fat and skin. Return meat to the soup and simmer until heated through. Season with salt and pepper to taste.

4. Ladle into heated bowls and garnish with parsley.

> ▶ **Health Tip**
>
> Navy beans pack some protein and are high in fiber.

Nutrients per 1 of 8 servings	
Calories	315
Fat	6 g
Carbohydrate	33 g
Protein	31 g
Vitamin C	5 mg
Vitamin D	0 IU
Vitamin E	0 mg
Niacin	6 mg
Folate	177 mcg
Vitamin B$_6$	0.7 mg
Vitamin B$_{12}$	0.7 mcg
Zinc	3.6 mg
Selenium	39 mcg

Salads

Everyday Salad

This salad is a quickly prepared standby that delivers more than a full serving of fresh vegetables for each person.

Tip

For the dried herbs, try dried Italian seasoning. You can also use basil or thyme, or a combination.

4 cups	packed baby spinach (about 6 oz/175 g)	1 L
½ cup	shredded red cabbage	125 mL
½ cup	sliced peeled cucumber	125 mL
½ cup	chopped yellow bell pepper	125 mL
¼ cup	chopped red bell pepper	60 mL
20	cherry tomatoes	20
2 tbsp	balsamic vinegar	30 mL
1½ tbsp	extra virgin olive oil	22 mL
1 tsp	dried herbs (see tip, at left)	5 mL
	Salt and freshly ground black pepper	

1. In a large bowl, combine spinach, cabbage, cucumber, yellow pepper, red pepper and tomatoes.

2. In a small bowl, whisk together vinegar, oil and herbs. Drizzle over salad and toss to coat. Season to taste with salt and pepper.

▶ **Health Tip**

The spinach and bell peppers deliver a host of carotenoids, which have major antioxidant roles to play in the body and are best consumed as a mixed carotenoid package, as they naturally occur in foods.

Nutrients per serving	
Calories	89
Fat	6 g
Carbohydrate	9 g
Protein	2 g
Vitamin C	63 mg
Vitamin D	0 IU
Vitamin E	2 mg
Niacin	1 mg
Folate	89 mcg
Vitamin B$_6$	0.2 mg
Vitamin B$_{12}$	0.0 mcg
Zinc	0.4 mg
Selenium	0 mcg

Spinach Salad with Oranges and Mushrooms

Toasted almonds and water chestnuts give this salad a crunch factor.

Makes 6 servings

Tips

Use 1½ cups (375 mL) canned drained mandarins to replace the orange.

Oyster mushrooms and other wild mushrooms are exceptionally tasty.

Prepare salad early in the day and keep it refrigerated. Prepare dressing up to 2 days ahead. Pour over salad just before serving.

Salad

8 cups	packed fresh spinach, washed, dried and torn into bite-sized pieces	2 L
1½ cups	sliced mushrooms	375 mL
¾ cup	sliced water chestnuts	175 mL
½ cup	sliced red onion	125 mL
¼ cup	raisins	60 mL
2 tbsp	sliced or chopped almonds, toasted	30 mL
1	orange, peeled and sections cut into pieces	1

Dressing

3 tbsp	olive oil	45 mL
3 tbsp	balsamic vinegar	45 mL
2 tbsp	orange juice concentrate, thawed	30 mL
1 tbsp	liquid honey	15 mL
1 tsp	grated orange zest	5 mL
1 tsp	minced garlic	5 mL

1. *Salad:* In a large serving bowl, combine spinach, mushrooms, water chestnuts, red onion, raisins, almonds and orange pieces; toss well.

2. *Dressing:* In small bowl, whisk together olive oil, balsamic vinegar, orange juice concentrate, honey, orange zest and garlic; pour over salad and toss.

▶ Health Tip

Although drying somewhat decreases the antioxidant powers of raisins versus the grapes they started out as, the beneficial molecules, including flavanols, are still present in valuable amounts.

Nutrients per serving	
Calories	163
Fat	8 g
Carbohydrate	22 g
Protein	3 g
Vitamin C	33 mg
Vitamin D	1 IU
Vitamin E	3 mg
Niacin	2 mg
Folate	107 mcg
Vitamin B_6	0.2 mg
Vitamin B_{12}	0.0 mcg
Zinc	0.5 mg
Selenium	1 mcg

Sweet Cinnamon Waldorf Salad

Nothing complements a special meal like a good Waldorf salad, and this recipe is a winner.

Makes 6 to 8 servings

Tips

For a nice change, use a combination of peas and apples to total 2½ cups (625 mL).

Prepare salad early in the day and refrigerate. Toss well just before serving. Keeps well for 2 days in tho rofrigorator.

Salad

2½ cups	diced apples	625 mL
¾ cup	diced celery	175 mL
1 cup	red or green seedless grapes, quartered	250 mL
1 cup	chopped red or green bell peppers	250 mL
⅓ cup	raisins	75 mL
½ cup	canned mandarin oranges, drained	125 mL
2 tbsp	finely chopped pecans	30 mL

Dressing

¼ cup	light mayonnaise	60 mL
¼ cup	light (1%) sour cream	60 mL
2 tbsp	liquid honey	30 mL
1 tbsp	freshly squeezed lemon juice	15 mL
½ tsp	ground cinnamon	2 mL

1. *Salad:* In a serving bowl, combine apples, celery, grapes, bell peppers, raisins, mandarin oranges and pecans.

2. *Dressing:* In small bowl, combine mayonnaise, sour cream, honey, lemon juice and cinnamon; mix thoroughly. Pour over salad and toss.

> ▶ **Health Tip**
>
> Pecans may have cholesterol-lowering effects and cinnamon has a blood-sugar-stabilizing effect.

Nutrients per 1 of 8 servings	
Calories	128
Fat	5 g
Carbohydrate	22 g
Protein	1 g
Vitamin C	33 mg
Vitamin D	1 IU
Vitamin E	1 mg
Niacin	0 mg
Folate	16 mcg
Vitamin B$_6$	0.1 mg
Vitamin B$_{12}$	0.0 mcg
Zinc	0.3 mg
Selenium	1 mcg

Green Bean, Pecan and Pomegranate Salad

This is a good departure from lettuce-based salad, which we love but can become repetitive. Pomegranate and green beans give this salad flavor and crunch — add the olives for a more Mediterranean take.

Makes 4 servings

Tip

Do not be tempted to cook the beans for more than 3 minutes, or they will soften too much.

Salad

1 lb	green beans, cut into 2-inch (5 cm) pieces	500 g
½ cup	diced red onion	125 mL
1 cup	whole pecans	250 mL
1 cup	pomegranate seeds	250 mL
¼ cup	chopped green olives (optional)	60 mL

Pomegranate Dressing

⅓ cup	olive oil	75 mL
3 tbsp	pomegranate molasses	45 mL
1 tbsp	chopped fresh parsley	15 mL

1. *Salad:* In a pot of boiling salted water, cook green beans for 3 minutes. Drain and rinse with cold water. Let cool to room temperature. In a bowl, combine green beans, red onion, pecans, pomegranate seeds and olives (if using).

2. *Dressing:* Meanwhile, in a jar with a tight-fitting lid, combine oil, molasses and parsley. Shake well to combine and drizzle over salad.

> ▶ **Health Tip**
>
> The concentrate of pomegranate juice in the molasses of the dressing packs a powerful dose of vascular-protective molecules.

Nutrients per serving	
Calories	451
Fat	37 g
Carbohydrate	32 g
Protein	5 g
Vitamin C	21 mg
Vitamin D	0 IU
Vitamin E	4 mg
Niacin	1 mg
Folate	64 mcg
Vitamin B$_6$	0.4 mg
Vitamin B$_{12}$	0.0 mcg
Zinc	1.6 mg
Selenium	5 mcg

Avocado Salad

This easy-to-prepare salad will satisfy the growing number of avocado fans and create some new ones.

Makes 2 servings

Tip

Hass avocados (sometimes called Haas avocados) are dark-skinned avocados with a nutty, buttery flesh and a longer shelf life than other varieties, making them the most popular avocado in North America. To determine whether a Hass avocado is ripe, look for purple-black skin and gently press the top — a ripe one will give slightly.

1 tbsp	freshly squeezed lime juice	15 mL
1	ripe avocado	1
1/4 cup	slivered red bell pepper	60 mL
1/4 cup	slivered red onion	60 mL
2 tbsp	vegetable oil	30 mL
	Salt and freshly ground black pepper	
	Few sprigs fresh coriander, chopped	
	Pico de gallo	
	Corn chips	

1. Put lime juice in a small bowl. Peel avocado and cut into slices (or scoop out with a small spoon) and add to the lime juice. Toss gently until well coated. Add red pepper and onion; drizzle with oil. Toss gently until all ingredients are thoroughly combined. Season to taste with salt and pepper.

2. Transfer salad to a serving plate and spread out attractively. Garnish with chopped coriander and serve within 1 hour, accompanied by pico de gallo and corn chips.

> ▶ **Health Tip**
>
> Not only are the oils and fats in avocado nutritious in their own right, they enhance absorption of other nutrients, such as the carotenoids from bell peppers.

Nutrients per serving	
Calories	298
Fat	29 g
Carbohydrate	12 g
Protein	2 g
Vitamin C	37 mg
Vitamin D	0 IU
Vitamin E	5 mg
Niacin	2 mg
Folate	93 mcg
Vitamin B$_6$	0.3 mg
Vitamin B$_{12}$	0.0 mcg
Zinc	0.7 mg
Selenium	1 mcg

Roasted Beet and Beet Greens Salad

For beet lovers, this dish has the sour factor from vinegar but adds the sweetness and tanginess of orange, along with ample garlic.

Makes 4 servings

Tip

Any type of beet (red, golden or red-and-white-striped Chioggia) is great in this salad. To avoid stained hands, wear plastic gloves when peeling dark-colored beets.

- **Preheat oven to 400°F (200°C)**
- **Large rimmed baking sheet**

4	beets, with greens attached (about 1½ lbs/750 g)	4
2	oranges	2
2	cloves garlic, minced	2
½ cup	thinly sliced red onion	125 mL
½ tsp	fine sea salt	2 mL
2 tbsp	extra virgin olive oil	30 mL
1 tbsp	red wine vinegar	15 mL

1. Trim greens from beets. Cut off and discard stems, then coarsely chop leaves. Set beet greens aside.

2. Tightly wrap each beet in foil and place on baking sheet. Roast in preheated oven for about 90 minutes or until tender when pierced with a fork. Let cool completely in foil on baking sheet.

3. Meanwhile, in a large saucepan of boiling water, cook beet greens for 2 to 3 minutes or until tender. Drain, then let cool completely.

4. Peel beets and cut each into 8 wedges. Place beets in a medium bowl.

5. Squeeze beet greens to remove any excess water, then add to beets.

6. Grate 1 tsp (5 mL) zest from oranges. Add to beet mixture, along with garlic, red onion, salt, oil and vinegar.

7. Using a sharp knife, cut peel and pith from oranges. Working over the beet mixture, cut between membranes to release segments. Squeeze the membranes to release any remaining juice. Gently toss to coat. Let stand for at least 30 minutes or overnight to blend the flavors.

Nutrients per serving	
Calories	115
Fat	7 g
Carbohydrate	13 g
Protein	2 g
Vitamin C	50 mg
Vitamin D	0 IU
Vitamin E	1 mg
Niacin	0 mg
Folate	8 mcg
Vitamin B_6	0.1 mg
Vitamin B_{12}	0.0 mcg
Zinc	0.2 mg
Selenium	1 mcg

▶ **Health Tip**

Beet greens contain lutein, a great protector of blood vessels and the retina, and beet roots are a liver-friendly food.

Insalata Caprese

This is a salad favorite, and this version definitely qualifies as "Mediterranean diet" with the addition of kalamata olives.

Tip

Bocconcini are fresh, golf-ball-sized mozzarella curds that must be kept in water until they are needed. They are widely available. In supermarkets, they usually sit in plastic tubs right by the ricotta and other Italian dairy products.

1 lb	ripe tomatoes, sliced ½ inch (1 cm) thick (about 4 tomatoes)	500 g
¼ cup	thinly sliced red onion	60 mL
¼ cup	thinly sliced green bell pepper	60 mL
¼ cup	extra virgin olive oil	60 mL
2 tbsp	balsamic vinegar	30 mL
	Salt and freshly ground black pepper	
6 oz	bocconcini (see tip, at left)	175 g
¼ cup	kalamata olives (about 8)	60 mL
12	large fresh basil leaves	12

1. On a large presentation plate, arrange tomato slices in one layer. Scatter sliced onion and green pepper evenly over the tomatoes.

2. In a small bowl, whisk together oil, vinegar, salt and pepper until emulsified. Pour dressing evenly over the tomatoes.

3. Drain and pat dry the bocconcini. Slice into rounds ¼ inch (0.5 cm) thick. Put at least one slice of cheese on top of each tomato slice.

4. Place olives decoratively among the tomatoes. Garnish with the basil leaves, and serve within 30 minutes.

▸ **Health Tip**

Olives pack a remarkable array of beneficial phytonutrients and may be part of the reason why the Mediterranean diet is consistently proving itself beneficial.

Nutrients per serving	
Calories	282
Fat	22 g
Carbohydrate	9 g
Protein	13 g
Vitamin C	24 mg
Vitamin D	6 IU
Vitamin E	3 mg
Niacin	1 mg
Folate	26 mcg
Vitamin B$_6$	0.2 mg
Vitamin B$_{12}$	0.4 mcg
Zinc	1.6 mg
Selenium	7 mcg

Broccoli Carrot Slaw with Cranberries and Sunflower Seeds

This dish is a great way to get the health benefits of broccoli, sweetened and brightened by the other ingredients in this upbeat salad.

Makes 6 servings

Tip

Agave nectar (a.k.a. agave syrup) is a plant-based sweetener derived from the agave cactus, native to Mexico. Agave juice produces a light golden syrup.

¼ cup	nonfat plain Greek yogurt	60 mL
2 tbsp	freshly squeezed lemon juice	30 mL
1 tbsp	agave nectar or liquid honey	15 mL
2 tsp	Dijon mustard	10 mL
⅛ tsp	fine sea salt	0.5 mL
3 cups	shredded peeled broccoli stems (from 1 large bunch)	750 mL
2 cups	shredded peeled carrots	500 mL
½ cup	chopped green onions	125 mL
⅓ cup	dried cranberries, chopped	75 mL
¼ cup	lightly salted roasted sunflower seeds	60 mL

1. In a small bowl, whisk together yogurt, lemon juice, agave nectar, mustard and salt.

2. In a large bowl, combine broccoli, carrots, green onions and cranberries. Add dressing and gently toss to coat. Cover and refrigerate for at least 30 minutes, until chilled, or for up to 2 hours. Just before serving, sprinkle with sunflower seeds.

> ▶ **Health Tip**
>
> Broccoli contains compounds that switch on the body's anti-cancer and detoxification molecules.

Nutrients per serving	
Calories	105
Fat	3 g
Carbohydrate	18 g
Protein	3 g
Vitamin C	36 mg
Vitamin D	0 IU
Vitamin E	2 mg
Niacin	1 mg
Folate	71 mcg
Vitamin B$_6$	0.2 mg
Vitamin B$_{12}$	0.0 mcg
Zinc	0.6 mg
Selenium	5 mcg

Cranberry Mandarin Coleslaw with Walnuts and Raisins

This is no ordinary coleslaw — it has plenty of sweetness and lots of crunch, and a checklist of healthy ingredients.

Makes 8 to 10 servings

Tip

Pepitas are pumpkin seeds with the white hull removed, leaving the flat, dark green inner seed. They are subtly sweet and nutty, with a slightly chewy texture.

3 cups	shredded red and/or green cabbage	750 mL
2 cups	shredded carrots	500 mL
1 cup	chopped celery	250 mL
1/2 cup	chopped green onions	125 mL
1 tbsp	freshly squeezed lemon juice	15 mL
1/2 cup	raisins	125 mL
1/2 cup	raw green pumpkin seeds (pepitas)	125 mL
1/2 cup	fresh cranberries	125 mL
1/2 cup	walnut halves	125 mL
6 tbsp	extra virgin olive oil	90 mL
1/4 cup	brown or natural rice vinegar	60 mL
1	can (10 oz/284 mL) mandarin oranges, drained	1

1. In a large bowl, combine cabbage, carrots, celery and green onions. Drizzle with lemon juice and toss to coat. Toss in raisins, pumpkin seeds, cranberries and walnuts.

2. In a small bowl, whisk together oil and vinegar. Drizzle over salad and toss to coat. Top with mandarin oranges. Cover and refrigerate overnight to blend the flavors.

▶ **Health Tip**

Just 1/4 cup (60 mL) walnuts has nearly all of the recommended daily amount of brain-nourishing omega-3 fats.

Nutrients per 1 of 10 servings	
Calories	199
Fat	15 g
Carbohydrate	16 g
Protein	4 g
Vitamin C	22 mg
Vitamin D	0 IU
Vitamin E	1 mg
Niacin	1 mg
Folate	30 mcg
Vitamin B_6	0.1 mg
Vitamin B_{12}	0.0 mcg
Zinc	0.9 mg
Selenium	1 mcg

Grilled Mediterranean Vegetable and Lentil Salad

Using the grill keeps the kitchen cool in the summertime, but the vegetables may be roasted in the oven (see tip, below).

Makes 4 to 6 servings

Tip

To roast vegetables in the oven, place on a lightly oiled rimmed baking sheet and roast in a 400°F (200°C) oven for 30 minutes or until soft.

▶ Health Tip

This is a great way to get at least one of the several servings of vegetables we ought to incorporate into our diet daily.

Nutrients per 1 of 6 servings	
Calories	205
Fat	14 g
Carbohydrate	17 g
Protein	5 g
Vitamin C	37 mg
Vitamin D	0 IU
Vitamin E	3 mg
Niacin	2 mg
Folate	105 mcg
Vitamin B$_6$	0.3 mg
Vitamin B$_{12}$	0.0 mcg
Zinc	0.8 mg
Selenium	2 mcg

- **Preheat barbecue grill to high**
- **2 grilling baskets, lightly oiled**

Grilled Vegetables

1	red bell pepper, cut in half	1
2	small zucchini	2
2 tbsp	olive oil, divided	30 mL
1	eggplant, cut into ½-inch (1 cm) rounds	1

Dressing

¼ cup	olive oil	60 mL
1 tbsp	freshly squeezed lemon juice	15 mL
1 tbsp	balsamic vinegar	15 mL
1 tbsp	tamari or soy sauce	15 mL
1	clove garlic, minced	1
1 tbsp	chopped fresh oregano	15 mL
1 tbsp	chopped fresh mint or tarragon	15 mL

Salad

½	red onion, thinly sliced	½
½	cucumber, diced	½
1 cup	cooked lentils or black-eyed peas, drained and rinsed	250 mL
	Sea salt and freshly ground pepper	

1. *Grilled Vegetables:* Arrange red pepper halves and zucchini in a prepared grilling basket. Brush with 1 tbsp (15 mL) oil and grill for 8 to 10 minutes or until tender when pierced with the tip of a knife. Arrange eggplant in the remaining basket and brush with the remaining oil. Grill for 3 to 4 minutes or until tender. Let vegetables cool enough to handle. Peel and slice red pepper and cut zucchini and eggplant into chunks.

2. *Dressing:* Meanwhile, in a large bowl, whisk together oil, lemon juice, vinegar, tamari, garlic, oregano and mint.

3. *Salad:* Add red onion, cucumber and lentils to dressing. Add grilled vegetables and stir to combine well. Taste and season with salt and pepper, if required.

Greek-Style Potato Salad

Roasted fingerling potatoes combine with all the ingredients of a classic Greek salad to make one memorable dish.

Makes 4 servings

Tip

Either whole olives with pits or pitted olives are fine in this recipe.

- **Preheat oven to 375°F (190°C)**
- **Shallow 11- by 7-inch (2 L) baking dish**

Roasted Vegetables

1½ lbs	fingerling potatoes, scrubbed	750 g
6	cloves garlic (unpeeled)	6
1 tbsp	dried oregano, divided	15 mL
¼ cup	olive oil	60 mL
	Salt and freshly ground black pepper	

Vinaigrette

¼ cup	white wine vinegar	60 mL
1 tbsp	liquid honey	15 mL
1 tbsp	dried oregano	15 mL
½ tsp	salt	2 mL
Pinch	hot pepper flakes	Pinch
¾ cup	extra virgin olive oil	175 mL

Salad

1	red onion, thinly sliced	1
1	small seedless cucumber, peeled, halved and sliced into bite-size chunks	1
1 cup	kalamata olives (see tip, at left)	250 mL
8 oz	grape or cherry tomatoes	250 g
8	hearts of romaine lettuce	8
⅓ cup	chopped fresh flat-leaf (Italian) parsley leaves	75 mL
8 oz	feta cheese, broken into chunks	250 g

1. *Roasted Vegetables:* In baking dish, toss together potatoes, garlic, oregano and olive oil to coat. Season to taste with salt and freshly ground pepper. Roast in preheated oven for 30 minutes or until potatoes are tender. Remove from oven and set aside until garlic is cool enough to handle.

Variation

You can also grill the fingerlings: parboil for about 10 minutes, toss in olive oil and place on preheated grill, turning once or twice, until golden brown and cooked through, about 8 minutes. The garlic cloves can be threaded onto a soaked wooden skewer, drizzled with a bit of olive oil and grilled alongside the potatoes for the same length of time, until browned and tender.

2. *Vinaigrette:* Squeeze garlic cloves out of their skins, transfer to a bowl and, using a fork, mash into a paste. Whisk in vinegar, honey, oregano, salt, and hot pepper flakes. Whisk in oil. Taste and add vinegar or seasoning to taste, then whisk again.

3. *Salad:* In a large bowl, gently toss potatoes, onion, cucumber, olives and tomatoes. Drizzle with three-quarters of the vinaigrette and toss.

4. Slice each heart of romaine in half vertically. Place, cut side up, on a large platter. Arrange potato mixture evenly over lettuce. Sprinkle with parsley, then feta. Drizzle with the remaining vinaigrette.

> ### ▶ Health Tip
> Oregano provides a high amount of antioxidant activity.

Tabbouleh

This is one of the healthiest salads around, and a great example of how flavor can meet nutritional value.

Tips

If you prefer a sweeter taste, add 2 tbsp (30 mL) more oil.

Leftover tabbouleh can be kept in the refrigerator, covered, for up to 3 days. Be sure to bring it back up to room temperature before serving.

2 cups	packed chopped fresh parsley	500 mL
1	onion, finely chopped	1
1	tomato, finely chopped	1
1/2 cup	bulgur (about 4 oz/125 g)	125 mL
6 tbsp	freshly squeezed lemon juice	90 mL
1/4 cup	olive oil	60 mL
	Salt and freshly ground black pepper	

1. In a bowl, combine parsley, onion and tomato. Mix well. Set aside.

2. In a saucepan, boil bulgur wheat in plenty of water for 6 to 8 minutes, until tender. Drain and refresh with cold water. Drain again completely and add cooked bulgur to the vegetables in the bowl. Mix well.

3. Sprinkle lemon juice and olive oil over the salad. Add salt and pepper to taste. Toss to mix thoroughly. Transfer to a serving plate. The salad can be served immediately, although it'll be better if it waits up to 2 hours, covered and unrefrigerated.

> ▶ **Health Tip**
>
> Parsley contains compounds that have a natural diuretic effect on the body, and it is a fantastic source of vitamin K.

Nutrients per serving	
Calories	139
Fat	9 g
Carbohydrate	13 g
Protein	2 g
Vitamin C	37 mg
Vitamin D	0 IU
Vitamin E	2 mg
Niacin	1 mg
Folate	42 mcg
Vitamin B_6	0.1 mg
Vitamin B_{12}	0.0 mcg
Zinc	0.5 mg
Selenium	0 mcg

Couscous Salad with Basil and Pine Nuts

This couscous recipe packs in vegetables and the flavor of orange zest, as well as garlic.

Tips

Tender basil leaves bruise easily when chopped. Stack the leaves one on top of the other, roll up into a cigar shape and, using a sharp knife, cut into fine, thin shreds.

If you can't find fresh basil, substitute 1/4 cup (60 mL) chopped fresh parsley and 1 tsp (5 mL) dried basil.

1 cup	couscous	250 mL
1 cup	ready-to-use low-sodium chicken or vegetable broth	250 mL
4	green onions, chopped	4
1	red bell pepper, finely chopped	1
1	zucchini, diced	1
1/4 cup	raisins	60 mL
1/4 cup	olive oil	60 mL
2 tbsp	red wine vinegar	30 mL
1 tsp	grated orange zest	5 mL
2 tbsp	freshly squeezed orange juice	30 mL
1	large garlic clove, minced	1
1/2 tsp	salt (optional)	2 mL
	Freshly ground black pepper	
1/4 cup	chopped fresh basil (see tip, at left)	60 mL
1/4 cup	toasted pine nuts	60 mL

1. Place couscous in a large bowl; pour broth over. Cover with a dinner plate and let stand for 5 minutes. Fluff with a fork to break up any lumps. Let cool to room temperature. Add green onions, red pepper, zucchini and raisins.

2. In a small bowl, whisk together oil, vinegar, orange zest, orange juice, garlic, salt (if using) and pepper to taste. Pour over salad; toss well. Just before serving, stir in basil and pine nuts. Serve salad at room temperature.

> ▶ **Health Tip**
>
> Pine nuts contain pinolenic acid, which may work to curb appetite.

Nutrients per serving	
Calories	394
Fat	20 g
Carbohydrate	46 g
Protein	9 g
Vitamin C	46 mg
Vitamin D	0 IU
Vitamin E	3 mg
Niacin	3 mg
Folate	34 mcg
Vitamin B_6	0.2 mg
Vitamin B_{12}	0.1 mcg
Zinc	1.2 mg
Selenium	0 mcg

Quinoa Salad

The versatile supergrain appears once again, this time as a side salad with a full complement of vegetables and herbs.

Tip

To keep quinoa as fresh as possible, store it in an airtight container in the refrigerator for up to 6 months or in the freezer for up to 1 year.

Variation

If you're making this salad for non-vegetarians, you can substitute reduced-sodium chicken or turkey broth for the vegetable broth.

1¼ cups	ready-to-use reduced-sodium vegetable broth	300 mL
¾ cup	quinoa, rinsed	175 mL
½ cup	thawed frozen peas	125 mL
¼ cup	finely chopped orange bell pepper	60 mL
¼ cup	finely chopped yellow bell pepper	60 mL
1 tbsp	finely chopped red onion	15 mL
2 tbsp	extra virgin olive oil	30 mL
1 tbsp	chopped fresh parsley	15 mL
1 tsp	dried thyme	5 mL
1 tsp	freshly squeezed lemon juice	5 mL
	Salt and freshly ground black pepper	

1. In a saucepan, bring broth to a boil over high heat. Add quinoa, reduce heat to low, cover and simmer for 20 minutes or until quinoa is tender and liquid is almost absorbed. Remove from heat and let stand, covered, for 5 minutes or until liquid is absorbed.

2. In a large bowl, combine quinoa, peas, orange pepper, yellow pepper and red onion.

3. In a small bowl, whisk together oil, parsley, thyme and lemon juice. Drizzle over salad and toss to coat. Season to taste with salt and pepper. Serve warm or cover and refrigerate for 1 hour, until chilled, and serve cold.

▶ **Health Tip**

Quinoa, unlike many other grains, can be considered a complete protein.

Nutrients per serving	
Calories	201
Fat	9 g
Carbohydrate	25 g
Protein	6 g
Vitamin C	29 mg
Vitamin D	0 IU
Vitamin E	2 mg
Niacin	1 mg
Folate	79 mcg
Vitamin B_6	0.2 mg
Vitamin B_{12}	0.0 mcg
Zinc	1.2 mg
Selenium	3 mcg

Meatless Mains

Jerusalem Artichoke Stew

This vegetarian stew draws on vegetable broth and wine to create a basic stock and then adds a variety of vegetables.

Tips

When Jerusalem artichokes are not available, use potatoes instead.

You can use 2 cups (500 mL) cooked white beans, drained and rinsed, instead of canned.

1 tbsp	olive oil	15 mL
1	onion, chopped	1
2	stalks celery, chopped	2
2	cloves garlic, finely chopped	2
4 cups	ready-to-use vegetable broth or water	1 L
2 cups	diced Jerusalem artichokes or potatoes	500 mL
1	carrot, diced	1
½ cup	shredded rutabaga or green cabbage	125 mL
¼ cup	dry white wine	60 mL
1	can (14 to 19 oz/398 to 540 mL) cannellini beans or flageolets, drained and rinsed	1
3 tbsp	chopped fresh parsley	45 mL
2 tbsp	freshly squeezed lemon juice	30 mL
	Sea salt and freshly ground pepper	

1. In a large saucepan, heat oil over medium heat. Add onion and celery and cook, stirring occasionally, for 6 to 8 minutes or until soft. Add garlic and cook, stirring frequently, for 2 minutes. Add broth. Increase heat to high and bring to a boil. Add Jerusalem artichokes, carrot, rutabaga and white wine. Cover, reduce heat to medium-low and simmer, stirring once or twice, for 15 minutes or until vegetables are tender when pierced with the tip of a knife.

2. Add beans, parsley and lemon juice and heat through. Season to taste with salt and pepper. Using a potato masher, mash some of the vegetables to thicken the stew.

> ▶ **Health Tip**
>
> Jerusalem artichokes are a good source of minerals, supplying magnesium, potassium and iron — all important for the nervous system and transportation of oxygen to the nervous system.

Nutrients per serving	
Calories	146
Fat	3 g
Carbohydrate	25 g
Protein	5 g
Vitamin C	12 mg
Vitamin D	0 IU
Vitamin E	1 mg
Niacin	1 mg
Folate	46 mcg
Vitamin B_6	0.2 mg
Vitamin B_{12}	0.0 mcg
Zinc	0.5 mg
Selenium	1 mcg

Braised Beets with Roquefort Gratin

This dish features a combination of sweet beets, robust mushrooms and in-your-face Roquefort cheese. If you prefer more timid cheeses, make this using soft goat cheese. Serve with brown rice for a complete meal.

Makes 4 to 6 servings

Tips

If you prefer, transfer beet mixture to an ovenproof serving dish before adding the bread-crumb mixture.

To make ahead, complete steps 1 and 2. Cover and refrigerate for up to 2 days. When you're ready to cook, complete the recipe.

- **Medium (about 4-quart) slow cooker**

1	package (½ oz/14 g) dried mushrooms, such as porcini	1
2 cups	hot water	500 mL
2 tbsp	vegetable oil	30 mL
1 cup	chopped shallots	250 mL
4	cloves garlic, minced	4
2 tsp	dried tarragon	10 mL
1 tsp	salt	5 mL
½ tsp	cracked black peppercorns	2 mL
4	large beets, peeled and thinly sliced (about 2 lbs/1 kg)	4
1 cup	fresh bread crumbs	250 mL
½ cup	crumbled Roquefort or soft goat cheese	125 mL
1 tbsp	melted butter	15 mL

1. In a bowl, combine dried mushrooms and hot water. Let stand for 30 minutes. Strain through a fine sieve, reserving liquid. Remove stems. Pat mushrooms dry and chop finely. Set mushrooms and liquid aside separately.

2. In a skillet, heat oil over medium heat. Add shallots and cook, stirring, until softened, about 3 minutes. Add garlic, tarragon, salt, peppercorns and reserved mushrooms; cook, stirring, for 1 minute. Stir in reserved mushroom-soaking liquid. Transfer to slow cooker stoneware.

3. Stir in beets. Cover and cook on Low for 6 hours or on High for 3 hours, until beets are tender.

4. Preheat broiler. In a bowl, combine bread crumbs and cheese. Stir well. Spread evenly over beets and drizzle with melted butter. Broil until crumbs begin to brown and cheese melts. Serve immediately.

> ▶ **Health Tip**
>
> Beets are a great source of folate.

Nutrients per 1 of 6 servings	
Calories	252
Fat	14 g
Carbohydrate	26 g
Protein	8 g
Vitamin C	6 mg
Vitamin D	1 IU
Vitamin E	1 mg
Niacin	2 mg
Folate	99 mcg
Vitamin B$_6$	0.2 mg
Vitamin B$_{12}$	0.2 mcg
Zinc	1.0 mg
Selenium	9 mcg

Louisiana Ratatouille

Eggplant, tomato and okra stew is a classic Southern dish that probably owes its origins to the famous Mediterranean mélange ratatouille.

Makes 6 servings

Tips

Choose young okra pods, 2 to 4 inches (5 to 10 cm) long, that don't feel sticky to the touch. Gently scrub the pods and cut off the top and tail.

To sweat eggplant: Place cubed eggplant in a colander, sprinkle liberally with salt, toss well and set aside for 30 to 60 minutes. Rinse thoroughly in fresh cold water and, using your hands, squeeze out excess moisture. Pat dry with paper towels.

- **Medium (about 4-quart) slow cooker**

2	eggplants, peeled, cut into 2-inch (5 cm) cubes, sweated and drained of excess moisture (see tip, at left)	2
2 tbsp	vegetable oil	30 mL
2	onions, finely chopped	2
4	cloves garlic, minced	4
1 tsp	dried oregano	5 mL
1 tsp	salt	5 mL
½ tsp	cracked black peppercorns	2 mL
1	can (28 oz/796 mL) tomatoes, with juice, coarsely chopped	1
2 tbsp	red wine vinegar	30 mL
1 lb	okra, trimmed and cut into 1-inch (2.5 cm) lengths (about 2 cups/500 mL)	500 g
1	green bell pepper, cut into ¼-inch (0.5 cm) pieces	1

1. In a skillet, heat oil over medium-high heat. Add eggplant, in batches, and cook, stirring, until lightly browned. Transfer to slow cooker stoneware.

2. Reduce heat to medium. Add onions to pan and cook, stirring, until softened, about 3 minutes. Add garlic, oregano, salt and peppercorns and cook, stirring, for 1 minute. Stir in tomatoes, with juice, and red wine vinegar and bring to a boil. Transfer to slow cooker stoneware.

3. Cover and cook on Low for 6 hours or on High for 3 hours, until hot and bubbly. Add okra and bell pepper. Cover and cook on High for 30 minutes, until okra is tender.

> ▶ **Health Tip**
>
> This recipe is a great way to pack nutritious vegetables into a flavorful dish.

Nutrients per serving	
Calories	152
Fat	5 g
Carbohydrate	24 g
Protein	5 g
Vitamin C	49 mg
Vitamin D	0 IU
Vitamin E	2 mg
Niacin	2 mg
Folate	110 mcg
Vitamin B$_6$	0.4 mg
Vitamin B$_{12}$	0.0 mcg
Zinc	0.8 mg
Selenium	2 mcg

Broccoli and Quinoa Enchiladas

This high-protein dish is meatless but not short on taste.

Tip

To keep quinoa as fresh as possible, store it in an airtight container in the refrigerator for up to 6 months or in the freezer for up to 1 year.

- **Preheat oven to 350°F (180°C)**
- **8- or 9-inch (20 or 23 cm) square glass baking dish or metal baking pan, sprayed with nonstick cooking spray**

2 tsp	olive oil	10 mL
1¼ cups	chopped onions	300 mL
2 cups	finely chopped broccoli florets	500 mL
1 tsp	ground cumin	5 mL
1½ cups	picante sauce, divided	375 mL
1½ cups	cooked quinoa, cooled	375 mL
1 cup	cottage or ricotta cheese	250 mL
1 cup	shredded sharp (old) white Cheddar cheese, divided	250 mL
8	8-inch (20 cm) multigrain tortillas, warmed	8

1. In a large skillet, heat oil over medium heat. Add onions and cook, stirring, for 6 to 8 minutes or until softened. Add broccoli, cumin and ⅓ cup (75 mL) of the picante sauce; cook, stirring, for 1 minute. Remove from heat and stir in quinoa, cottage cheese and ⅓ cup (75 mL) of the Cheddar.

2. Spoon about ⅓ cup (75 mL) of the quinoa mixture along the center of each warmed tortilla. Roll up like a cigar and place, seam side down, in prepared baking dish. Spoon the remaining picante sauce over top.

3. Cover and bake in preheated oven for 20 to 25 minutes or until heated through. Sprinkle with the remaining Cheddar. Bake, uncovered, for 5 minutes or until cheese is bubbling.

> ▶ **Health Tip**
>
> With a history dating back thousands of years, cumin has some potent antioxidant molecules and has been used for digestive ailments.

Nutrients per serving	
Calories	268
Fat	7 g
Carbohydrate	38 g
Protein	13 g
Vitamin C	18 mg
Vitamin D	1 IU
Vitamin E	1 mg
Niacin	2 mg
Folate	85 mcg
Vitamin B$_6$	0.2 mg
Vitamin B$_{12}$	0.3 mcg
Zinc	1.1 mg
Selenium	16 mcg

Three-Pepper Tamale Pie

This satisfying, chile-spiced dish provides a break from animal sources of protein.

Tip

Vegan hard margarine, such as Earth Balance Vegan Buttery Flavor Sticks, has almost half as much saturated fat as regular butter and no cholesterol. Where butter is called for in a recipe, vegan hard margarine can be a heart-healthy, delicious alternative.

- **8-cup (2 L) glass baking dish, lightly oiled**

2 tbsp	olive oil	30 mL
1	onion, chopped	1
1	red bell pepper, chopped	1
2	cloves garlic, minced	2
1½ cups	drained cooked pinto beans	375 mL
1 cup	drained cooked kidney beans	250 mL
1 cup	frozen roasted corn kernels	250 mL
1	can (4 oz/127 mL) diced roasted mild green chiles	1
1 cup	canned diced tomatoes, with juice	250 mL
1 cup	tomato sauce	250 mL
2 tsp	New Mexico red chile powder	10 mL
2 tsp	ground cumin	10 mL
¾ tsp	salt	3 mL

Topping

¾ cup	cornmeal	175 mL
2 cups	water	500 mL
¾ tsp	salt	3 mL
¾ tsp	chipotle chile powder (optional)	3 mL
2 tbsp	vegan hard margarine	30 mL
½ cup	pitted black olives	125 mL

1. Place a large, heavy-bottomed skillet over medium heat and let pan get hot. Add oil and tip pan to coat. Add onion, bell pepper and garlic and cook, stirring, until softened and slightly browned, 6 to 8 minutes.

2. Increase heat to medium-high. Stir in pinto beans, kidney beans, corn, green chiles, tomatoes, tomato sauce, chile powder, cumin and salt; bring just to a boil. Reduce heat and simmer until thickened, 20 to 25 minutes. Transfer to baking dish. Preheat oven to 375°F (190°C).

Nutrients per 1 of 6 servings

Calories	309
Fat	11 g
Carbohydrate	46 g
Protein	9 g
Vitamin C	38 mg
Vitamin D	20 IU
Vitamin E	3 mg
Niacin	3 mg
Folate	142 mcg
Vitamin B_6	0.3 mcg
Vitamin B_{12}	0.0 mcg
Zinc	1.2 mg
Selenium	8 mcg

Variation

For a spicier tamale pie, add 2 chopped chipotle chiles and 1 tbsp (15 mL) adobo sauce from canned chipotles when you add the green chiles.

3. *Topping:* In a small saucepan, whisk together cornmeal and water. Whisk in salt and chipotle chile powder (if using). Bring to a boil over medium-high heat. Reduce heat and simmer, stirring frequently, until thickened, 8 to 10 minutes. Whisk in margarine. Spread mixture evenly over filling and dot top with olives.

4. Bake in preheated oven until filling is bubbly and top is golden brown, 35 to 45 minutes. Let tamale pie cool slightly before cutting and serving.

> ### ▶ Health Tip
>
> Chiles are members of the capsicum family and have numerous health benefits, including cancer prevention and cardiovascular uses, because of the presence of capsaicin (the heat-producing compound).

Spinach and Tomato Quiche

Although this quiche is somewhat untraditional, given the cracker-crumb crust, the cream-based filling is easy to prepare and the results are very tasty. Serve with a tossed green salad for brunch, lunch or a light supper.

Tip

To make ahead, complete step 1. Cover and freeze for up to 2 days. When you're ready to cook, complete the recipe.

- **6-cup (1.5 L) baking or soufflé dish, lined with greased heavy-duty foil**
- **Large (minimum 5-quart) oval slow cooker**
- **Food processor**

Crust

1 cup	cracker crumbs (about 20 crackers)	250 mL
2 tbsp	melted butter	30 mL

Filling

3	large eggs	3
1 cup	heavy or whipping (35%) cream	250 mL
2 cups	packed baby spinach leaves	500 mL
1	can (14 oz/398 mL) diced tomatoes, with juice	1
½ cup	finely grated Parmesan cheese	125 mL
⅓ cup	finely chopped shallots	75 mL

1. *Crust:* In a bowl, mix together crumbs and butter. Press mixture into bottom of prepared dish. Place in freezer until ready to use.

2. *Filling:* In food processor, combine eggs and cream. Process until blended. Add spinach, tomatoes, Parmesan and shallots; pulse until spinach is chopped and ingredients are blended. Pour into chilled crust. Cover dish tightly with foil and secure with a string. Place in slow cooker stoneware and pour in enough boiling water to reach 1 inch (2.5 cm) up the sides of the dish.

3. Cover and cook on High for 3 to 4 hours, until a tester inserted into the center of the custard comes out clean. Let cool slightly. Serve warm.

> ▶ **Health Tip**
>
> Tomatoes are a source of lycopene, an antioxidant that can support cardiovascular and eye health.

Nutrients per 1 of 6 servings

Calories	306
Fat	24 g
Carbohydrate	15 g
Protein	9 g
Vitamin C	10 mg
Vitamin D	36 IU
Vitamin E	2 mg
Niacin	1 mg
Folate	58 mcg
Vitamin B_6	0.2 mg
Vitamin B_{12}	0.5 mcg
Zinc	1.0 mg
Selenium	10 mcg

Falafel Burgers with Creamy Sesame Sauce

Prepare the burgers early in the day and refrigerate until ready to cook. Prepare the sauce up to a day ahead.

Tips

Replace the cilantro with dill or parsley.

Peanut butter can replace the tahini.

Nutrients per serving	
Calories	318
Fat	14 g
Carbohydrate	39 g
Protein	10 g
Vitamin C	12 mg
Vitamin D	1 IU
Vitamin E	1 mg
Niacin	2 mg
Folate	113 mcg
Vitamin B$_6$	0.6 mg
Vitamin B$_{12}$	0.1 mcg
Zinc	2.2 mg
Selenium	11 mcg

- **Food processor**

2 cups	drained canned chickpeas	500 mL
1/4 cup	chopped green onion	60 mL
1/4 cup	chopped fresh cilantro	60 mL
1/4 cup	finely chopped carrot	60 mL
1/4 cup	dry bread crumbs	60 mL
3 tbsp	freshly squeezed lemon juice	45 mL
3 tbsp	water	45 mL
2 tbsp	tahini	30 mL
2 tsp	minced garlic	10 mL
1/4 tsp	freshly ground black pepper	1 mL

Creamy Sesame Sauce

1/4 cup	light sour cream	60 mL
2 tbsp	tahini	30 mL
2 tbsp	chopped fresh cilantro	30 mL
2 tbsp	water	30 mL
2 tsp	freshly squeezed lemon juice	10 mL
1/2 tsp	minced garlic	2 mL
2 tsp	vegetable oil, divided	10 mL

1. In food processor, combine chickpeas, green onion, cilantro, carrot, bread crumbs, lemon juice, water, tahini, garlic and black pepper; pulse until finely chopped. With wet hands, form each 1/4 cup (60 mL) into a patty.

2. *Sauce:* In a small bowl, whisk together sour cream, tahini, cilantro, water, lemon juice and garlic.

3. In a nonstick skillet sprayed with vegetable spray, heat 1 tsp (5 mL) oil over medium heat. Add 4 patties and cook for 3 1/2 minutes or until golden; turn and cook for 3 1/2 minutes longer or until golden and hot inside. Remove from pan. Heat the remaining oil and cook the remaining patties. Serve with sesame sauce.

> ▶ **Health Tip**
>
> Sesame contains a substance called sesamol, which is a potent antioxidant.

Vegetable Cheese Loaf with Lemon Tomato Sauce

This meat(less) loaf packs plenty of flavor and is topped with a tangy sauce.

Makes 6 servings

Tip

When buying celery, look for heads that are tight. Avoid any that are discolored or cracked, as they are not fresh. In this recipe, celery is used to flavor the vegetable loaf. But celery is also one of the all-time great healthy snacks. Keep plenty on hand, as it keeps well, refrigerated.

- **Preheat oven to 350°F (180°C)**
- **9- by 5-inch (23 by 12.5 cm) loaf pan, lightly greased**

¾ cup	finely chopped onion	175 mL
3 tbsp	butter or margarine	45 mL
¾ cup	finely chopped celery	175 mL
2	carrots, peeled and grated	2
2 cups	small-curd cottage cheese	500 mL
2 cups	fresh bread crumbs	500 mL
2	large eggs, well beaten	2
	Zest and juice of ½ lemon	
1 tsp	salt	5 mL
½ tsp	freshly ground black pepper	2 mL
¼ tsp	dried basil	1 mL

Lemon Tomato Sauce

2½ cups	tomato juice, divided	625 mL
1	onion, cut in half	1
4	sprigs fresh parsley	4
1	bay leaf	1
1	whole clove	1
½ tsp	dried basil	2 mL
½ tsp	granulated sugar	2 mL
⅓ cup	butter or margarine	75 mL
¼ cup	all-purpose flour	60 mL
	Juice of ½ lemon	

1. In a medium skillet over medium heat, cook onion in melted butter for about 5 minutes or until tender. Add celery and carrots; cook for 1 minute.

2. In a large bowl, combine cottage cheese, bread crumbs, eggs, lemon zest and juice, salt, pepper and basil. Add vegetable mixture; stir.

3. Place in prepared loaf pan. Bake in preheated oven for 35 to 40 minutes or until knife inserted in center comes out clean. Remove loaf from pan.

Nutrients per serving	
Calories	327
Fat	19 g
Carbohydrate	24 g
Protein	15 g
Vitamin C	37 mg
Vitamin D	26 IU
Vitamin E	1 mg
Niacin	1 mg
Folate	61 mcg
Vitamin B$_6$	0.2 mg
Vitamin B$_{12}$	0.7 mcg
Zinc	0.8 mg
Selenium	15 mcg

To keep parsley fresh, wrap it in several layers of paper towels and place in a plastic bag. Store in the warmest part of your refrigerator — in the butter keeper, for example, or the door.

4. *Sauce:* In a medium saucepan, combine $1\frac{1}{2}$ cups (375 mL) tomato juice, onion, parsley, bay leaf, clove, basil and sugar. Bring to a boil, reduce heat and simmer for 15 to 20 minutes. Press mixture through a sieve. Reserve sieved tomato mixture.

5. In a small saucepan, melt butter and blend in flour; cook for 1 to 2 minutes. Gradually add remaining tomato juice. Cook, stirring constantly, for 4 to 5 minutes or until smooth and thickened. Add reserved tomato mixture and lemon juice. Reheat to serving temperature. To serve, slice loaf; pour sauce over slices.

▶ **Health Tip**

Lycopene, from tomatoes, has been shown to be one of the more useful cancer-prevention phytochemicals.

This recipe courtesy of Margaret McIntyre.

Vegetable Moussaka

Moussaka is a favorite in Balkan and Mediterranean cooking. Many readers will have had moussaka at their favorite Greek restaurant, but this version is meatless — and good.

Tip

To vary the flavors in this tasty dish and transform it into a great party pleaser, add grilled peppers and zucchini to the eggplant layer.

- **Preheat oven to 350°F (180°C)**
- **Baking sheets, greased**
- **Food processor**
- **13- by 9-inch (33 by 23 cm) baking pan, greased**

2	eggplants	2
1½ tsp	salt, divided	7 mL
1	onion, chopped	1
1	clove garlic, minced	1
1	can (19 oz/540 mL) chickpeas, drained and rinsed	1
1	can (28 oz/796 mL) tomatoes	1
1 tbsp	dried oregano	15 mL
1 tbsp	dried basil	15 mL
½ tsp	ground cinnamon	2 mL
½ tsp	freshly ground black pepper	2 mL
¼ cup	freshly grated Parmesan cheese	60 mL

Topping

1 lb	tofu	500 g
1	onion, quartered	1
2	large egg whites	2
Pinch	ground nutmeg	Pinch

1. Slice eggplants lengthwise into ¼-inch (5 mm) thick slices; sprinkle with 1 tsp (5 mL) salt. Drain in colander for 30 minutes. Arrange in a single layer on prepared baking sheets. Bake in preheated oven for 15 minutes. Turn and bake for 15 minutes.

2. In a nonstick skillet sprayed with nonstick cooking spray, cook onion and garlic, stirring, for 2 minutes. Add chickpeas, mashing slightly. Stir in tomatoes, oregano, basil, cinnamon, pepper and the remaining salt; bring to a boil. Reduce heat and simmer, uncovered, for 20 minutes, stirring occasionally. Process in food processor until mixture resembles coarse meal.

Nutrients per serving	
Calories	246
Fat	7 g
Carbohydrate	34 g
Protein	17 g
Vitamin C	15 mg
Vitamin D	1 IU
Vitamin E	1 mg
Niacin	2 mg
Folate	102 mcg
Vitamin B$_6$	0.5 mg
Vitamin B$_{12}$	0.1 mcg
Zinc	2.2 mg
Selenium	15 mcg

Is cutting onions
bringing you to tears?
Try placing them in the
freezer for 10 minutes
before chopping.

3. In prepared baking pan, layer half of the eggplant, then all of the chickpea mixture, half of the Parmesan, then remaining eggplant.

4. *Topping:* In food processor, purée tofu, onion, egg whites and nutmeg until smooth. Spread over moussaka. Sprinkle with remaining Parmesan. Bake in preheated oven for 30 minutes.

> **▶ Health Tip**
>
> Chickpeas are an excellent source of fiber — key to the health of the gastrointestinal system.

This recipe courtesy of chef Mark Mogensen and dietitian Marsha Rosen.

Lunch Box Peachy Sweet Potato and Couscous

Here is a convenient and nutritious hot lunch with minimal prep time.

Tip

Pack up the ingredients you need for this meal the night before and, if you have access to a microwave, cook the meal at work or at school.

Variation

For a change, substitute curry powder for the ginger and cinnamon. Add some leftover cooked pork strips, if desired.

- **3-cup (750 mL) microwave-safe glass or ceramic container**

1	small sweet potato (about 6 oz/175 g)	1
¼ cup	couscous	60 mL
2 tbsp	raisins	30 mL
1 tsp	chicken or vegetable bouillon powder	5 mL
¼ tsp	ground ginger	1 mL
⅛ tsp	ground cinnamon (optional)	0.5 mL
1	can (5 oz/142 g) diced peaches, with juice	1
¼ cup	water	60 mL

1. Microwave sweet potato on High for 2 to 2½ minutes or until just cooked. Let cool; peel and dice into 1-inch (2.5 cm) pieces. Place in microwave-safe container.

2. Add couscous, raisins, chicken bouillon, ginger and cinnamon (if using). Refrigerate for up to 1 day.

3. When you are ready to cook, stir in peaches and water. Microwave, loosely covered, on High for 3 minutes. Stir, cover and let stand for 2 to 3 minutes. Fluff with a fork.

> ▶ **Health Tip**
>
> Sweet potatoes are loaded with carotenoids, beneficial antioxidants that can also be converted to vitamin A in the body.

This recipe courtesy of dietitians Bev Callaghan and Lynn Roblin.

Nutrients per serving	
Calories	317
Fat	1 g
Carbohydrate	75 g
Protein	6 g
Vitamin C	10 mg
Vitamin D	0 IU
Vitamin E	1 mg
Niacin	3 mg
Folate	31 mcg
Vitamin B$_6$	0.5 mg
Vitamin B$_{12}$	0.0 mcg
Zinc	0.8 mg
Selenium	13 mcg

Quinoa Vegetable Cakes

In this dish, the quinoa vegetable cakes are baked, eliminating any greasy aftertaste while delivering the goods in flavor and nutrition.

Tips

If you prefer, an equal amount of chopped fresh cilantro, basil or flat-leaf (Italian) parsley may be used in place of the dill.

Store the quinoa cakes wrapped in foil or in an airtight container in the refrigerator for up to 2 days. Reheat in the microwave on Medium (50%) for 45 to 60 seconds or until warmed through.

Nutrients per serving	
Calories	308
Fat	7 g
Carbohydrate	47 g
Protein	17 g
Vitamin C	10 mg
Vitamin D	21 IU
Vitamin E	3 mg
Niacin	1 mg
Folate	193 mcg
Vitamin B$_6$	0.4 mg
Vitamin B$_{12}$	0.6 mcg
Zinc	2.9 mg
Selenium	18 mcg

- **Preheat oven to 400°F (200°C)**
- **Large rimmed baking sheet, sprayed with nonstick cooking spray (preferably olive oil)**

2	cloves garlic, minced	2
1	package (10 oz/300 g) frozen chopped spinach, thawed and squeezed dry	1
3 cups	cooked quinoa, cooled	750 mL
¾ cup	finely shredded carrots	175 mL
½ cup	finely chopped green onions	125 mL
¼ cup	quinoa flour	60 mL
1 tbsp	dried Italian seasoning	15 mL
1 tsp	baking powder	5 mL
	Fine sea salt and freshly cracked black pepper	
2	large eggs, lightly beaten	2
1 tbsp	chopped fresh dill	15 mL
1 cup	plain yogurt	250 mL
1 tbsp	freshly squeezed lemon juice	15 mL

1. In a large bowl, combine garlic, spinach, quinoa, carrots, green onions, quinoa flour, Italian seasoning, baking powder, ½ tsp (2 mL) salt, ½ tsp (2 mL) pepper and eggs.

2. Scoop 8 equal mounds of quinoa mixture onto prepared baking sheet. Using a spatula, flatten mounds to ½-inch (1 cm) thickness.

3. Bake in preheated oven for 15 minutes. Turn cakes over and bake for 8 to 12 minutes or until golden brown and hot in the center.

4. Meanwhile, in a small bowl, whisk together dill, yogurt and lemon juice. Season to taste with salt and pepper.

5. Serve warm quinoa cakes with yogurt sauce drizzled on top or served alongside.

> ▶ **Health Tip**
>
> Quinoa is not only rich in many nutrients, it is also very high in fiber, even for a whole grain.

Tomato Dal

As the name implies, this tasty dal is enhanced with lots of tomatoes.
Serve with rice.

Makes 6 to 8 servings

1 cup	dried red lentils	250 mL
2½ cups	chopped tomatoes (about 3)	625 mL
¼ tsp	ground turmeric	1 mL
1½ tsp	salt (or to taste)	7 mL
½ cup	packed fresh cilantro, chopped	125 mL
1 tsp	minced gingerroot	5 mL
1 tsp	minced garlic	5 mL
1 tbsp	vegetable oil	15 mL
½ tsp	mustard seeds	2 mL
½ tsp	cumin seeds	2 mL
2	dried red Indian chile peppers, broken in half	2
8 to 10	fresh curry leaves (optional)	8 to 10

1. Clean and pick through lentils for any small stones and grit. Rinse several times in cold water until water is fairly clear. Soak in 4 cups (1 L) water in a large saucepan for 10 minutes.

2. Bring to a boil over medium-high heat, skimming froth off surface. Stir in tomatoes and turmeric. Reduce heat to medium-low and cook for 20 minutes. Sprinkle in salt and cook until dal is soft, about 10 minutes. With an immersion blender or in a blender, blend and return to a gentle boil. Stir in cilantro, ginger and garlic.

3. Meanwhile, in a small saucepan, heat oil over high heat until a couple of mustard seeds thrown in start to sputter. Add the remaining mustard seeds and cover immediately. When seeds stop popping after a few seconds, uncover and reduce heat to medium. Add cumin seeds, chiles and curry leaves, if using. Sauté for 30 seconds. Pour immediately into dal. Cover and simmer for 10 minutes.

> ▶ **Health Tip**
>
> The gingerroot in this dish is a natural digestive aid, as are the cumin seeds.

Nutrients
per 1 of 8 servings

Calories	116
Fat	3 g
Carbohydrate	18 g
Protein	7 g
Vitamin C	24 mg
Vitamin D	0 IU
Vitamin E	1 mg
Niacin	1 mg
Folate	60 mcg
Vitamin B_6	0.2 mg
Vitamin B_{12}	0.0 mcg
Zinc	1.1 mg
Selenium	2 mcg

Red Lentil Curry with Coconut and Cilantro

This dish turns up the spices with the aromatic tastes of curry.

Makes 6 servings

Tips

Choose enriched coconut milk to increase your intake of calcium and vitamin D.

Traditionally, Indian lentil dishes such as this one are served very loose and almost soupy. You can adjust the texture to your taste by adding more water or simmering longer to thicken.

Leftovers will thicken considerably upon cooling. If reheating in the microwave or a saucepan, add boiling water before heating to return to desired consistency.

Nutrients per serving	
Calories	291
Fat	20 g
Carbohydrate	23 g
Protein	10 g
Vitamin C	3 mg
Vitamin D	0 IU
Vitamin E	1 mg
Niacin	1 mg
Folate	77 mcg
Vitamin B_6	0.2 mg
Vitamin B_{12}	0.0 mcg
Zinc	1.7 mg
Selenium	3 mcg

2 tbsp	vegetable oil	30 mL
1	small onion, finely chopped	1
2	cloves garlic, minced	2
1 tbsp	minced gingerroot	15 mL
	Salt	
1 tsp	ground coriander	5 mL
1 tsp	ground cumin	5 mL
1/4 tsp	ground turmeric	1 mL
1 cup	dried red lentils, rinsed	250 mL
1	can (14 oz/400 mL) coconut milk	1
1 cup	water	250 mL
1/4 cup	torn fresh cilantro leaves	60 mL
	Garam masala	

1. In a saucepan, heat oil over medium heat. Add onion and cook, stirring, until softened and starting to brown, about 5 minutes. Add garlic, ginger, 1 tsp (5 mL) salt, coriander, cumin and turmeric; cook, stirring, until softened and fragrant, about 2 minutes.

2. Stir in lentils until coated with spices. Stir in coconut milk and water; bring to a boil, scraping up bits stuck to pan and stirring to prevent lumps. Reduce heat to low, partially cover and simmer, stirring often, until lentils are very soft and mixture is thick, about 15 minutes.

3. Remove from heat, cover and let stand for 5 minutes. Season to taste with salt. Stir in all but a few leaves of cilantro. Serve sprinkled with remaining cilantro and garam masala.

Variation

Add 1 or 2 hot chile peppers, minced, with the garlic.

▶ **Health Tip**

The array of spices in this dish provides a substantial dose of antioxidants and anti-inflammatory compounds, not the least of which come from the turmeric.

Brown Chickpea Curry

This is as aromatic and pungent a dish of chickpeas as you'll find, and the touch of coconut makes it extra-special.

Makes 4 to 6 servings

Tips

Sambhar powder, a South Indian spice blend, includes fenugreek, peppercorns, red chiles, coriander, cumin, mustard seeds, turmeric, curry leaves and asafetida, among other spices. It will stay fresh for 1 year if stored in the refrigerator.

Indian poppy seeds are pale-colored and will not discolor the dish as dark poppy seeds tend to do. However, if you only have dark ones, they can be substituted.

• Blender

1 cup	chickpeas	250 mL
1 tsp	salt (or to taste)	5 mL
1/3 cup	fresh or frozen grated coconut	75 mL
2 tbsp	unsalted Thai tamarind purée	30 mL
1 tbsp	sambhar powder (see tip, at left)	15 mL
1 tsp	Indian poppy seeds (see tip, at left)	5 mL

1. Pick through and rinse chickpeas 2 to 3 times. Add water to cover by 3 inches (7.5 cm) and soak at room temperature in a bowl for 6 hours or overnight.

2. Drain chickpeas. Place in a saucepan with 4 cups (1 L) fresh water. Bring to a boil over high heat. Reduce heat to low and boil gently until chickpeas are tender, 20 to 25 minutes. Add salt just before chickpeas are ready, then remove from heat.

3. With a slotted spoon, transfer 1/2 cup (125 mL) of the cooked chickpeas to blender. Add coconut, tamarind, sambhar powder and poppy seeds. Add 1/2 cup (125 mL) of the chickpea liquid and blend to a purée.

4. Pour purée into remaining chickpeas in saucepan and cook over medium-low heat, stirring occasionally, until gravy thickens to the consistency you prefer, 6 to 8 minutes. If not serving immediately, allow a little extra liquid to remain, as the curry thickens considerably as it cools.

> ▶ **Health Tip**
>
> Coconut has a large amount of medium-chain fatty acids, which are heart-friendly and are not processed in the body the same way as long-chain fatty acids.

Nutrients per 1 of 6 servings	
Calories	147
Fat	4 g
Carbohydrate	23 g
Protein	7 g
Vitamin C	2 mg
Vitamin D	0 IU
Vitamin E	0 mg
Niacin	1 mg
Folate	188 mcg
Vitamin B$_6$	0.2 mg
Vitamin B$_{12}$	0.0 mcg
Zinc	1.2 mg
Selenium	3 mcg

Winter Greens with Split Yellow Peas

For anyone who has been turned off greens by mushy, nondescript victims of the saucepan, this dish will put them back on your favorites list.

Tip

Greens, when cooked, reduce drastically in volume, so a little bit more or a little bit less will not change the dish.

▶ Health Tip

Collard greens and mustard greens have compounds that help support the body's detoxification systems, and they are phenomenal sources of vitamin K.

Nutrients per serving	
Calories	158
Fat	5 g
Carbohydrate	22 g
Protein	9 g
Vitamin C	65 mg
Vitamin D	0 IU
Vitamin E	3 mg
Niacin	2 mg
Folate	273 mcg
Vitamin B$_6$	0.3 mg
Vitamin B$_{12}$	0.0 mcg
Zinc	1.2 mg
Selenium	5 mcg

1 cup	split yellow peas	250 mL
½ tsp	ground turmeric	2 mL
2½ tsp	salt (or to taste), divided	12 mL
6 to 7 cups	spinach, rinsed and chopped (see tip, at left)	1.5 to 1.75 L
6 to 7 cups	turnip greens, rinsed and chopped	1.5 to 1.75 L
6 to 7 cups	mustard or collard greens, rinsed and chopped	1.5 to 1.75 L
2 tbsp	vegetable oil	30 mL
2 tbsp	slivered gingerroot	30 mL
1 tbsp	minced green chile peppers, preferably serranos	15 mL
2 tbsp	dark mustard seeds, coarsely pounded	30 mL
1 tbsp	cumin seeds	15 mL
2 tbsp	freshly squeezed lime or lemon juice (or to taste)	30 mL

1. Clean and pick through peas for any small stones and grit. Rinse several times in cold water until water is fairly clear. Soak in 2½ cups (625 mL) water in a saucepan for 15 minutes.

2. Bring peas to a boil over medium heat. Reduce heat to low. Stir in turmeric and boil gently, partially covered, until peas are soft but not mushy and water is absorbed, 20 to 25 minutes. Add 1 tsp (5 mL) of the salt in the last 5 minutes of cooking. Set aside.

3. In a large pot, combine spinach, turnip and mustard greens and 2 tbsp (30 mL) water. Cover and cook over low heat until water is absorbed, about 5 minutes.

4. Meanwhile, in a large skillet, heat oil over medium heat. Add ginger and chiles and sauté for 1 minute. Add mustard and cumin and sauté, stirring continuously, for 2 minutes.

5. Add spinach mixture, peas and remaining salt. Mix well and heat through. Add lime juice to taste. Serve with Indian bread.

Quinoa Chili

Quinoa makes a terrific centerpiece in this chili along with the wonderful smokiness of chipotle pepper.

Tip

Like most whole-grain dishes, this chili soaks up liquid if left to sit, so keep some extra vegetable broth on hand to add if you're reheating leftovers.

▶ Health Tip

Quinoa is a source of iron, so in fact this vegetarian dish comes complete with iron, along with many other nutrients.

Nutrients per serving	
Calories	306
Fat	6 g
Carbohydrate	56 g
Protein	13 g
Vitamin C	52 mg
Vitamin D	0 IU
Vitamin E	3 mg
Niacin	3 mg
Folate	193 mcg
Vitamin B$_6$	0.7 mg
Vitamin B$_{12}$	0.0 mcg
Zinc	2.2 mg
Selenium	8 mcg

1 tbsp	olive oil	15 mL
2	onions, finely chopped	2
2	stalks celery, diced	2
1	carrot, peeled and diced	1
1	green bell pepper, finely chopped	1
4	cloves garlic, minced	4
2 tbsp	chili powder	30 mL
1	chipotle pepper in adobo sauce, minced	1
1	can (28 oz/796 mL) no-salt-added diced tomatoes, with juice	1
2 cups	ready-to-use reduced-sodium vegetable broth	500 mL
	Salt and freshly ground black pepper	
1 cup	quinoa, rinsed	250 mL
2 cups	drained rinsed cooked or canned pinto beans (see variation, below)	500 mL
1 cup	corn kernels	250 mL

1. In a large, deep skillet with a tight-fitting lid, heat oil over medium heat for 30 seconds. Add onions, celery, carrot, bell pepper and garlic and stir well. Reduce heat to low. Cover and cook until vegetables are softened, about 10 minutes.

2. Increase heat to medium. Add chili powder and chipotle pepper and cook, stirring, for 1 minute. Add tomatoes and broth and bring to a boil. Season to taste with salt and black pepper. Add quinoa, beans and corn and cook, stirring, until mixture returns to a boil. Reduce heat to low. Cover and simmer until quinoa is tender, about 20 minutes.

Variations

Millet Chili: Substitute an equal quantity of toasted millet for the quinoa. Increase the quantity of vegetable broth to 2$\frac{1}{2}$ cups (625 mL) and increase the cooking time to about 25 minutes.

Substitute red kidney, cranberry or small red beans for the pinto beans.

Southwest Butternut Squash Tortilla Bake

This easy casserole, filled with traditional flavors of the Southwest, is a wonderful way to showcase butternut squash.

Makes 6 servings

Tips

For more heat, use 2 jalapeños and leave in the seeds. But be careful — the ribs and seeds really add to the heat!

Butternut squash is easier to dice if you microwave it on High for about 2 minutes before peeling.

▶ Health Tip

In addition to being flavorful, squash contains carotenoids, including beta carotene, a vitamin A precursor.

Nutrients per serving	
Calories	300
Fat	7 g
Carbohydrate	52 g
Protein	12 g
Vitamin C	30 mg
Vitamin D	1 IU
Vitamin E	2 mg
Niacin	4 mg
Folate	133 mcg
Vitamin B$_6$	0.4 mg
Vitamin B$_{12}$	0.1 mcg
Zinc	1.4 mg
Selenium	4 mcg

- **Preheat oven to 400°F (200°C)**
- **8-cup (2 L) round casserole dish**

2 tbsp	olive oil, divided	30 mL
1	onion, thinly sliced	1
2	cloves garlic, minced	2
1	jalapeño pepper, seeded and minced	1
1 tsp	paprika	5 mL
1 tsp	ground cumin	5 mL
1 tsp	dried oregano	5 mL
1	can (16 oz/454 mL) crushed tomatoes	1
1 lb	butternut squash, peeled, seeded and diced	500 g
1 cup	ready-to-use vegetable broth	250 mL
1	can (14 to 19 oz/398 to 540 mL) black beans, drained and rinsed	1
1½ cups	corn kernels (thawed if frozen)	375 mL
¼ tsp	salt	1 mL
¼ tsp	freshly ground black pepper	1 mL
8	6-inch (15 cm) corn tortillas, cut into ¾-inch (2 cm) strips	8
½ cup	shredded reduced-fat sharp (old) Cheddar cheese	125 mL

1. In a large nonstick skillet, heat half the oil over medium heat. Sauté onion for 5 to 7 minutes or until softened. Add garlic and jalapeño; sauté for 1 minute. Add paprika, cumin and oregano; sauté for 1 minute. Add tomatoes, squash and broth; bring to a simmer. Reduce heat to low, cover and simmer for about 10 minutes or until squash is just tender. Stir in beans, corn, salt and pepper.

2. Spoon squash mixture into casserole dish. Layer tortilla strips over top. Brush with the remaining oil.

3. Bake in preheated oven for 25 to 30 minutes or until topping is golden brown and filling is bubbling. Sprinkle with cheese and bake for 3 minutes or until cheese is melted.

Three-Bean Chili

Who doesn't like a good bowl of chili? This version will give you all the benefits from beans, garlic, onion and spices, without the saturated fats.

Tips

Because can sizes vary, we provide a range of amounts for beans in our recipes. If you're using 19-oz (540 mL) cans, add a bit more chili powder to taste.

Use diced tomatoes with or without seasonings.

1 tbsp	vegetable oil	15 mL
1	large onion, coarsely chopped	1
1	red bell pepper, cut into 1-inch (2.5 cm) cubes	1
2	cloves garlic, minced (about 2 tsp/10 mL)	2
1½ tbsp	chili powder	22 mL
1½ tsp	ground cumin	7 mL
½ tsp	dried oregano	2 mL
½ tsp	ground cinnamon	2 mL
½ tsp	ground allspice	2 mL
¼ tsp	hot pepper flakes	1 mL
2 cups	ready-to-use vegetable broth	500 mL
½ cup	tomato paste	125 mL
1	can (14 to 19 oz/398 to 540 mL) black beans, drained and rinsed	1
1	can (14 to 19 oz/398 to 540 mL) red kidney beans, drained and rinsed	1
1	can (14 to 19 oz/398 to 540 mL) navy or white kidney beans, drained and rinsed	1
1	can (28 oz/796 mL) diced tomatoes, with juices (see tip, at left)	1
1 tbsp	red wine vinegar	15 mL

1. In a large pot, heat oil over medium heat for 30 seconds. Add onion and red pepper and cook, stirring, for 3 minutes or until softened. Add garlic and cook, stirring, for 1 minute. Add chili powder, cumin, oregano, cinnamon, allspice and hot pepper flakes; cook, stirring, for 1 minute.

Nutrients per 1 of 8 servings	
Calories	213
Fat	3 g
Carbohydrate	38 g
Protein	11 g
Vitamin C	36 mg
Vitamin D	0 IU
Vitamin E	2 mg
Niacin	3 mg
Folate	92 mcg
Vitamin B$_6$	0.4 mg
Vitamin B$_{12}$	0.0 mcg
Zinc	1.3 mg
Selenium	4 mcg

Tip

Store leftovers in an airtight container in the refrigerator for up to 4 days, or in the freezer for up to 2 months.

Variation

For a more substantial version of this chili, add 6 oz (175 g) soy ground meat alternative. In a skillet, heat 1 tbsp (15 mL) olive oil over medium-high heat. Add meat alternative and reduce heat to medium. Cook, stirring frequently, for 5 minutes or until heated through. Add to chili along with the vinegar.

2. Add vegetable broth and increase heat to medium-high. Bring to a simmer and cook for 5 minutes or until pepper is very soft. Add tomato paste and stir well. Add black, red kidney and navy beans, tomatoes and vinegar. Return to a boil. Reduce heat to low, cover and simmer for 35 minutes or until thickened.

> ### ▶ Health Tip
>
> Oregano has antioxidant and antibacterial volatile oils such as thymol, pinene, limonene, carvacrol, ocimene and caryophyllene.

Fragrant Rice-Stuffed Peppers

This dish uses pleasing-to-the-senses jasmine rice, along with crunchy walnuts, to create a delicious stuffed pepper.

Makes 4 servings

Tips

Leaves and the tender top stems of beets are often trimmed and tossed away. These leaves, also referred to as beet greens, are delicious and a source of nutritious antioxidants.

Toast walnut halves in a dry skillet over low heat, stirring constantly, for 3 to 4 minutes or until fragrant. Transfer the toasted nuts to a plate and let cool before chopping.

- **Preheat oven to 425°F (220°C)**
- **Baking sheet, lined with parchment paper**
- **13- by 9-inch (33 by 23 cm) baking dish, lightly oiled**

Filling

1 cup	brown jasmine rice	250 mL
1¾ cups	ready-to-use vegetable broth	425 mL
8	beets, trimmed and peeled, beet greens reserved	8
5 tbsp	olive oil, divided	75 mL
3½ tsp	balsamic vinegar, divided	17 mL
½ tsp	salt, divided	2 mL
½ tsp	freshly ground black pepper, divided	2 mL
2	green onions, white and green parts, thinly sliced	2
2	cloves garlic, minced	2
¾ cup	coarsely chopped toasted walnuts	175 mL
4	yellow or red bell peppers	4

1. *Filling:* In a small saucepan over medium-high heat, combine rice and vegetable broth and bring to a boil. Reduce heat, cover and simmer for 50 minutes.

2. Cut beets into ¼-inch (0.5 cm) pieces and toss with 1 tbsp (15 mL) of the olive oil, 3 tsp (15 mL) of the balsamic vinegar, ¼ tsp (1 mL) of the salt and ¼ tsp (1 mL) of the black pepper. Spread beets on prepared baking sheet and roast in preheated oven until softened and slightly browned, 20 to 25 minutes.

Nutrients per serving

Calories	588
Fat	31 g
Carbohydrate	69 g
Protein	13 g
Vitamin C	351 mg
Vitamin D	0 IU
Vitamin E	3 mg
Niacin	2 mg
Folate	236 mcg
Vitamin B_6	0.6 mg
Vitamin B_{12}	0.0 mcg
Zinc	1.7 mg
Selenium	6 mcg

Variation

Add 1 cup (250 mL) cooked lentils or black beans to add protein to this meal.

3. Remove and discard tough stems from beet greens, coarsely chop greens and set aside. Place a large skillet over medium-high heat and let pan get hot. Add 2 tbsp (30 mL) oil and tip pan to coat. Add green onions and garlic and cook, stirring frequently, until softened, about 1 minute. Add beet greens, $\frac{1}{2}$ tsp (2 mL) balsamic vinegar, $\frac{1}{4}$ tsp (1 mL) salt and $\frac{1}{4}$ tsp (1 mL) black pepper; cook until most of the liquid has evaporated, 2 to 3 minutes. Remove from heat and stir in cooked rice, roasted beets and toasted walnuts, mixing to incorporate. Taste and adjust seasonings.

4. Cut tops off peppers and reserve. Remove and discard seeds and membranes and slice a thin strip off pepper bottoms to level. Arrange peppers in prepared baking dish and spoon in filling. Replace tops and drizzle peppers with remaining 2 tbsp (30 mL) oil. Bake in preheated oven until peppers are tender and slightly charred, about 30 minutes.

> ### ▶ Health Tip
>
> Consuming walnuts has been shown to improve working memory.

Emerald Summer Pizza

The bright green veggies that adorn this pizza give it its name.

Tip

If you're in a rush, use a purchased parbaked pizza shell instead of fresh dough.

Variations

Replace half the ricotta with feta cheese.

Use half radicchio and half arugula.

- **Preheat oven to 400°F (200°C)**
- **12-inch (30 cm) pizza pan, lightly greased**

½	recipe Big-Batch Whole Wheat Pizza Dough (see recipe, opposite)	½
3 tbsp	basil pesto	45 mL
2 cups	chopped kale	500 mL
½ cup	cooked fresh or drained thawed frozen green peas	125 mL
1 cup	light ricotta cheese	250 mL
¾ cup	thinly sliced onion	175 mL
½ tsp	freshly ground black pepper	2 mL
1 cup	torn arugula leaves	250 mL

1. Roll out dough to a 12-inch (30 cm) diameter and fit into prepared pan. Spread pesto evenly over crust to within ½ inch (1 cm) of edge. Arrange kale and peas evenly over pesto. Drop ricotta by spoonfuls over top and spread slightly. Sprinkle with onion and pepper.

2. Bake in preheated oven for 14 to 16 minutes or until cheese has spread slightly, onions are lightly browned and crust is golden and crisp. Remove from oven and arrange arugula over pizza.

> ▶ **Health Tip**
>
> Kale is a good source of calcium and complements other calcium sources (such as ricotta cheese).

This recipe courtesy of dietitian Honey Bloomberg.

Nutrients per serving	
Calories	236
Fat	8 g
Carbohydrate	31 g
Protein	12 g
Vitamin C	34 mg
Vitamin D	3 IU
Vitamin E	1 mg
Niacin	3 mg
Folate	83 mcg
Vitamin B_6	0.2 mg
Vitamin B_{12}	0.2 mcg
Zinc	1.7 mg
Selenium	20 mcg

Tip

If you do not have an electric mixer with a dough hook, you can use a food processor.

Big-Batch Whole Wheat Pizza Dough

A homemade crust, when you have time to prepare it, will make a huge difference to the taste of your pizza and provides added nutrition.

- **Electric mixer with dough hook**

2	packages (each ¼ oz/7 g) instant yeast	2
2 cups	whole wheat flour	500 mL
1 cup	all-purpose flour	250 mL
1 tsp	salt	5 mL
½ tsp	granulated sugar	2 mL
1½ cups	lukewarm water	375 mL
½ tsp	olive oil	2 mL

1. In mixer bowl, combine yeast, whole wheat flour, all-purpose flour, salt and sugar. Attach dough hook and mixer bowl to mixer. With mixer running on low speed, gradually add water; knead until dough is smooth and elastic, about 10 minutes. Turn mixer off and pour oil down side of bowl. Set to low speed for 15 seconds to coat inside of bowl and cover dough lightly with oil. Remove mixer bowl and cover loosely with plastic wrap.

2. Let dough rise in a warm, draft-free place until doubled in bulk, about 2 hours.

3. Punch down dough and cut in half to make two balls. Place each ball in an airtight freezer bag and store for up to 3 months, or roll out for immediate use.

4. To make crust, place dough ball on a floured work surface and form into a circle. Roll out until dough reaches a 12- to 15-inch (30 to 38 cm) diameter. Pierce dough with a fork before adding toppings.

This recipe courtesy of Eileen Campbell.

Nutrients per ⅙ pizza crust	
Calories	112
Fat	1 g
Carbohydrate	23 g
Protein	4 g
Vitamin C	0 mg
Vitamin D	0 IU
Vitamin E	0 mg
Niacin	2 mg
Folate	56 mcg
Vitamin B$_6$	0.1 mg
Vitamin B$_{12}$	0.0 mcg
Zinc	0.7 mg
Selenium	13 mcg

Spaghetti with Sun-Dried Tomatoes and Broccoli

This truly Mediterranean dish muscles up on the broccoli for even more taste and health benefits.

Tips

Instead of hot pepper flakes, use 1/8 tsp (0.5 mL) cayenne pepper.

Buy dry-pack sun-dried tomatoes, not those marinated in oil.

Prepare pasta up to 2 hours ahead, leaving it at room temperature. loss before serving.

8 oz	spaghetti	250 g
1/2 cup	sun-dried tomatoes	125 mL
2 cups	chopped broccoli	500 mL
2 1/2 cups	chopped tomatoes	625 mL
2 tbsp	olive oil	30 mL
1 1/2 tsp	crushed garlic	7 mL
Pinch	hot pepper flakes	Pinch
1/2 cup	chopped fresh basil (or 2 tsp/10 mL dried)	125 mL
3 tbsp	grated Parmesan cheese	45 mL

1. Cook pasta in boiling water according to package instructions or until firm to the bite. Drain and place in a serving bowl

2. Pour boiling water over sun-dried tomatoes. Let soak for 15 minutes. Drain, then chop. Add to pasta.

3. Blanch broccoli in boiling water just until barely tender. Rinse with cold water, drain and add to pasta. Add tomatoes, oil, garlic, hot pepper flakes, basil and cheese. Toss.

> ▶ **Health Tip**
>
> Tomatoes contain hydroxycinnamic acids such as caffeic acid and ferulic acid — important antioxidants.

Nutrients per serving	
Calories	346
Fat	10 g
Carbohydrate	54 g
Protein	12 g
Vitamin C	58 mg
Vitamin D	1 IU
Vitamin E	2 mg
Niacin	6 mg
Folate	188 mcg
Vitamin B_6	0.3 mg
Vitamin B_{12}	0.1 mcg
Zinc	1.5 mg
Selenium	38 mcg

Rice Noodles with Roasted Mediterranean Vegetables

Rice noodles have a wonderful ability to absorb flavors and sauces, and this dish provides them with plenty of inspiration.

Makes 4 servings

Tip

Toasted sesame oil has a dark brown color and a rich, nutty flavor. It only needs to be used sparingly to add a tremendous amount of flavor.

- **Preheat oven to 375°F (190°C)**
- **Roasting pan, lightly oiled**

2	zucchini, trimmed and cut into 1-inch (2.5 cm) pieces	2
2	large tomatoes, halved	2
2	onions, quartered	2
1	eggplant, trimmed and cut into 1-inch (2.5 cm) pieces	1
1	red bell pepper, thickly sliced	1
2	cloves garlic	2
1/4 cup	tamari or soy sauce	60 mL
2 tbsp	olive oil	30 mL
2 tbsp	freshly squeezed lime or lemon juice	30 mL
1 tbsp	toasted sesame oil	15 mL
8 oz	dried wide rice noodles	250 g

1. In prepared roasting pan, combine zucchini, tomatoes, onions, eggplant, red pepper and garlic.

2. In a bowl, whisk together tamari, olive oil, lime juice and sesame oil. Toss with vegetables in roasting pan. Bake in preheated oven, stirring once or twice, for 30 to 40 minutes or until vegetables are tender when pierced with the tip of a knife. Do not turn the oven off.

3. Meanwhile, in a bowl, cover rice noodles with hot water. Soak for 15 to 20 minutes or according to package directions, until al dente. Drain and set aside. When vegetables are cooked, toss drained noodles with roasted vegetables. Return to the oven for 10 minutes to heat through.

Nutrients per serving	
Calories	393
Fat	11 g
Carbohydrate	70 g
Protein	6 g
Vitamin C	76 mg
Vitamin D	0 IU
Vitamin E	3 mg
Niacin	3 mg
Folate	93 mcg
Vitamin B_6	0.6 mg
Vitamin B_{12}	0.0 mcg
Zinc	1.2 mg
Selenium	6 mcg

> ▶ **Health Tip**
>
> Rice noodles are good evidence that gluten-free noodles are easy to come by.

Egg Noodles with Vegetables

This recipe uses fresh egg noodles, but softened rice noodles can be substituted. For a vegetarian version, replace the oyster sauce with vegetarian (mushroom) oyster sauce.

Makes 4 servings

1/4 cup	ready-to-use chicken broth or water	60 mL
2 tbsp	oyster sauce	30 mL
1 tbsp	soy sauce	15 mL
1 tbsp	freshly squeezed lime juice	15 mL
1 tsp	granulated sugar	5 mL
1/4 tsp	freshly ground black pepper	1 mL
2 tbsp	vegetable oil	30 mL
4	cloves garlic, chopped	4
1/2	bunch broccoli (about 8 oz/250 g), cut into florets, stems peeled and sliced	1/2
1	red bell pepper, cut into 1-inch (2.5 cm) pieces	1
2	stalks celery, sliced	2
4 oz	snow peas, trimmed (about 1 cup/250 mL)	125 g
8 oz	fresh egg noodles, rinsed under hot water and loosened	250 g
1 cup	bean sprouts	250 mL
3	green onions, thinly sliced	3
1	small fresh red chile pepper, seeded and thinly sliced	1
2 tbsp	fresh cilantro leaves	30 mL

1. In a small bowl or measuring cup, combine broth, oyster sauce, soy sauce, lime juice, sugar and pepper.

2. Heat a wok or large skillet over medium-high heat and add oil. Add garlic and stir-fry for 30 seconds. Add broccoli, red pepper, celery and snow peas. Increase heat to high and stir-fry for 3 minutes, or until crisp.

3. Add noodles and reserved sauce, tossing to combine with vegetables. Cook for 3 to 4 minutes, or until noodles are tender but not mushy. Add bean sprouts and green onions and toss with noodles. Serve garnished with chile slices and cilantro.

Nutrients per serving	
Calories	240
Fat	10 g
Carbohydrate	31 g
Protein	10 g
Vitamin C	145 mg
Vitamin D	2 IU
Vitamin E	3 mg
Niacin	3 mg
Folate	167 mcg
Vitamin B_6	0.5 mg
Vitamin B_{12}	0.1 mcg
Zinc	1.2 mg
Selenium	17 mcg

▶ **Health Tip**

Egg noodles are best served a bit firm. The addition of egg to the wheat raises the protein content.

Fish and Seafood

Parmesan Herb Baked Fish Fillets

Just a touch of cayenne, basil and Parmesan cheese make these fish fillets more than just another grilled fish.

Makes 4 servings

Tips

For convenience and speed, this recipe uses frozen fish fillets, but fresh fish may also be used. If you prefer a thicker fish fillet, such as salmon or halibut, increase the cooking time by about 5 minutes.

If available, substitute 1 to 2 tbsp (15 to 30 mL) chopped fresh basil for the dried basil.

Remember to use dry bread crumbs in this recipe; fresh bread crumbs will make the dish too soggy.

- **Preheat oven to 400°F (200°C)**
- **11- by 7-inch (28 by 18 cm) baking dish, greased**

1	package (1 lb/500 g) frozen fish fillets, thawed and patted dry	1
1/4 cup	light mayonnaise	60 mL
1/4 cup	freshly grated Parmesan cheese	60 mL
2 tbsp	chopped green onion	30 mL
1 tbsp	chopped pimiento or red bell pepper	15 mL
	Cayenne pepper	
1/2 cup	dry bread crumbs	125 mL
1/2 tsp	dried basil	2 mL
	Freshly ground black pepper	

1. Place fish fillets in a single layer in bottom of prepared baking dish. Set aside.

2. In a small bowl, stir together mayonnaise, Parmesan cheese, onion, pimiento and cayenne to taste. Spread mixture evenly over fish fillets.

3. In a separate bowl, combine bread crumbs, basil and pepper to taste; sprinkle over top of fish. Bake in preheated oven for 10 to 12 minutes or until fish is opaque and flakes easily with a fork.

▶ Health Tip

Fish is a great source of omega-3 fats. To minimize consumption of higher-mercury-content fish, try to rotate your selections.

This recipe courtesy of Marilena Rutka.

Nutrients per serving	
Calories	290
Fat	18 g
Carbohydrate	5 g
Protein	25 g
Vitamin C	8 mg
Vitamin D	2 IU
Vitamin E	2 mg
Niacin	10 mg
Folate	45 mcg
Vitamin B$_6$	0.5 mg
Vitamin B$_{12}$	1.6 mcg
Zinc	0.8 mg
Selenium	44 mcg

Turmeric Fried Fish

The brilliant color of turmeric gives dishes a bright, sunny appearance. For a colorful display, serve the fish surrounded by sliced lettuce, tomatoes and cucumbers.

Makes 4 to 5 servings

Tip

When working with turmeric, protect work surfaces and clothing, as it will stain (though it will wash off your hands).

3	cloves garlic, minced	3
2 tsp	ground turmeric	10 mL
1 tsp	freshly ground black pepper	5 mL
1 tsp	granulated sugar	5 mL
½ tsp	salt	2 mL
3 tbsp	vegetable oil, divided	45 mL
1½ lbs	fish fillets (such as tilapia, catfish, grouper or cod)	750 g
¾ cup	tapioca starch, cornstarch or all-purpose flour	175 mL
2 tbsp	fish sauce (nam pla)	30 mL
2 tbsp	rice vinegar	30 mL
½ tsp	hot pepper flakes	2 mL

1. In a bowl, combine garlic, turmeric, pepper, sugar, salt and 1 tbsp (15 mL) oil.

2. Arrange fish fillets in a shallow dish in a single layer. Spoon marinade over fish and rub into surface.

3. Spread tapioca starch in a shallow pan. Coat both sides of fish, shaking off excess.

4. In a nonstick skillet, heat the remaining oil over medium-high heat. Add fish and cook for 3 to 4 minutes per side, or until golden and cooked through.

5. In a small bowl, combine fish sauce, vinegar and hot pepper flakes. Serve with fish.

> ▶ **Health Tip**
>
> Turmeric is known for its anti-inflammatory properties, which are helpful for supporting joint health.

Nutrients per 1 of 5 servings	
Calories	303
Fat	11 g
Carbohydrate	24 g
Protein	28 g
Vitamin C	1 mg
Vitamin D	169 IU
Vitamin E	2 mg
Niacin	6 mg
Folate	38 mcg
Vitamin B_6	0.3 mg
Vitamin B_{12}	2.2 mcg
Zinc	0.6 mg
Selenium	58 mcg

Baked Fish Fillets with Yogurt Topping

An easy but impressive dish, this recipe has a topping that keeps the fish moist while imparting outstanding flavor.

Makes 6 to 8 servings

Tip

Is cutting onions bringing you to tears? Try placing them in the freezer for 10 minutes before chopping.

- **Preheat oven to 400°F (200°C)**
- **Baking sheet, lined with foil**

2 to 2½ lbs	catfish fillets, or any other similarly thick fillet, such as cod or red snapper	1 to 1.25 kg
½ tsp	ground turmeric	2 mL
2½ tsp	salt (or to taste), divided	12 mL
5 tbsp	vegetable oil, divided	75 mL
3 cups	chopped red onions	750 mL
3 cups	plain yogurt, well drained	750 mL
2 tsp	ground coriander	10 mL
1 tsp	cayenne pepper	5 mL
½ tsp	garam masala	2 mL
1 cup	packed fresh cilantro, coarsely chopped	250 mL
2 tsp	minced gingerroot	10 mL
2 tsp	minced garlic	10 mL
1 cup	chopped plum (Roma) tomato	250 mL
3 to 4 tbsp	freshly squeezed lemon juice Cucumber slices	45 to 60 mL

1. Rinse fish and pat dry. Rub turmeric and 1½ tsp (7 mL) salt into fish and set aside for 15 minutes. (It can be refrigerated for several hours.)

2. In a skillet, heat 2 tbsp (30 mL) oil over medium-high heat. Sauté onions until softened and no moisture is left, 6 to 8 minutes. Let cool. Stir onions and any oil remaining in pan into yogurt. Add coriander, cayenne pepper, garam masala, cilantro, ginger, garlic and tomato. Stir in lemon juice and the remaining salt. Mix well.

Nutrients per 1 of 8 servings	
Calories	306
Fat	17 g
Carbohydrate	14 g
Protein	23 g
Vitamin C	11 mg
Vitamin D	11 IU
Vitamin E	3 mg
Niacin	3 mg
Folate	38 mcg
Vitamin B$_6$	0.3 mg
Vitamin B$_{12}$	3.8 mcg
Zinc	1.5 mg
Selenium	13 mcg

Tip

The yogurt topping can be made up to 2 days ahead and refrigerated.

3. In same skillet, heat the remaining oil. Partially fry fish on each side, but do not cook through. Transfer to prepared baking sheet. Spread yogurt mixture over fish. Bake in preheated oven for 30 minutes if fillets are large, or 20 to 25 minutes if smaller. Test center of fillets with fork to see if fish flakes easily, and cook longer, if necessary.

4. Transfer to a serving platter and garnish with cucumber slices.

> ▶ **Health Tip**
>
> Fish is a great source of protein and healthy fats.

Crisp Potato-Wrapped Halibut

Like brown paper packages tied up with string, these lovely little golden brown potato parcels hold a special prize inside: moist snow-white halibut with all its natural flavors intact, thanks to being encased in paper-thin slices of potato. This may be a little tricky for the novice cook, but even a less than perfect attempt will be delicious.

Makes 4 servings

Tips

You really do need a mandoline for this recipe to achieve the ultra-thin slices of potato. If they are sliced too thickly, they won't be wrappable.

If you prefer, very lightly steam the potato slices beforehand to make them a little more pliable — just don't cook them through.

Nutrients per serving	
Calories	882
Fat	58 g
Carbohydrate	57 g
Protein	34 g
Vitamin C	60 mg
Vitamin D	303 IU
Vitamin E	4 mg
Niacin	12 mg
Folate	93 mcg
Vitamin B$_6$	1.7 mg
Vitamin B$_{12}$	1.7 mcg
Zinc	1.5 mg
Selenium	67 mcg

* **Mandoline**

3 to 4	large floury or all-purpose potatoes, peeled and halved lengthwise	3 to 4
3 tbsp	olive oil, divided	45 mL
	Salt and freshly ground black pepper	
4	halibut fillets (each about 5 oz/150 g), skinned and lightly seasoned with salt and freshly ground black pepper	4
½ cup	clarified butter (see tip, opposite), divided	125 mL
2	large leeks (white and light green parts only), trimmed and finely chopped (see tip, opposite)	2
½ tsp	curry powder	2 mL
¼ cup	dry white wine	60 mL
1 cup	heavy or whipping (35%) cream	250 mL

1. Using mandoline and slicing lengthwise, cut potatoes into slices that are thin enough to fold without snapping but not so thin that they are completely translucent (see tip, at left). On a piece of plastic wrap, lay out 5 or 6 slices in a row, slightly overlapping the long edges. Then make another, identical row, overlapping the short ends of the slices in the first row so that the slices form a rectangle. Lightly brush with a little of the oil. Season to taste with salt and freshly ground pepper.

2. Center a seasoned fish fillet on the rectangle. Then, using the plastic wrap to help, fold over the potato slices to enclose the fish, pressing down to adhere them to the fish. Wrap parcel tightly in the plastic. Transfer to a baking sheet. Repeat with the remaining potato slices and fish. Refrigerate for 1 hour to chill and set.

Tips

Clarified butter (also known as drawn butter) is easy to make. Since you will lose about a quarter of your original amount during the process, you'll need ¾ cup (175 mL) butter to make the amount required for this recipe. Place butter in a small saucepan and melt over low heat until milk solids accumulate on the bottom of the pan and the pure butterfat has risen to the top. Carefully pour off clear butterfat and discard remaining water and milk solids. Clarified butter will keep, tightly covered, in the refrigerator for about 1 month.

Make sure to wash the leeks thoroughly by slitting them open lengthwise and spreading them apart while rinsing clean under cold running water.

Variation

Use cod, haddock or sea bass in place of the halibut.

3. In a skillet, heat about 2 tbsp (30 mL) clarified butter over medium heat. Add leeks, season to taste with salt and freshly ground pepper and cook gently, stirring, for 5 to 7 minutes or until softened. Just before the leeks have softened completely, stir in curry powder and wine and cook for 2 minutes. Season to taste with salt and freshly ground pepper. Stir in cream and simmer for 5 minutes or until reduced and thickened into a sauce. Remove from heat and keep warm.

4. Preheat oven to 140°F (60°C). Heat a large, preferably nonstick skillet over medium-high heat. Add 3 to 4 tbsp (45 to 60 mL) clarified butter. Working with two parcels at a time, remove plastic wrap and place in pan, seam side down. Cook for about 4 minutes or until bottoms are golden brown. Using a metal spatula, carefully turn over and cook for 2 to 3 minutes or until golden and crisp. Transfer to a platter lined with paper towels and keep warm in preheated oven. Repeat with the remaining butter and parcels.

5. Spoon a mound of the leek mixture onto each of four individual serving plates. Top each with a fish parcel, seam side down, and serve immediately.

> ### ▶ Health Tip
>
> Halibut is a great source of protein and is a mild fish that most people find appetizing.

Salmon over White and Black Bean Salsa

Salsas are a popular dressing for fish, and you'll see why with this salmon entrée.

Makes 4 servings

Tip

Prepare bean mixture early in the day and keep refrigerated. Stir before serving.

- **Preheat barbecue to high or preheat oven to 425°F (220°C)**

1 cup	rinsed drained canned black beans	250 mL
1 cup	rinsed drained canned white navy beans	250 mL
¾ cup	chopped tomatoes	175 mL
½ cup	chopped green bell pepper	125 mL
¼ cup	chopped red onion	60 mL
¼ cup	chopped fresh cilantro	60 mL
2 tbsp	balsamic vinegar	30 mL
2 tbsp	freshly squeezed lemon juice	30 mL
1 tbsp	olive oil	15 mL
1 tsp	minced garlic	5 mL
1 lb	salmon steaks	500 g

1. In a bowl, combine black beans, navy beans, tomatoes, green pepper, red onion and cilantro. In a small bowl, whisk together vinegar, lemon juice, olive oil and garlic; pour over bean mixture and toss to combine.

2. Barbecue fish or bake uncovered for approximately 10 minutes for each 1-inch (2.5 cm) thickness of fish, or until fish flakes with a fork. Serve fish over bean salsa.

> ▶ **Health Tip**
> Salmon is a very good source of omega-3 fats, but try to stick to wild and sustainable salmon.

Nutrients per serving	
Calories	313
Fat	9 g
Carbohydrate	25 g
Protein	31 g
Vitamin C	23 mg
Vitamin D	493 IU
Vitamin E	1 mg
Niacin	10 mg
Folate	99 mcg
Vitamin B_6	0.8 mg
Vitamin B_{12}	4.7 mcg
Zinc	1.3 mg
Selenium	37 mcg

Open-Face Salmon Salad Sandwich with Apple and Ginger

Here is another use for canned salmon, which fits many budgets but still delivers the benefits of this nutritious fish.

Makes 4 servings

Tip

Stir the salmon mixture gently if you like your salad flaky; stir vigorously for a smoother texture.

Variation

Use canned tuna instead of salmon.

Nutrients per serving	
Calories	299
Fat	10 g
Carbohydrate	37 g
Protein	17 g
Vitamin C	4 mg
Vitamin D	248 IU
Vitamin E	1 mg
Niacin	6 mg
Folate	56 mcg
Vitamin B$_6$	0.1 mg
Vitamin B$_{12}$	2.6 mcg
Zinc	1.1 mg
Selenium	35 mcg

- **Preheat broiler**

1	can (7$^1/_2$ oz/213 g) salmon, drained	1
$^1/_4$ cup	light mayonnaise	60 mL
2 tbsp	finely chopped green onion	30 mL
$^1/_4$ cup	finely chopped apple	60 mL
1 tbsp	freshly squeezed lemon juice	15 mL
1 tsp	finely grated gingerroot	5 mL
2 tsp	curry powder	10 mL
$^1/_2$ tsp	cayenne pepper	2 mL
4	thin whole-grain hamburger buns, split	4
3 tbsp	ginger marmalade	45 mL
1	apple, peeled and cut into 8 slices (optional)	1
1 tbsp	liquid honey (optional)	15 mL

1. In a small bowl, combine salmon, mayonnaise, green onion, chopped apple, lemon juice, ginger, curry powder and cayenne.

2. Place hamburger buns cut side up on a baking sheet. Spread each half with about 1 tsp (5 mL) ginger marmalade. Divide salmon mixture evenly on top. If desired, place 1 apple slice on top of salmon mixture and brush with honey.

3. Broil for 4 to 5 minutes or until salmon mixture is warm.

> ▶ **Health Tip**
>
> Ginger is an anti-inflammatory and anti-nausea agent and activates digestion even in people who are healthy.

This recipe courtesy of dietitian Mary Sue Waisman.

Tuna Salad Melt

This is a great use of water-packed tuna, and can turn this simple fare into a delicious weekend lunch or quick dinner.

Tips

The tuna mixture also makes a great filling for sandwiches, wraps and pita bread, as well as a great topping for salad greens or spinach.

If desired, substitute salmon for the tuna.

▶ Health Tip

Yogurt and cheese can deliver some of the calcium we need in a form that many people who don't tolerate cow's milk well can do just fine with.

Nutrients per serving	
Calories	196
Fat	3 g
Carbohydrate	24 g
Protein	17 g
Vitamin C	7 mg
Vitamin D	1 IU
Vitamin E	0 mg
Niacin	6 mg
Folate	7 mcg
Vitamin B$_6$	0.2 mg
Vitamin B$_{12}$	1.3 mcg
Zinc	0.5 mg
Selenium	36 mcg

- **Preheat broiler**
- **Large baking sheet**

2	cans (6 oz/170 g) water-packed tuna, drained	2
¼ cup	finely chopped celery	60 mL
¼ cup	finely chopped sweet pickle or sweet relish	60 mL
¼ cup	finely chopped red or green bell pepper (optional)	60 mL
¼ cup	light mayonnaise	60 mL
2 tbsp	lower-fat plain yogurt	30 mL
1 tbsp	lemon juice or pickle juice	15 mL
1	French stick (baguette)	1
½ cup	shredded Cheddar cheese	125 mL

1. In a bowl, stir together tuna, celery, pickle, red pepper (if using), mayonnaise, yogurt and lemon juice. Blend well.

2. Slice French stick in half lengthwise. Cut each half into 4 equal portions, making 8 pieces; place on baking sheet. Toast under preheated broiler for 1 to 2 minutes or until golden.

3. Remove from broiler; spread tuna mixture evenly over each piece. Sprinkle with cheese. Broil for 2 to 3 minutes or until cheese is melted and golden.

Variations

Hot Tuna Salad Wrap: Fill flour tortillas with tuna mixture and shredded cheese. Fold up and microwave on High for 30 to 45 seconds or until cheese is melted.

Cold Tuna Salad Wrap: Add any shredded or grated vegetable, such as purple cabbage, carrot, zucchini, arugula, mustard greens, kale or spinach, to the tuna mixture. Roll in a tortilla and serve.

This recipe courtesy of dietitian Bev Callaghan.

Tuna Casserole

A 21st-century take on a North American classic — supergrain quinoa and brown rice take the place of refined pasta shells in a way that transforms it.

Tip

Vegan hard margarine, such as Earth Balance Vegan Buttery Flavor Sticks, has almost half as much saturated fat as regular butter and no cholesterol. Where butter is called for in a recipe, vegan hard margarine can be a heart-healthy, delicious alternative.

Variation

Add ½ cup (125 mL) frozen peas with the rice.

- **Preheat oven to 350°F (180°C)**
- **10- by 8-inch (25 by 20 cm) casserole dish with lid, lightly greased**

1 tsp	grapeseed oil	5 mL
1 cup	chopped onion	250 mL
1 cup	chopped celery	250 mL
1 tbsp	chopped fresh parsley	15 mL
1 tsp	vegan hard margarine or butter	5 mL
1	can (6 oz/170 g) water-packed flaked tuna, drained	1
½ cup	long-grain brown rice	125 mL
½ cup	quinoa, rinsed	125 mL
2 cups	fortified gluten-free non-dairy milk or lactose-free 1% milk	500 mL

1. In a skillet, heat oil over medium-high heat. Sauté onion, celery and parsley for 3 to 5 minutes or until onion is starting to brown. Stir in margarine. Remove from heat.

2. In prepared baking dish, combine tuna, rice, quinoa and milk. Stir in onion mixture.

3. Cover and bake in preheated oven for 45 minutes or until rice and quinoa are tender and liquid is absorbed. Uncover and bake for 5 minutes or until top is browned.

> ▶ **Health Tip**
>
> Whole grains such as brown rice and quinoa combined with tuna deliver a major source of brain fuel to the body, along with a great deal of protein.

Nutrients per serving	
Calories	304
Fat	6 g
Carbohydrate	42 g
Protein	20 g
Vitamin C	5 mg
Vitamin D	57 IU
Vitamin E	2 mg
Niacin	8 mg
Folate	75 mcg
Vitamin B$_6$	0.5 mg
Vitamin B$_{12}$	2.3 mcg
Zinc	1.9 mg
Selenium	45 mcg

Lobster and Potato Supper Salad

This salad is a great choice when lobsters are seasonally priced and more readily available. If fresh lobster is not an option, it will also happily come together with frozen (thawed and drained) or even canned lobster.

Tip

Don't "over-mayo" the salad; you want to be able to really taste the lobster and potatoes.

Variation

Grill four or five lobster tails, cool, then remove the meat from the shells and chop coarsely. Substitute for the lobster meat.

5 cups	cooled cooked diced new potatoes	1.25 L
3 cups	coarsely chopped cooked lobster meat	750 mL
8 oz	snow peas, cut diagonally into thin slices	250 g
4	green onions, trimmed and chopped	4
	Salt and freshly ground black pepper	
1 cup	mayonnaise (approx.)	250 mL
3 tbsp	freshly squeezed lemon juice	45 mL
1/2 cup	chopped fresh dill	125 mL
1 to 2	heads red oak-leaf lettuce, separated	1 to 2

1. In a large bowl, combine potatoes, lobster, snow peas and green onions. Season to taste with salt and freshly ground pepper. Toss to combine.

2. In another bowl, whisk together mayonnaise and lemon juice until blended. Add to potato mixture and toss to coat (if it needs more mayonnaise, add a little more and toss again). Add dill and toss again.

3. Cover with plastic wrap and refrigerate for 1 hour or up to 3 hours. Divide leaf lettuce evenly among individual serving plates and top with potato mixture.

> ▶ **Health Tip**
>
> Lobster is a good source of vitamin B_{12}.

Nutrients per 1 of 6 servings	
Calories	337
Fat	14 g
Carbohydrate	34 g
Protein	18 g
Vitamin C	39 mg
Vitamin D	1 IU
Vitamin E	1 mg
Niacin	4 mg
Folate	59 mcg
Vitamin B_6	0.6 mg
Vitamin B_{12}	1.0 mcg
Zinc	3.5 mg
Selenium	55 mcg

Pasta with Shrimp and Peas

This is a simple gluten-free pasta dish that will come in handy at the end of a hectic day and still be worth looking forward to.

Tip

If you have fresh basil and parsley on hand, use 1 tbsp (15 mL) of each in place of dried, adding them with the Romano cheese.

12 oz	gluten-free penne or spiral pasta	375 g
3 tbsp	olive oil	45 mL
3 to 4	cloves garlic, minced	3 to 4
1 tsp	dried basil	5 mL
1 tsp	dried parsley	5 mL
Pinch	cayenne pepper	Pinch
8 oz	cooked frozen peeled shrimp	250 g
1 cup	frozen green peas	250 mL
1/4 cup	grated Romano cheese	60 mL
	Salt and freshly ground black pepper	

1. In a large pot of boiling water, cook pasta according to package instructions until tender but firm (al dente). Drain, reserving 2 cups (500 mL) of the pasta cooking water. Return pasta to the pot.

2. In a skillet, heat oil over low heat. Add garlic to taste, basil, parsley and cayenne; sauté for 3 to 5 minutes or until garlic is softened and fragrant. Add shrimp and peas; sauté for about 5 minutes or until heated through.

3. Add shrimp mixture to pasta. Add enough of the reserved pasta cooking water to moisten to desired consistency, tossing gently to coat. Stir in Romano cheese and season to taste with salt and pepper.

> ▶ **Health Tip**
>
> Make sure you buy organic or wild/sustainable shrimp, as some farm-raised shrimp come from unhealthy conditions and have many antibiotics added to their "pens."

Nutrients per 1 of 6 servings	
Calories	352
Fat	10 g
Carbohydrate	47 g
Protein	19 g
Vitamin C	5 mg
Vitamin D	2 IU
Vitamin E	2 mg
Niacin	6 mg
Folate	156 mcg
Vitamin B_6	0.4 mg
Vitamin B_{12}	0.6 mcg
Zinc	1.6 mg
Selenium	5 mcg

Shrimp, Vegetables and Whole Wheat Pasta

This is a dish that has many of the Mediterranean diet's outstanding features and is easy to make.

Variations

Change some of the vegetables for variety. You can try sugar snap peas, snow peas or spinach instead of the broccoli, or yellow pepper or carrot instead of the red pepper. Or use a frozen vegetable blend.

This dish does not have a lot of sauce. If you prefer a saucier dish, add a little pesto or a creamy tomato sauce. If using pesto, omit the Italian seasoning.

4 cups	whole wheat pasta (such as fusilli or penne)	1 L
1 tbsp	olive oil	15 mL
3	cloves garlic, minced	3
1	bunch broccoli, chopped	1
1	red bell pepper, sliced	1
2 cups	grape tomatoes, halved	500 mL
12 oz	shrimp, peeled, deveined and halved	375 g
1 tsp	dried Italian herb seasoning	5 mL
½ tsp	salt	2 mL
½ tsp	freshly ground black pepper	2 mL

1. Cook pasta according to package directions until al dente (tender to the bite). Drain.

2. Meanwhile, heat a large skillet over medium-high heat. Add oil and swirl to coat pan. Sauté garlic for 1 minute, being careful not to burn it. Add broccoli, red pepper and tomatoes; sauté for 5 to 7 minutes or until vegetables are tender-crisp. Add shrimp and cook, turning once, until opaque and slightly browned, about 4 minutes. Stir in pasta, Italian seasoning, salt and pepper.

> ▶ **Health Tip**
>
> A whole grain, olive oil, bell pepper, broccoli and garlic in one dish add up to cardiovascular-healthy eating — which is important for long-term brain health.

This recipe courtesy of dietitian Beth Gould.

Nutrients per serving	
Calories	331
Fat	4 g
Carbohydrate	59 g
Protein	20 g
Vitamin C	59 mg
Vitamin D	1 IU
Vitamin E	2 mg
Niacin	5 mg
Folate	86 mcg
Vitamin B$_6$	0.4 mg
Vitamin B$_{12}$	0.6 mcg
Zinc	2.5 mg
Selenium	18 mcg

Shrimp Risotto with Artichoke Hearts and Parmesan

The firm, nutty texture of properly cooked Arborio rice perfectly complements the meatiness of shrimp in this classic dish.

Tip

If you haven't got the time or ingredients necessary to make seafood broth from scratch, you can buy it canned or in powdered form (1 tsp/5 mL in 1 cup/250 mL boiling water yields 1 cup/250 mL broth). Keep in mind, however, that these broths are often loaded with sodium. To cut back on the sodium, try using only $\frac{1}{2}$ tsp (2 mL) powder.

3 cups	ready-to-use seafood or chicken broth	750 mL
$\frac{1}{2}$ cup	chopped onion	125 mL
2 tsp	minced garlic	10 mL
1 cup	Arborio rice	250 mL
1 tsp	dried basil	5 mL
$\frac{1}{2}$	can (14 oz/398 mL) artichoke hearts, drained and chopped	$\frac{1}{2}$
8 oz	shrimp, peeled, deveined and chopped	250 g
$\frac{1}{4}$ cup	chopped green onion	60 mL
$\frac{1}{4}$ cup	freshly grated low-fat Parmesan cheese	60 mL
$\frac{1}{4}$ tsp	freshly ground black pepper	1 mL

1. In a saucepan over medium-high heat, bring broth to a boil; reduce heat to low. In another, nonstick saucepan sprayed with vegetable spray, cook onion and garlic over medium-high heat for 3 minutes or until softened. Add rice and basil; cook for 1 minute.

2. Using a ladle, add $\frac{1}{2}$ cup (125 mL) hot broth to rice; stir constantly to keep rice from sticking to pan. When liquid is absorbed, add another $\frac{1}{2}$ cup (125 mL) broth. Reduce heat if necessary to maintain a slow, steady simmer. Repeat this process, ladling in hot broth and stirring constantly, for 15 minutes, reducing amount of broth added to $\frac{1}{4}$ cup (60 mL) near end of cooking time.

3. Add artichokes and shrimp; cook, adding more broth as necessary, for 3 minutes or until shrimp turn pink and rice is tender but firm. Add green onions, Parmesan cheese and pepper. Serve immediately.

> ▶ **Health Tip**
>
> Artichokes have been shown to have a cholesterol-lowering effect.

Nutrients per serving	
Calories	303
Fat	4 g
Carbohydrate	49 g
Protein	18 g
Vitamin C	6 mg
Vitamin D	2 IU
Vitamin E	1 mg
Niacin	6 mg
Folate	171 mcg
Vitamin B$_6$	0.3 mg
Vitamin B$_{12}$	0.9 mcg
Zinc	1.7 mg
Selenium	25 mcg

Peppery Shrimp with Quinoa

Saffron gives this dish a signature flavor. Quinoa and shrimp make it a meal in itself.

Tips

Saffron is expensive, but you never need a lot of it to make something really special.

To keep quinoa as fresh as possible, store it in an airtight container in the refrigerator for up to 6 months or in the freezer for up to 1 year.

2 tbsp	olive oil, divided	30 mL
1	onion, diced	1
1	green bell pepper, finely chopped	1
1/4 tsp	crumbled saffron threads, dissolved in 2 tbsp (30 mL) boiling water	1 mL
1/2 cup	water or ready-to-use reduced-sodium vegetable broth	125 mL
1	can (14 oz/398 mL) no-salt-added diced tomatoes, with juice	1
3/4 cup	quinoa, rinsed	175 mL
12 oz	shrimp, peeled and deveined, thawed if frozen	375 g
4	cloves garlic, minced	4
1 tsp	finely grated lemon zest	5 mL
1/4 tsp	cayenne pepper	1 mL
	Freshly ground black pepper	
1/2 cup	dry white wine	125 mL
2 tbsp	freshly squeezed lemon juice	30 mL
1 cup	cooked green peas	250 mL
	Salt (optional)	

1. In a saucepan, heat 1 tbsp (15 mL) of the oil over medium heat for 30 seconds. Add onion and bell pepper and cook, stirring, until softened, about 5 minutes. Add saffron liquid, water and tomatoes and bring to a boil. Stir in quinoa. Reduce heat to low. Cover and cook until quinoa is tender, about 15 minutes. Remove from heat and let stand, covered, for 5 minutes. Fluff with a fork.

Nutrients per serving	
Calories	331
Fat	10 g
Carbohydrate	37 g
Protein	20 g
Vitamin C	43 mg
Vitamin D	2 IU
Vitamin E	4 mg
Niacin	4 mg
Folate	115 mcg
Vitamin B_6	0.6 mg
Vitamin B_{12}	0.9 mcg
Zinc	2.3 mg
Selenium	29 mcg

Variation

Peppery Shrimp with Millet: Substitute an equal quantity of millet for the quinoa. For the best flavor, before using in the recipe, toast the rinsed millet in a dry skillet, stirring until fragrant, about 5 minutes. Stir millet into tomato mixture (step 1) and return to a boil. Cover and simmer over low heat for 20 minutes, then remove from heat and let stand for 10 minutes.

2. In a skillet, heat remaining 1 tbsp (15 mL) oil over medium-high heat. Add shrimp and cook, stirring, just until they turn pink and opaque, 3 to 5 minutes. Add garlic, lemon zest, cayenne and black pepper to taste. Cook, stirring, for 1 minute. Add white wine and lemon juice and bring to a boil. Stir in peas until heated through. Season to taste with salt (if using).

3. On a deep platter, arrange quinoa in a ring around the edge, leaving the center hollow. Arrange shrimp in the center.

▶ Health Tip

Green peas are a legume but not just a starch or carb source: pisumsaponins I and II and pisomosides A and B are anti-inflammatory compounds almost exclusive to peas.

Curry Shrimp and Shaved Carrots

Carrots peeled into ribbons give this dish an elegant appearance and an interesting texture. Serve atop fluffy brown rice with steamed asparagus as an attractive color contrast.

Tips

Test your peeling skills on a carrot before making this for guests.

Shrimp are packaged and sold according to size. The number on the package indicates the number of shrimp per lb (454 g). For example, a bag labeled "21 to 25" has 21 to 25 shrimp per lb (454 g); these will be fairly large. In a bag of shrimp labeled "51 to 60," the shrimp will be much smaller.

Nutrients per serving	
Calories	143
Fat	5 g
Carbohydrate	8 g
Protein	16 g
Vitamin C	4 mg
Vitamin D	2 IU
Vitamin E	3 mg
Niacin	3 mg
Folate	34 mcg
Vitamin B$_6$	0.3 mg
Vitamin B$_{12}$	1.3 mcg
Zinc	1.3 mg
Selenium	34 mcg

2 lbs	large shrimp, peeled and deveined	1 kg
6	cloves garlic, minced	6
3 tbsp	curry powder	45 mL
1 tbsp	canola oil	15 mL
6	carrots	6
1	can (14 oz/398 mL) light coconut milk	1
	Juice of $\frac{1}{2}$ lime	
$\frac{1}{4}$ cup	finely chopped fresh cilantro	60 mL

1. In a large bowl, combine shrimp, garlic, curry powder and oil, making sure shrimp are well coated. Marinate at room temperature for 30 minutes.

2. Meanwhile, peel outer layer from carrots. Using the vegetable peeler, press firmly against one side of a carrot to cut large ribbons. Turn carrot and continue to cut ribbons. Discard the inner core of the carrot if it seems tough. Repeat with the remaining carrots. You should have about 6 cups (1.5 L) loosely packed carrot curls.

3. Heat a large skillet over medium-high heat. Add half the shrimp and cook for 1 to 2 minutes or until shrimp turn pink. Turn shrimp over and cook for 1 to 2 minutes or until almost firm. Transfer to a plate and keep warm. Repeat with the remaining shrimp.

4. Return all shrimp to the skillet and add carrot ribbons and coconut milk; bring to a boil. Reduce heat and simmer for 2 minutes or until carrots are tender and shrimp are opaque. Sprinkle with lime juice and serve garnished with cilantro.

> **▶ Health Tip**
>
> Cilantro is known in herbal medicine as a "carminative" — it aids digestion and relaxes the stomach after a meal.

This recipe courtesy of Candace Ivanco-Boutot.

Shrimp Omelet

This seafood omelet makes a quick brunch or supper dish. Serve it with a simple green salad.

Makes 2 servings

Variation

Oyster Omelet:
Replace the shrimp with 6 shucked oysters, drained and patted dry. Stir-fry for 1 minute, or until just set, before adding eggs.

3	large eggs	3
2 tbsp	water	30 mL
2 tsp	fish sauce (nam pla)	10 mL
1 tbsp	vegetable oil	15 mL
2	cloves garlic, chopped	2
1	shallot, chopped	1
1	green onion, chopped	1
8 oz	shrimp, diced	250 g

1. In a bowl, beat together eggs, water and fish sauce.

2. Heat oil in an 8- to 10-inch (20 to 25 cm) skillet over medium-high heat. Add garlic, shallot and green onion and stir-fry for 30 seconds. Add shrimp and stir-fry for 1 minute.

3. Add egg mixture. Swirl around shrimp and cook for 2 to 3 minutes, or until eggs are firm and golden brown on bottom. Flip omelet and cook for 2 minutes on second side.

> ▶ **Health Tip**
>
> Shrimp are a good source of zinc, copper and protein. Try to purchase wild-caught shrimp or responsibly raised farmed shrimp from a clean source of water.

Nutrients per serving	
Calories	258
Fat	15 g
Carbohydrate	3 g
Protein	25 g
Vitamin C	2 mg
Vitamin D	64 IU
Vitamin E	4 mg
Niacin	2 mg
Folate	62 mcg
Vitamin B_6	0.4 mg
Vitamin B_{12}	2.0 mcg
Zinc	2.1 mg
Selenium	58 mcg

Pad Thai

Here is the classic and perhaps most familiar Thai dish to many North Americans. This version requires some specialty ingredients, but they give it authentic Thai flavor.

Tips

To get the most juice from citrus fruits, let them warm up for about 15 minutes, then roll them on the counter a few times before juicing.

For 3 tbsp (45 mL) lime juice, you'll need 2 to 3 medium limes.

8 oz	dried medium rice noodles	250 g
3 tbsp	ready-to-use chicken broth, ketchup or tomato sauce	45 mL
3 tbsp	freshly squeezed lime juice or tamarind paste	45 mL
2 tbsp	fish sauce (nam pla)	30 mL
2 tbsp	palm sugar or packed brown sugar	30 mL
½ tsp	hot chili sauce	2 mL
3 tbsp	vegetable oil, divided	45 mL
2	large eggs, beaten	2
3	cloves garlic, chopped	3
4 oz	shrimp, peeled, deveined and cut into small pieces	125 g
4 oz	boneless chicken or pork, cut into small pieces	125 g
2 cups	bean sprouts, divided	500 mL
2	green onions, chopped	2
¼ cup	chopped peanuts	60 mL
¼ cup	chopped fresh cilantro leaves	60 mL
	Fresh red chile peppers, cut into strips (optional)	
1	lime, cut into wedges	1

1. To soften noodles, place in a large bowl. Cover with very hot water and let stand for 10 to 12 minutes or until softened but still firm (pinch them to check). Rinse well with cold water and drain.

2. In a small bowl or measuring cup, combine broth, lime juice, fish sauce, sugar and chili sauce.

3. Heat a wok or large skillet over medium-high heat and add 1 tbsp (30 mL) oil. Add beaten eggs to hot pan and swirl to coat bottom of pan. Cook until starting to set, then stir to break into pieces. Remove from wok and reserve.

Nutrients per serving	
Calories	579
Fat	25 g
Carbohydrate	67 g
Protein	26 g
Vitamin C	16 mg
Vitamin D	23 IU
Vitamin E	4 mg
Niacin	8 mg
Folate	113 mcg
Vitamin B$_6$	0.5 mg
Vitamin B$_{12}$	0.7 mcg
Zinc	2.7 mg
Selenium	31 mcg

Tip

Make sure you buy organic or wild/ sustainable shrimp, as some farm-raised shrimp come from unhealthy conditions and have many antibiotics added to their "pens."

4. Add remaining oil to wok. When hot, add garlic, shrimp and chicken and stir-fry for 2 minutes, or until shrimp and chicken are just cooked. Stir in noodles and reserved sauce mixture and cook for 1 to 2 minutes, or until noodles are soft but not mushy.

5. Add 1 cup (250 mL) bean sprouts and cooked eggs and toss to combine.

6. Turn noodles onto a serving platter. Sprinkle with remaining bean sprouts, green onions, peanuts, cilantro and chiles (if using). Garnish with lime wedges.

> **▶ Health Tip**
>
> Tamarind has traditionally been used for gastrointestinal and liver problems.

Steamed Shrimp-Stuffed Tofu with Broccoli

If you want to eat more tofu for its health benefits, this adaptation of a classic Cantonese recipe should convince you that it can also be delicious.

Makes 4 servings

Tip

Before placing the tofu on the plate, make sure it will fit in your steamer.

• **Preheat steamer over medium-high heat**

8 oz	shrimp, coarsely chopped	250 g
1 tsp	minced gingerroot	5 mL
½ cup	water chestnuts, finely chopped	125 mL
2 tbsp	finely chopped green onion	30 mL
1	large egg white, beaten	1
¼ tsp	salt	1 mL
1 tbsp	cornstarch	15 mL
1 lb	soft tofu, drained	500 g
2 cups	broccoli florets, cut into bite-sized pieces	500 mL
2 tbsp	soy sauce	30 mL
1 tbsp	ready-to-use chicken broth	15 mL
2 tsp	sesame oil	10 mL
Pinch	granulated sugar	Pinch

1. In a mixing bowl, combine shrimp, gingerroot, water chestnuts, green onion, egg white, salt and cornstarch; mix well and set aside.

2. Gently cut tofu in half lengthwise, then slice each half into ½-inch (1 cm) thick slices. Pat dry with paper towels. Lay tofu in a single layer in the center of a plate (see tip, at left) and line the outside with a ring of broccoli florets. Spoon a portion (about 1 tbsp/15 mL) of shrimp stuffing onto each slice of tofu, pressing gently with the back of the spoon so it sticks to the tofu. Place plate in preheated steamer, cover and steam for 5 minutes or until shrimp mixture is firm to the touch.

3. In a small saucepan over medium-high heat, combine soy sauce, broth, sesame oil and sugar; heat just until boiling. Pour sauce evenly over cooked tofu and broccoli; serve immediately.

> ▶ **Health Tip**
>
> Tofu is a source of genistein, a compound that may promote cardiovascular health.

Nutrients per serving	
Calories	175
Fat	7 g
Carbohydrate	11 g
Protein	18 g
Vitamin C	35 mg
Vitamin D	1 IU
Vitamin E	1 mg
Niacin	2 mg
Folate	93 mcg
Vitamin B$_6$	0.3 mg
Vitamin B$_{12}$	0.6 mcg
Zinc	1.6 mg
Selenium	30 mcg

Meaty Mains

Rosemary Chicken Breasts with Sweet Potatoes and Onions

This dish makes good use of fragrant rosemary, added two ways.

Makes 4 servings

Tips

Make extra batches of rosemary butter, shape into small logs, wrap in plastic wrap and store in the freezer. Cut into slices and use to tuck under the breast skin of whole roasting chickens or Cornish hens, or to top grilled meats.

If you purchased whole breasts with backs on, cut away the backbone using poultry shears.

This recipe can easily be halved to serve 2.

Nutrients per serving	
Calories	251
Fat	9 g
Carbohydrate	15 g
Protein	26 g
Vitamin C	5 mg
Vitamin D	10 IU
Vitamin E	1 mg
Niacin	13 mg
Folate	16 mcg
Vitamin B$_6$	1.1 mg
Vitamin B$_{12}$	0.3 mcg
Zinc	0.9 mg
Selenium	38 mcg

- **Preheat oven to 375°F (190°C)**
- **13- by 9-inch (33 by 23 cm) baking dish, greased**

2	sweet potatoes (about 1½ lbs/750 g)	2
1	onion	1
1½ tsp	chopped fresh rosemary (or ½ tsp/ 2 mL dried rosemary, crumbled)	7 mL
	Salt and freshly ground black pepper	
4	skin-on bone-in chicken breasts	4

Rosemary Butter

2 tbsp	butter	30 mL
1	large clove garlic, minced	1
1 tsp	grated lemon zest	5 mL
2 tsp	chopped fresh rosemary (or ¾ tsp/ 3 mL dried rosemary, crumbled)	10 mL
¼ tsp	salt	1 mL
¼ tsp	freshly ground black pepper	1 mL

1. Peel sweet potatoes and onion; cut into thin slices. Layer in prepared baking dish. Season with rosemary and salt and pepper to taste.

2. *Rosemary Butter:* In a small bowl, mash together butter, garlic, lemon zest, rosemary, salt and pepper. Divide into four portions.

3. Place chicken breasts, skin side up, on work surface. Remove any fat deposits under skin. Press down on breast bone to flatten slightly. Carefully loosen the breast skin and tuck rosemary butter under skin, patting to distribute evenly.

4. Arrange chicken on top of vegetables in baking dish. Roast for 45 to 55 minutes or until vegetables are tender and chicken is nicely colored.

> ▶ **Health Tip**
> Rosemary contains rosmarinic acid, a compound that helps the body carry out detoxificiation reactions.

Three-Spice Chicken with Potatoes

Chicken thighs tend to stay moist while cooking — all the better to absorb the rich spice flavors in this dish.

Makes 8 servings

Tips

To toast coriander seeds, spread them in a dry heavy skillet. Cook over medium heat, shaking skillet occasionally to toast evenly, until seeds are a little darker and aromatic, 4 to 5 minutes. Let cool. Grind to a powder in a spice grinder.

A quick way to seed cardamoms is to put the whole pods into a spice grinder or blender jar. With a few on-off pulse motions, the skins will come loose. Remove and discard skins.

Nutrients per serving	
Calories	349
Fat	13 g
Carbohydrate	28 g
Protein	30 g
Vitamin C	32 mg
Vitamin D	7 IU
Vitamin E	2 mg
Niacin	11 mg
Folate	43 mcg
Vitamin B$_6$	0.8 mg
Vitamin B$_{12}$	0.5 mcg
Zinc	3.3 mg
Selenium	20 mcg

6	potatoes	6
16	boneless skinless chicken thighs (about 4 lbs/2 kg)	16
¼ cup	vegetable oil	60 mL
⅓ cup	coriander seeds, freshly toasted and powdered in spice grinder (see tip, at left)	75 mL
¼ cup	cardamom seeds, coarsely pounded (see tip, at left)	60 mL
1 tbsp	black peppercorns, coarsely pounded	15 mL
1¼ tsp	salt (or to taste)	6 mL
	Cherry tomatoes, halved	

1. In a saucepan of boiling water, cook whole potatoes with skins on until tender, 20 to 25 minutes. Drain. When cool enough to handle, peel and cut into quarters. Set aside.

2. Rinse chicken and pat dry. In a large wok or saucepan with a tight-fitting lid, heat oil over medium-high heat. Add chicken.

3. Mix together coriander powder, cardamom seeds, pepper and salt. Sprinkle evenly over chicken. Reduce heat to medium. Cover and cook, shaking pan occasionally to prevent sticking. Do not stir. (There will be a fair amount of liquid from the chicken as it cooks.) After 8 to 10 minutes, when there is no more liquid, add potatoes. Brown chicken and potatoes gently. If chicken is not cooked, add 2 to 3 tbsp (30 to 45 mL) water. Cover and cook over low heat until potatoes are tender and chicken is no longer pink inside, 10 to 12 minutes.

4. *To serve:* Mound on a platter and garnish with halved cherry tomatoes.

> ▶ **Health Tip**
>
> In Ayurvedic medicine, cardamom has been used for centuries to treat indigestion.

Chicken Paprika with Noodles

If you haven't tried chicken paprika yet (or chicken paprikash, in a Hungarian restaurant), you're missing out. This recipe will get you started.

Makes 4 servings

Tip

When ground chicken or turkey is browned in a skillet, it doesn't turn into a fine crumble like other ground meats. Overcome the problem by placing the cooked chicken in a food processor and chopping it using on-off turns to break up lumps.

1 lb	lean ground chicken or turkey	500 g
1 tbsp	butter	15 mL
1	onion, chopped	1
8 oz	mushrooms, sliced	250 g
1 tbsp	paprika	15 mL
2 tbsp	all-purpose flour	30 mL
1⅓ cups	ready-to-use chicken broth	325 mL
½ cup	sour cream	125 mL
2 tbsp	chopped fresh dill or parsley	30 mL
	Salt and freshly ground black pepper	
8 oz	fettuccine or broad egg noodles	250 g

1. In a large nonstick skillet over medium-high heat, cook chicken, breaking up with a wooden spoon, for 5 minutes or until no longer pink. Transfer to a bowl.

2. Melt butter in skillet. Add onion, mushrooms and paprika; cook, stirring often, for 3 minutes or until vegetables are softened.

3. Sprinkle with flour; stir in broth and return chicken to skillet. Bring to a boil; cook, stirring, until thickened. Reduce heat, cover and simmer for 5 minutes. Remove from heat and stir in sour cream (it may curdle if added over the heat) and dill; season with salt and pepper to taste.

4. Meanwhile, cook pasta in a large pot of boiling salted water until tender but firm. Drain well. Return to pot and toss with chicken mixture. Serve immediately.

> ▶ **Health Tip**
>
> Paprika comes from members of the capsicum family, but most varieties used or sold as spice are not very hot (though some can be). It is loaded with carotenoids such as lutein and zeaxanthin.

Nutrients per serving	
Calories	501
Fat	17 g
Carbohydrate	56 g
Protein	32 g
Vitamin C	2 mg
Vitamin D	7 IU
Vitamin E	1 mg
Niacin	16 mg
Folate	178 mcg
Vitamin B$_6$	0.8 mg
Vitamin B$_{12}$	0.9 mcg
Zinc	3.2 mg
Selenium	50 mcg

Garlic Chicken

In Thailand, this recipe would be made with whole chicken pieces with skin, but this version uses boneless skinless chicken breasts. Serve any leftover chicken in salads or sandwiches.

Makes 4 servings

Variation

Garlic Tofu: Replace chicken with 12 oz (375 g) firm tofu cut into ½-inch (1 cm) slices. For a vegetarian version, replace fish sauce with soy sauce. Marinate for up to 3 hours. Grill for 3 to 4 minutes per side, or until golden.

- **Food processor**

4	cloves garlic, peeled	4
2	shallots, peeled	2
1 cup	packed fresh cilantro leaves, stems and roots	250 mL
3 tbsp	freshly squeezed lime or lemon juice	45 mL
2 tsp	fish sauce (nam pla)	10 mL
1 tsp	freshly ground black pepper	5 mL
4	boneless skinless chicken breasts (each about 6 oz/175 g)	4

1. In food processor, combine garlic, shallots, cilantro, lime juice, fish sauce and pepper; process until smooth.

2. Place chicken breasts in a shallow dish. Pour marinade over chicken and turn to coat. Cover and marinate in refrigerator for 2 hours or overnight.

3. Preheat barbecue grill to high.

4. Remove chicken from marinade, discarding marinade. Grill chicken for 6 minutes per side or until no longer pink inside, being careful not to overcook. Serve hot, warm or cold.

> ▶ **Health Tip**
>
> Garlic has some beneficial effects on blood cholesterol, especially fresh garlic that was chopped just before using.

Nutrients per serving	
Calories	205
Fat	5 g
Carbohydrate	3 g
Protein	37 g
Vitamin C	7 mg
Vitamin D	9 IU
Vitamin E	0 mg
Niacin	18 mg
Folate	10 mcg
Vitamin B$_6$	1.3 mg
Vitamin B$_{12}$	0.4 mcg
Zinc	1.1 mg
Selenium	55 mcg

Red Curry Chicken with Snap Peas and Cashews

This dish is a delicious and spicy way to satisfy a craving for Thai curry.

Makes 4 servings

Tips

If lime leaves aren't available, substitute 1/2 tsp (2 mL) finely grated lime zest and add with the lime juice in step 2.

The cashews give the best texture to the sauce if pulsed in a food processor to a coarse meal (without processing too much, into butter). You may need to use more than 1/4 cup (60 mL), depending on the size of your food processor. Extra ground nuts can be frozen for future use.

1 tbsp	vegetable oil	15 mL
1	red or yellow bell pepper, thinly sliced	1
1 cup	sugar snap peas or frozen green peas	250 mL
2	wild lime leaves (see tip, at left)	2
1/4 cup	salted roasted cashews, ground or finely chopped (see tip, at left)	60 mL
1 tbsp	packed brown sugar or palm sugar	15 mL
1	can (14 oz/400 mL) coconut milk	1
1/4 cup	water	60 mL
1 tbsp	Thai red curry paste	15 mL
1 lb	boneless skinless chicken breasts or thighs, cut into thin strips	500 g
2 tbsp	freshly squeezed lime juice	30 mL
	Salt	
	Salted roasted cashews	
	Chopped fresh mint and/or Thai basil	
	Lime wedges	

1. In a large skillet, heat oil over medium heat. Add red pepper, peas and lime leaves; cook, stirring, until pepper is starting to soften, about 1 minute. Add ground cashews, brown sugar, coconut milk, water and curry paste; bring to a boil, stirring until blended. Reduce heat and boil gently, stirring often, until slightly thickened, about 2 minutes.

2. Stir in chicken and return to a simmer, stirring. Reduce heat and simmer gently, stirring often, until chicken is no longer pink inside and peas are tender-crisp, about 5 minutes. Discard lime leaves, if desired. Stir in lime juice and season to taste with salt. Serve sprinkled with cashews, mint and/or basil and garnished with lime wedges to squeeze over top.

> ▶ **Health Tip**
>
> Coconut milk provides a useful vehicle for absorption of the beneficial compounds in the curry paste.

Nutrients per serving	
Calories	328
Fat	29 g
Carbohydrate	16 g
Protein	5 g
Vitamin C	47 mg
Vitamin D	0 IU
Vitamin E	1 mg
Niacin	2 mg
Folate	52 mcg
Vitamin B$_6$	0.2 mg
Vitamin B$_{12}$	0.0 mcg
Zinc	1.4 mg
Selenium	2 mcg

Curried Chicken Salad Wraps

Chicken salad has never been so lively — it's amazing what a bit of curry can do.

Makes 10 wraps

Tips

Stuff this chicken mixture into mini pita breads for a tasty appetizer. It also makes a great sandwich filling for pumpernickel bread.

If you don't have any cooked chicken on hand, pick up a cooked chicken at the grocery store. One cooked deli chicken yields about 3 cups (750 mL) cubed cooked chicken.

You can substitute cooked turkey for the chicken — a great way to use up Christmas or Thanksgiving leftovers.

3 cups	cubed cooked chicken	750 mL
1 cup	chopped celery	250 mL
1 cup	halved seedless red or green grapes	250 mL
½ cup	toasted slivered almonds	125 mL
1 tbsp	freshly squeezed lemon juice	15 mL
¾ tsp	curry powder	3 mL
⅔ cup	light mayonnaise	150 mL
	Salt and freshly ground black pepper	
10	lettuce leaves	10
10	large (10-inch/25 cm) flour tortillas	10

1. In a large bowl, stir together chicken, celery, grapes, almonds, lemon juice, curry powder and mayonnaise. Season to taste with salt and pepper.

2. Place 1 lettuce leaf on each tortilla. Divide chicken mixture evenly along center of each lettuce leaf. Fold up bottom and roll up tortilla.

> ▶ **Health Tip**
>
> Curcuminoids from the turmeric in the curry powder are very beneficial (anti-inflammatory), and a food with fatty acids in it — mayonnaise in this case — is excellent for their absorption, as is the ground pepper.

This recipe courtesy of Cheryl Wren.

Nutrients per wrap	
Calories	403
Fat	15 g
Carbohydrate	46 g
Protein	21 g
Vitamin C	5 mg
Vitamin D	3 IU
Vitamin E	2 mg
Niacin	9 mg
Folate	107 mcg
Vitamin B_6	0.3 mg
Vitamin B_{12}	0.1 mcg
Zinc	1.2 mg
Selenium	29 mcg

Turkey Cutlets in Gingery Lemon Gravy with Cranberry Rice

This dish combines two foods — cranberry and turkey — that many of us have great associations with, but it does so in a way that is unique, gluten-free and chock-full of valuable phytonutrients.

Makes 4 servings

Tips

If you prefer a bit of heat, use hot rather than sweet paprika when dredging the turkey.

One medium orange yields about 1 1/2 tbsp (22 mL) zest and 1/3 to 1/2 cup (75 to 125 mL) juice.

Cranberry Rice

1 1/4 cups	water or ready-to-use reduced-sodium chicken broth	300 mL
1 tsp	grated orange zest	5 mL
2 tbsp	freshly squeezed orange juice	30 mL
3/4 cup	long-grain brown rice, rinsed and drained	175 mL
1/3 cup	dried cranberries	75 mL

Turkey Cutlets

2 tbsp	sorghum flour	30 mL
1 tbsp	cornstarch	15 mL
1 tsp	paprika	5 mL
1/2 tsp	freshly ground black pepper	2 mL
4	turkey cutlets (about 12 oz/375 g total)	4
2 tbsp	olive oil, divided	30 mL
1 tbsp	butter, divided	15 mL
2	cloves garlic, minced	2
1 tbsp	minced gingerroot	15 mL
1 cup	ready-to-use reduced-sodium chicken broth	250 mL
1 tbsp	freshly squeezed lemon juice	15 mL

1. *Cranberry Rice:* In a heavy saucepan with a tight-fitting lid, bring water and orange juice to a boil over medium heat. Stir in rice and return to a boil. Reduce heat to low. Cover and simmer until rice is tender and water has been absorbed, about 50 minutes. Remove from heat and fluff with a fork. Stir in cranberries and orange zest and keep warm.

2. *Turkey Cutlets:* On a plate or in a plastic bag, combine sorghum flour, cornstarch, paprika and pepper. Add turkey and toss until well coated with mixture. Reserve any excess.

Nutrients per serving	
Calories	385
Fat	13 g
Carbohydrate	43 g
Protein	25 g
Vitamin C	7 mg
Vitamin D	2 IU
Vitamin E	2 mg
Niacin	8 mg
Folate	18 mcg
Vitamin B_6	0.7 mg
Vitamin B_{12}	0.5 mcg
Zinc	2.2 mg
Selenium	29 mcg

Variation

Chicken Cutlets in Gingery Lemon Gravy with Cranberry Rice: Substitute an equal quantity of chicken cutlets for the turkey.

3. In a large skillet, heat 1 tbsp (15 mL) of the oil and $1\frac{1}{2}$ tsp (7 mL) of the butter over medium-high heat until butter has melted. Add 2 cutlets and cook until browned, about 2 minutes. Turn and cook until no longer pink inside, about 2 minutes more. Transfer to a warm platter and keep warm. Repeat with remaining cutlets, oil and butter. Reduce heat to medium.

4. Add garlic and ginger to pan and cook, stirring, for 1 minute. Add reserved flour mixture and cook, stirring, for 1 minute. Add broth, lemon juice and any turkey juices that have accumulated on the platter; cook, stirring, until thickened, about 2 minutes. Pour over cutlets. Serve on a bed of Cranberry Rice.

▶ Health Tips

Cranberries are packed with brain-protecting antioxidants.

In addition to being protein-rich, turkey is also a good source of important B vitamins — niacin, B_6 and B_{12} — as well as zinc, an immune-system protector that can be challenging to obtain from dietary sources. The body can utilize the zinc in turkey and other meats more readily than that from non-meat sources.

Barbecued Lemongrass Pork

This fragrant spiced take on pork will add some variety to your table.

Tip

If you're watching your sodium intake, look for reduced-sodium soy sauce, now readily available at grocery stores.

3 tbsp	coconut milk	45 mL
3 tbsp	finely chopped lemongrass (white part only)	45 mL
2	cloves garlic, minced	2
1	green onion, finely chopped	1
2 tbsp	fish sauce (nam pla)	30 mL
1 tbsp	soy sauce	15 mL
1 tbsp	granulated sugar	15 mL
2 tsp	sesame oil	10 mL
1/2 tsp	coarsely chopped fresh red chile peppers	2 mL
1/2 tsp	freshly ground black pepper	2 mL
1	pork tenderloin (about 12 oz/375 g), trimmed and cut crosswise into 1/2-inch (1 cm) slices	1

1. In a bowl, combine coconut milk, lemongrass, garlic, green onion, fish sauce, soy sauce, sugar, sesame oil, chiles and pepper.

2. Arrange pork slices in a shallow dish. Pour marinade over meat and turn pork to coat all sides. Cover and marinate, refrigerated, for several hours.

3. Grill pork for 4 to 6 minutes per side, or until no longer pink.

> ▶ **Health Tip**
>
> Lemongrass is full of essential oils that have numerous effects (antioxidant and anti-inflammatory) in the body.

Nutrients per serving	
Calories	168
Fat	8 g
Carbohydrate	6 g
Protein	19 g
Vitamin C	1 mg
Vitamin D	9 IU
Vitamin E	0 mg
Niacin	6 mg
Folate	11 mcg
Vitamin B_6	0.7 mg
Vitamin B_{12}	0.5 mcg
Zinc	1.8 mg
Selenium	27 mcg

Saucy Swiss Steak

Swiss steak evokes a memory of warm kitchens, hot ovens and comfort food on a cold winter's day. But you can enjoy this dish anytime.

Makes 8 servings

Tip

This dish can be partially prepared the night before. Complete step 2, heating 1 tbsp (15 mL) oil in pan before softening onions, carrot and celery. Cover and refrigerate mixture overnight. The next morning, brown steak (step 1), or skip this step and place steak directly in stoneware. Continue cooking as directed. Alternatively, cook steak overnight and refrigerate. When ready to serve, bring to a boil in a large skillet and simmer for 10 minutes, until meat is heated through and sauce is bubbling.

Nutrients per serving	
Calories	224
Fat	8 g
Carbohydrate	11 g
Protein	26 g
Vitamin C	14 mg
Vitamin D	0 IU
Vitamin E	2 mg
Niacin	8 mg
Folate	21 mcg
Vitamin B$_6$	0.9 mg
Vitamin B$_{12}$	4.9 mcg
Zinc	4.7 mg
Selenium	37 mcg

- **Slow cooker**

1 tbsp	vegetable oil	15 mL
2 lbs	round steak or simmering steak	1 kg
2	onions, finely chopped	2
1/4 cup	thinly sliced carrot	60 mL
1/4 cup	thinly sliced celery	60 mL
1/2 tsp	salt	2 mL
1/4 tsp	freshly ground black pepper	1 mL
2 tbsp	all-purpose flour	30 mL
1	can (28 oz/796 mL) tomatoes, drained and chopped, 1/2 cup (125 mL) juice reserved	1
1 tbsp	Worcestershire sauce	15 mL
1	bay leaf	1

1. In a skillet, heat oil over medium-high heat. Add steak, in pieces if necessary, and brown on both sides. Transfer to slow cooker stoneware.

2. Reduce heat to medium-low. Add onion, carrot, celery, salt and pepper to pan. Cover and cook until vegetables are softened, about 8 minutes. Sprinkle flour over vegetables and cook for 1 minute, stirring. Add tomatoes, reserved juice and Worcestershire sauce. Bring to a boil, stirring until slightly thickened. Add bay leaf.

3. Pour tomato mixture over steak and cook on Low for 8 to 10 hours or on High for 4 to 5 hours, until meat is tender. Discard bay leaf.

> ▶ **Health Tip**
>
> Although it's not necessary to eat beef every day, it's an excellent source of heme iron, which is easily absorbed and helps maintain normal hemoglobin levels in the body — especially important for elderly people and those with a history of anemia.

Beef with Broccoli

This classic stir-fry has the right seasonings, including the oyster sauce, to bring out the best in beef.

Makes 4 to 6 servings

Tip

When preparing food for stir-frying, cut it into small pieces of approximately equal size so that they will cook through rapidly and in the same length of time. Have the sauce and ingredients prepared and easily accessible before starting to cook.

1 lb	sirloin steak, cut into thin strips	500 g
1/4 cup	soy sauce	60 mL
2 tbsp	cornstarch, divided	30 mL
1	clove garlic, minced	1
1	thin slice gingerroot, minced	1
2 tbsp	safflower oil, divided	30 mL
2	onions, cut into wedges	2
3	large carrots, sliced into coins	3
1	head broccoli, cut into florets	1
1 1/4 cups	water, divided	300 mL
1 tbsp	oyster sauce	15 mL
1 tsp	granulated sugar	5 mL

1. Place steak in a medium bowl. In a separate bowl, combine soy sauce, 1 tbsp (15 mL) of the cornstarch, garlic and ginger; pour over steak.

2. In a wok or nonstick skillet, heat 1 tbsp (15 mL) of the oil over high heat. Add beef and stir-fry until browned. Set aside.

3. In wok, heat remaining oil over high heat. Add onions and stir-fry for 1 minute. Add carrots, broccoli and 1 cup (250 mL) of the water; cover and steam for 4 minutes.

4. Combine remaining water, oyster sauce, remaining cornstarch and sugar. Stir sauce into wok; cook until smooth and thickened. Return meat to wok. Reheat to serving temperature.

> ▶ **Health Tip**
>
> Broccoli has important cancer- and aging-preventive compounds, and this dish is a way to get a full serving.

This recipe courtesy of M. Kathy Dyck.

Nutrients per 1 of 6 servings	
Calories	216
Fat	8 g
Carbohydrate	17 g
Protein	21 g
Vitamin C	94 mg
Vitamin D	2 IU
Vitamin E	3 mg
Niacin	6 mg
Folate	87 mcg
Vitamin B$_6$	0.8 mg
Vitamin B$_{12}$	0.7 mcg
Zinc	3.6 mg
Selenium	26 mcg

Orange Ginger Beef

This dish balances the heaviness of beef with an array of aromatic spices, including fresh cilantro.

Tips

Eye of round is a lean cut of beef. Marinating it before cooking maximizes its tenderness.

Be sure not to crowd the beef while sautéing it, or it will steam instead of browning. You may need to brown it in three batches if you have a smaller skillet.

Variation

Use trimmed snow peas instead of mushrooms.

2 tbsp	minced gingerroot	30 mL
1 tbsp	minced garlic	15 mL
1 tsp	freshly ground black pepper	5 mL
2 tbsp	canola oil, divided	30 mL
1 tbsp	hoisin sauce	15 mL
1 lb	beef eye of round marinating steak, cut into 3- by 1/2-inch strips (7.5 by 1 cm)	500 g
1 tbsp	cornstarch	15 mL
1 tbsp	grated orange zest	15 mL
3/4 cup	orange juice	175 mL
2 cups	quartered mushrooms	500 mL
2 tbsp	chopped fresh cilantro	30 mL

1. In a shallow bowl, combine ginger, garlic, pepper, 1 tbsp (15 mL) of the oil and hoisin sauce. Add beef and stir to coat well. Cover and refrigerate for at least 4 hours or up to 12 hours.

2. Drain marinade from beef, discarding marinade. Pat beef strips dry with paper towels. Heat a large nonstick skillet over medium heat. Add half the beef and sauté for 3 to 4 minutes or until lightly browned. Transfer to a bowl and set aside. Repeat with the remaining beef.

3. In a small bowl, whisk together cornstarch and orange juice.

4. Add the remaining oil to skillet and sauté mushrooms for 3 to 4 minutes or until lightly browned. Return beef and accumulated juices to skillet. Stir in cornstarch mixture and cook, stirring, for about 3 minutes or until sauce is thickened. Serve garnished with orange zest and cilantro.

> ▶ **Health Tip**
>
> Cilantro contains helpful compounds called bioflavonoids.

This recipe courtesy of dietitian Jennifer Garus.

Nutrients per serving	
Calories	289
Fat	14 g
Carbohydrate	13 g
Protein	26 g
Vitamin C	26 mg
Vitamin D	2 IU
Vitamin E	1 mg
Niacin	10 mg
Folate	38 mcg
Vitamin B$_6$	0.9 mg
Vitamin B$_{12}$	4.9 mcg
Zinc	4.7 mg
Selenium	38 mcg

Shepherd's Pie
with Creamy Corn Filling

Shepherd's pie is an old-time favorite for many people. This version leaves behind the bland and brings out the flavor with black pepper, paprika and garlic.

Makes 6 servings

Tip

This dish can be partially prepared the night before it is cooked. Make mashed potatoes, cover and refrigerate. Complete steps 1 and 2, chilling cooked meat and onion mixture separately. Refrigerate overnight. The next morning, continue cooking as directed in step 3.

Nutrients per serving	
Calories	366
Fat	14 g
Carbohydrate	38 g
Protein	23 g
Vitamin C	21 mg
Vitamin D	19 IU
Vitamin E	1 mg
Niacin	7 mg
Folate	65 mcg
Vitamin B$_6$	0.6 mg
Vitamin B$_{12}$	1.9 mcg
Zinc	4.8 mg
Selenium	18 mcg

- **Slow cooker**

1 tbsp	vegetable oil	15 mL
1 lb	lean ground beef	500 g
2	onions, finely chopped	2
4	cloves garlic, minced	4
2 tsp	paprika	10 mL
1 tsp	salt (optional)	5 mL
1/2 tsp	cracked black peppercorns	2 mL
2 tbsp	all-purpose flour	30 mL
1 cup	condensed beef broth (undiluted)	250 mL
2 tbsp	tomato paste	30 mL
1	can (19 oz/540 mL) cream-style corn	1
4 cups	mashed potatoes, seasoned with 1 tbsp (15 mL) butter, 1/2 tsp (2 mL) salt (optional) and 1/4 tsp (1 mL) freshly ground black pepper	1 L
1/4 cup	shredded Cheddar cheese	60 mL

1. In a skillet, heat oil over medium-high heat. Add beef and cook, breaking up with the back of a spoon, until meat is no longer pink. Using a slotted spoon, transfer to slow cooker stoneware. Drain off liquid.

2. Reduce heat to medium. Add onions to pan and cook until softened. Add garlic, paprika, salt (if using) and pepper and cook, stirring, for 1 minute. Sprinkle flour over mixture, stir and cook for 1 minute. Add beef broth and tomato paste, stir to combine and cook, stirring, until thickened.

3. Transfer mixture to slow cooker stoneware. Spread corn evenly over mixture and top with mashed potatoes. Sprinkle cheese on top, cover and cook on Low for 4 to 6 hours or on High for 3 to 4 hours, until hot and bubbly.

> ### ▶ Health Tip
> Beef is very high in iron and the B vitamins, important for many functions in the body, including energy use in the brain.

Blue Cheese–Stuffed Sweet and Spicy Meatloaf

The heat from the cayenne is nicely offset by the creamy melted blue cheese in this modern take on a classic.

Makes 10 slices

Tips

Make sure the cayenne pepper is evenly distributed throughout the meat mixture.

If you're feeling adventurous, try using up to 4 tsp (20 mL) cayenne pepper.

This meatloaf makes great sandwiches for lunch. Keep your sandwich safe by packing it with a freezer pack in an insulated lunch box.

Variation

Use extra-lean ground pork instead of beef.

Nutrients per slice	
Calories	121
Fat	4 g
Carbohydrate	11 g
Protein	12 g
Vitamin C	0 mg
Vitamin D	2 IU
Vitamin E	1 mg
Niacin	3 mg
Folate	8 mcg
Vitamin B$_6$	0.2 mg
Vitamin B$_{12}$	1.1 mcg
Zinc	2.7 mg
Selenium	13 mcg

- **Preheat oven to 350°F (180°C)**
- **9- by 5-inch (23 by 12.5 cm) metal loaf pan**

1 lb	extra-lean ground beef	500 g
1	large egg, beaten	1
3/4 cup	natural bran	175 mL
1/3 cup	finely chopped dried cranberries	75 mL
1/3 cup	finely chopped dried apricots	75 mL
2 tsp	cayenne pepper	10 mL
1 tsp	freshly ground black pepper	5 mL
1/2 tsp	salt	2 mL
1 1/2 oz	blue cheese, cut into 6 pieces	45 g

1. In a large bowl, gently combine beef, egg, bran, cranberries, apricots, cayenne, black pepper and salt.

2. Lightly pack three-quarters of the beef mixture into the loaf pan. Make a valley 1 inch (2.5 cm) wide by 1/2 inch (1 cm) deep in the middle of the loaf. Arrange blue cheese pieces evenly along the valley and cover with the remaining beef mixture, encasing the blue cheese.

3. Bake in preheated oven for 25 to 30 minutes or until an instant-read thermometer inserted in the center of the meat (not touching the cheese layer) registers 160°F (71°C). Let stand for 10 minutes before cutting into slices.

> ▶ **Health Tip**
> Cranberries are a great source of antioxidants.

This recipe courtesy of dietitian Katherine Ng.

Peppery Meatloaf with Quinoa

With both ground beef and Italian sausage, this definitely qualifies as a meaty main dish, but the addition of quinoa and various spices and herbs takes it out of the realm of the ordinary daily special and into the 21st-century kitchen.

Tip

To enhance the pleasantly nutty flavor of the quinoa, toast it in a dry skillet (or the saucepan you are using for cooking) for about 4 minutes over medium heat, stirring constantly, until fragrant.

Variation

Substitute millet for the quinoa. For the best flavor, before using, toast it in a dry skillet, stirring until fragrant, about 5 minutes. Complete step 1, simmering the millet over low heat for 20 minutes, then remove from the heat and let stand for 10 minutes.

Nutrients per serving	
Calories	221
Fat	8 g
Carbohydrate	15 g
Protein	22 g
Vitamin C	27 mg
Vitamin D	12 IU
Vitamin E	2 mg
Niacin	4 mg
Folate	57 mcg
Vitamin B$_6$	0.5 mg
Vitamin B$_{12}$	1.7 mcg
Zinc	4.2 mg
Selenium	18 mcg

- **Preheat oven to 350°F (180°C)**
- **9- by 5-inch (23 by 12.5 cm) loaf pan**
- **Instant-read thermometer**

¾ cup	water	175 mL
½ cup	ready-to-use reduced-sodium beef broth or water	125 mL
¾ cup	quinoa, rinsed (see tip, at left)	175 mL
1 lb	extra-lean ground beef	500 g
8 oz	Italian sausage, removed from casings and crumbled	250 mL
1	onion, finely chopped	1
1	red bell pepper, finely chopped	1
½ cup	finely chopped fresh parsley	125 mL
2	large eggs, beaten	2
1 cup	reduced-sodium tomato sauce, divided	250 mL
1 tbsp	sweet paprika	15 mL
1 tbsp	ground cumin	15 mL
1 tsp	ground coriander	5 mL
½ tsp	salt	2 mL
¼ tsp	cayenne pepper	1 mL

1. In a saucepan, bring water and beef broth to a boil. Gradually stir in quinoa. Return to a boil. Cover and simmer over low heat for 15 minutes. Remove from heat, cover and set aside for 5 minutes. Fluff with a fork before using.

2. In a large bowl, combine ground beef, sausage, onion, bell pepper, parsley, eggs, all but 2 tbsp (30 mL) of the tomato sauce, paprika, cumin, coriander, salt, cayenne and quinoa. Using your hands, mix until well blended. Transfer to loaf pan and spread remaining 2 tbsp (30 mL) tomato sauce over top. Bake in preheated oven until temperature reaches 165°F (75°C) on thermometer, about 1 hour.

> ▶ **Health Tip**
>
> Spices help stimulate digestion — including the production of stomach acid and salivation in the mouth — which is very important when it comes to digesting a big serving of protein.

Beef and Quinoa Power Burgers

These burgers add some classic seasonings and the kick of quinoa.

Tips

Be careful to mix the beef mixture as little as possible; over-mixing can make the burgers tough.

Whenever possible, use whole-grain or multigrain hamburger buns.

Variation

Substitute lean ground turkey or extra-lean ground pork for the beef.

⅔ cup	quinoa, rinsed	150 mL
1 cup	water	250 mL
⅓ cup	barbecue sauce	75 mL
1 lb	extra-lean ground beef	500 g
½ cup	finely chopped green onions	125 mL
2 tsp	ground cumin	10 mL
½ tsp	fine sea salt	2 mL
¼ tsp	freshly cracked black pepper	1 mL
2 tsp	olive oil	10 mL
4	hamburger buns (gluten-free, if needed), split and toasted	4

Suggested Accompaniments

Thinly sliced cheese (such as sharp Cheddar or Gruyère) or crumbled goat cheese

Large tomato slices

Baby spinach, arugula or tender watercress sprigs

Additional barbecue sauce

1. In a medium saucepan, combine quinoa, water and barbecue sauce. Bring to a boil over medium-high heat. Reduce heat to low, cover and simmer for 12 to 15 minutes or until liquid is absorbed. Remove from heat and let cool to room temperature.

2. In a large bowl, combine quinoa, beef, green onions, cumin, salt and pepper. Form into four ¾-inch (2 cm) thick patties.

3. In a large, deep skillet, heat oil over medium-high heat. Add patties and cook for 4 minutes. Turn and cook for 4 to 5 minutes or until no longer pink inside.

4. Transfer patties to toasted buns. Top with any of the suggested accompaniments, as desired.

▶ **Health Tip**

Gluten-free buns vary in their composition. Look for those that have brown rice flour or teff flour and not just tapioca starch or rice starch, as these can be very high on the glycemic index.

Nutrients per serving	
Calories	441
Fat	12 g
Carbohydrate	49 g
Protein	33 g
Vitamin C	3 mg
Vitamin D	3 IU
Vitamin E	2 mg
Niacin	9 mg
Folate	106 mcg
Vitamin B$_6$	0.6 mg
Vitamin B$_{12}$	2.6 mcg
Zinc	7.0 mg
Selenium	31 mcg

Lamb Tagine with Chickpeas and Apricots

Lamb is a staple for some people and a rare treat for others. This sweet-and-spicy version brings out the best in lamb and adds wonderful phytonutrients in the process.

Makes 6 servings

Tips

Buy a 3-lb (1.5 kg) leg of lamb or shoulder roast to get 1½ lbs (750 g) boneless lamb.

Slow Cooker Method: Follow step 1 and transfer lamb to slow cooker. Follow step 2, then stir in tomatoes and broth; bring to a boil. Transfer to slow cooker. Cover and cook on Low for 6 hours or on High for 3 hours, until almost tender. Add chickpeas, apricots and honey. Cover and cook on Low for 1 hour or on High for 30 minutes.

Nutrients per serving	
Calories	419
Fat	11 g
Carbohydrate	52 g
Protein	31 g
Vitamin C	14 mg
Vitamin D	0 IU
Vitamin E	2 mg
Niacin	9 mg
Folate	106 mcg
Vitamin B₆	0.8 mg
Vitamin B₁₂	3.0 mcg
Zinc	5.8 mg
Selenium	30 mcg

2 tbsp	olive oil (approx.)	30 mL
1½ lbs	lean boneless lamb, cut into 1-inch (2.5 cm) cubes	750 g
5	carrots, peeled and thickly sliced	5
1	large onion, chopped	1
3	cloves garlic, finely chopped	3
1 tsp	each ground ginger, cumin, cinnamon and turmeric	5 mL
½ tsp	salt	2 mL
½ tsp	freshly ground black pepper	2 mL
1	can (14 oz/398 mL) diced tomatoes, with juice	1
1 cup	ready to use chicken broth (approx.)	250 mL
1	can (19 oz/540 mL) chickpeas, drained and rinsed	1
½ cup	dried apricots or figs, roughly chopped	125 mL
¼ cup	liquid honey	60 mL

1. In a Dutch oven, heat 1 tbsp (15 mL) oil over medium-high heat. Brown lamb, in batches, adding more oil as needed. Transfer to a plate as meat browns.

2. Reduce heat to medium. Add carrots, onion, garlic, ginger, cumin, cinnamon, turmeric, salt and pepper to pan; cook, stirring, for about 5 minutes or until onion is softened.

3. Add tomatoes, broth and lamb, along with any accumulated juices; bring to a boil. Reduce heat to medium-low, cover and simmer for 1½ hours or until lamb is just tender.

4. Add chickpeas, apricots and honey. Add more broth, if necessary. Cover and simmer for 30 minutes or until lamb is very tender.

> ▶ **Health Tip**
>
> Honey has cancer-prevention properties and contains a powerful antioxidant, caffeic acid phenethyl ester.

Side Dishes

Orange Broccoli with Red Pepper

Forget the salty cheese sauce — this fruit and vegetable combination beautifully complements broccoli.

Tip

While North American tastes are generally restricted to broccoli florets, Asian cooking also uses broccoli stalks extensively. So don't throw them away — trim the woody bottoms and peel the stalks using a paring knife; then cut the tender, mild interior into slices or strips.

1 tsp	grated orange zest	5 mL
1/3 cup	orange juice	75 mL
1/2 tsp	cornstarch	2 mL
1 tbsp	olive oil	15 mL
4 cups	small broccoli florets and stalks, cut into 1 1/2- by 1/2-inch (4 by 1 cm) lengths	1 L
1	red bell pepper, cut into 2- by 1/2-inch (5 by 1 cm) strips	1
1	clove garlic, minced	1
1/4 tsp	salt	1 mL
1/4 tsp	freshly ground black pepper	1 mL

1. In a glass measuring cup, stir together orange juice and cornstarch until smooth; reserve.

2. Heat oil in a large nonstick skillet over high heat. Add broccoli, red pepper and garlic; cook, stirring, for 2 minutes.

3. Add orange juice mixture; cover and cook 1 to 2 minutes or until vegetables are tender-crisp. Sprinkle with orange zest; season with salt and pepper. Serve immediately.

> ▶ **Health Tip**
>
> Broccoli and peppers are a winning combination, providing excellent sources of vitamins A and C and folate.

Nutrients per serving	
Calories	78
Fat	4 g
Carbohydrate	10 g
Protein	3 g
Vitamin C	113 mg
Vitamin D	0 IU
Vitamin E	2 mg
Niacin	1 mg
Folate	70 mcg
Vitamin B_6	0.2 mg
Vitamin B_{12}	0.0 mcg
Zinc	0.4 mg
Selenium	2 mcg

Green Beans and Carrots with Aromatic Spices

This dish has some heat, but for those who like some spice in their daily fare, it's a great way to bring a new twist to green beans and carrots.

Makes 6 to 8 servings

Tip

The important thing in Indian cooking is to use a chile with spirit. Fresh cayenne peppers, or any similar ones, will work very well. If using fresh Thai peppers, now readily available in North America, use only half the amount called for in the recipe. In a pinch, jalapeños can also be used.

2 tbsp	vegetable oil	30 mL
1 tsp	mustard seeds	5 mL
1 tsp	cumin seeds	5 mL
1 tbsp	minced garlic	15 mL
1 tbsp	minced green chile pepper (see tip, at left)	15 mL
¼ cup	coarsely crushed roasted peanuts	60 mL
¼ cup	grated unsweetened fresh or frozen coconut, divided	60 mL
½ tsp	ground turmeric	2 mL
½ tsp	cayenne pepper	2 mL
8 oz	green beans, cut into 2-inch (5 cm) sections	250 g
8 oz	carrots (2 to 3), peeled and sliced diagonally ¼ inch (0.5 cm) thick	250 g
1 tsp	salt (or to taste)	5 mL

1. In a large skillet with a tight-fitting lid, heat oil over high heat until a couple of mustard seeds thrown in start to sputter. Add remaining mustard seeds and cover quickly.

2. When seeds stop popping in a few seconds, uncover, reduce heat to medium and add cumin seeds. Sauté for 30 seconds. Add garlic, chile, peanuts and 3 tbsp (45 mL) of the coconut. Reduce heat slightly to prevent burning and stir-fry for 2 minutes. Add turmeric and cayenne. Sauté for 1 minute longer (add 1½ tsp/7 mL water if necessary). Do not allow masala to burn.

3. Stir in beans and carrots. Add salt and mix well. Sprinkle with 1 tbsp (15 mL) water. Cover and cook over medium heat for 5 minutes. Reduce heat to low and stir. Cook, covered, until vegetables are tender, 5 to 8 minutes.

4. Garnish with remaining coconut to serve.

Nutrients per 1 of 8 servings	
Calories	94
Fat	7 g
Carbohydrate	7 g
Protein	2 g
Vitamin C	6 mg
Vitamin D	0 IU
Vitamin E	1 mg
Niacin	1 mg
Folate	21 mcg
Vitamin B$_6$	0.1 mg
Vitamin B$_{12}$	0.0 mcg
Zinc	0.5 mg
Selenium	1 mcg

> ▶ **Health Tip**
>
> Chile and cayenne peppers are species of capsicum, which has circulatory and digestive support benefits.

Cauliflower and Beans with Turmeric

This flavorful, aromatic dish incorporates many healthy ingredients, such as garlic and turmeric.

Tip

For a spicier dish, add ½ tsp (2 mL) chopped fresh red or green chile pepper with the garlic.

2 tbsp	vegetable oil	30 mL
3	cloves garlic, chopped	3
3 cups	small cauliflower florets	750 mL
2 tbsp	chopped fresh cilantro leaves	30 mL
1 tbsp	fish sauce (nam pla)	15 mL
1 tsp	granulated sugar	5 mL
½ tsp	ground turmeric	2 mL
¼ cup	water	60 mL
1 cup	sliced green beans (1-inch/ 2.5 cm slices)	250 mL
4	green onions, sliced	4

1. Heat a wok or large skillet over medium-high heat and add oil. Add garlic and stir-fry for 15 seconds. Add cauliflower and stir-fry for 1 minute.

2. Add cilantro, fish sauce, sugar, turmeric and water. Cover and cook for 3 minutes. Add beans. Cover and cook for 2 to 3 minutes, or until vegetables are tender. Stir in green onions and cook for 1 minute.

> ▶ **Health Tip**
>
> Turmeric is a great antioxidant, and one of its compounds, curcumin, is being researched for its cancer-prevention properties.

Nutrients per serving	
Calories	101
Fat	7 g
Carbohydrate	8 g
Protein	3 g
Vitamin C	44 mg
Vitamin D	0 IU
Vitamin E	1 mg
Niacin	1 mg
Folate	60 mcg
Vitamin B$_6$	0.2 mg
Vitamin B$_{12}$	0.0 mcg
Zinc	0.4 mg
Selenium	1 mcg

Simple Stir-Fried Kale

This easy-to-prepare dish uses some basic Asian — and Middle Eastern — flavors to enliven one of our most nutritious greens.

Tips

Tahini is often used in Middle Eastern cooking and is an ingredient in hummus. It is made from ground sesame seeds and adds a nutty flavor to dishes.

Leave out the hot pepper sauce if your family does not like spice.

1 tbsp	vegetable oil	15 mL
1 tsp	sesame oil	5 mL
4 cups	julienned kale (tough center rib removed first)	1 L
2	leeks (white and light green parts only), julienned	2
1 tbsp	tahini	15 mL
2 tsp	hot pepper sauce	10 mL
2 tsp	soy sauce	10 mL
	Freshly ground white or black pepper	

1. In a wok or large skillet, heat vegetable oil and sesame oil over high heat. Add kale and leeks; stir-fry for 3 to 5 minutes or until limp.

2. Combine tahini, hot pepper sauce and soy sauce; pour over vegetables. Season to taste with pepper. Serve warm.

> ▶ **Health Tip**
>
> Sesame oil and tahini provide lots of the antioxidant compound sesamol.

This recipe courtesy of dietitian Gerry Kasten.

Nutrients per serving	
Calories	126
Fat	7 g
Carbohydrate	14 g
Protein	4 g
Vitamin C	88 mg
Vitamin D	0 IU
Vitamin E	1 mg
Niacin	1 mg
Folate	52 mcg
Vitamin B_6	0.3 mg
Vitamin B_{12}	0.0 mcg
Zinc	0.5 mg
Selenium	2 mcg

New Orleans Braised Onions

This dish takes its time, but since slow cookers allow you to do other tasks, the end result is well worth it.

**Makes
10 servings**

Tips

Onions are high in natural sugars, which long, slow simmering brings out, as does the orange juice in this recipe.

If you halve this recipe, use a 1½- to 3½-quart slow cooker, checking to make sure the whole onions will fit.

• **Minimum 5-quart slow cooker**

2 to 3	large Spanish onions	2 to 3
6 to 9	whole cloves	6 to 9
½ tsp	salt	2 mL
½ tsp	cracked black peppercorns	2 mL
Pinch	dried thyme	Pinch
	Grated zest and juice of 1 orange	
½ cup	ready-to-use vegetable broth	125 mL
	Finely chopped fresh parsley (optional)	
	Hot pepper sauce (optional)	

1. Stud onions with cloves. Place in slow cooker stoneware and sprinkle with salt, peppercorns, thyme and orange zest. Pour orange juice and vegetable broth over onions, cover and cook on Low for 8 hours or on High for 4 hours, until onions are tender.

2. Using a slotted spoon, transfer onions to a serving dish and keep warm in a 250°F (120°C) oven. Transfer liquid to a saucepan over medium heat. Cook until reduced by half.

3. When ready to serve, cut onions into quarters. Place on a deep platter and cover with sauce. Sprinkle with parsley, if desired, and pass the hot pepper sauce, if desired.

Nutrients per serving	
Calories	13
Fat	0 g
Carbohydrate	3 g
Protein	0 g
Vitamin C	2 mg
Vitamin D	0 IU
Vitamin E	0 mg
Niacin	0 mg
Folate	6 mcg
Vitamin B$_6$	0.0 mg
Vitamin B$_{12}$	0.0 mcg
Zinc	0.1 mg
Selenium	0 mcg

▶ **Health Tip**

As the beneficial flavonoids in onions tend to be located in the outer layers, peel off as little as possible of the edible portion when removing the paper-like layer.

Roasted Bell Peppers

The garlic on these peppers brings out a flavor that will have your guests asking for seconds.

Tips

These multipurpose peppers are always great to have on hand, as they can be used in a number of recipes. Use a variety of colored peppers, such as yellow, red, orange and green, to add vibrancy to pasta sauces and salads or to use in one of the variations.

If some of the skin adheres to the flesh after the peppers have cooled, use your fingers to peel it off.

Marinating peppers in balsamic vinegar extends their shelf life.

Nutrients per 1 of 4 servings

Calories	97
Fat	7 g
Carbohydrate	7 g
Protein	1 g
Vitamin C	114 mg
Vitamin D	0 IU
Vitamin E	3 mg
Niacin	1 mg
Folate	42 mcg
Vitamin B$_6$	0.3 mg
Vitamin B$_{12}$	0.0 mcg
Zinc	0.3 mg
Selenium	1 mcg

- **Preheat oven to 350°F (180°C)**
- **13- by 9-inch (33 by 23 cm) baking dish, greased**

3	bell peppers, seeds and ribs removed, peppers quartered	3
2 tbsp	garlic-infused oil	30 mL
1 tbsp	garlic powder	15 mL
	Salt and freshly ground black pepper	

1. Place peppers in prepared baking dish. Brush both sides of each pepper piece with garlic oil and sprinkle with garlic powder and salt and pepper to taste. Bake in preheated oven for 45 to 50 minutes or until very soft and wrinkled.

2. Transfer to a bowl, cover with a plate and let cool to room temperature. The skins will naturally separate from the flesh of the pepper (see tip, at left). Store in an airtight container and refrigerate for up to 4 days.

Variations

Balsamic Marinated Peppers: Cut peeled roasted peppers into quarters. Add 1/2 cup (125 mL) balsamic vinegar and toss to coat. Cover and refrigerate for 8 hours or for up to 1 week.

Garlic Marinated Peppers: Toss peeled roasted peppers with 2 cloves garlic, thinly sliced, and 1/4 cup (60 mL) extra virgin olive oil. Marinate for several hours or overnight, then remove the garlic. Add sea salt and freshly ground black pepper to taste and serve immediately.

> ▶ **Health Tip**
>
> *Allium sativa* — garlic — has numerous beneficial effects on cardiovascular health.

Stuffed Zucchini

This is a great side when entertaining, or just because it's something that you were craving.

Makes 4 servings

Tip

For convenience, look for vegetable broth in Tetra Paks. Once opened, these can be stored in the refrigerator for up to 1 week.

- **Preheat oven to 350°F (180°C)**

¾ cup	ready-to-use reduced-sodium vegetable broth	175 mL
2	small zucchini, halved lengthwise	2
2	green onions, chopped	2
2	cloves garlic, minced	2
1	tomato, diced	1
½ tsp	dried basil	2 mL
½ tsp	dried thyme	2 mL
¼ tsp	hot pepper sauce	1 mL
¾ cup	shredded Cheddar cheese	175 mL

1. In a large skillet over medium-high heat, bring broth to a boil. Reduce heat to medium and add zucchini halves, skin side up. Cook for 2 to 3 minutes or until tender. Remove zucchini and let cool. Discard excess liquid.

2. Using a spoon, scoop out zucchini flesh, leaving a shell. Chop zucchini flesh. In a large bowl, combine zucchini flesh, green onions, garlic, tomato, basil, thyme and hot pepper sauce. Fill zucchini shells with mixture and top with cheese. Place filled shells on a baking sheet.

3. Bake in preheated oven for 10 minutes or until heated through and cheese is melted.

> ▶ **Health Tip**
>
> Zucchini is rich in fiber, as well as magnesium and potassium.

This recipe courtesy of Laurie Evans.

Nutrients per serving	
Calories	107
Fat	7 g
Carbohydrate	5 g
Protein	6 g
Vitamin C	16 mg
Vitamin D	5 IU
Vitamin E	0 mg
Niacin	1 mg
Folate	25 mcg
Vitamin B$_6$	0.2 mg
Vitamin B$_{12}$	0.2 mcg
Zinc	0.9 mg
Selenium	3 mcg

Spaghetti Squash with Mushrooms

Spaghetti squash is known for its pasta-like texture. It cooks like other squashes and goes well with the pasta-style sauce given here.

Makes 6 servings

Tips

Spaghetti squash is easily recognized by its oblong shape and pale to bright yellow skin. It bakes and microwaves quite easily. To keep the strands intact, be sure to cut squash in half lengthwise.

Serve this dish over brown rice for a light meal.

Nutrients per serving

Calories	181
Fat	7 g
Carbohydrate	27 g
Protein	7 g
Vitamin C	14 mg
Vitamin D	24 IU
Vitamin E	1 mg
Niacin	5 mg
Folate	64 mcg
Vitamin B_6	0.4 mg
Vitamin B_{12}	0.3 mcg
Zinc	1.1 mg
Selenium	4 mcg

- **Preheat oven to 350°F (180°C)**

1	spaghetti squash (about 3½ lbs/1.5 kg)	1
2 tbsp	butter or margarine	30 mL
2 cups	sliced mushrooms	500 mL
1	green onion, sliced	1
1	small stalk celery, chopped	1
2 cups	chopped tomatoes (about 4 small)	500 mL
2 tbsp	all-purpose flour	30 mL
1 cup	milk	250 mL
½ cup	shredded Cheddar cheese	125 mL
1 tsp	dried oregano	5 mL
½ tsp	garlic powder	2 mL
½ tsp	salt	2 mL
¼ tsp	freshly ground black pepper	1 mL
	Grated Parmesan cheese	

1. Cut squash in half lengthwise. Bake cut side down on a baking sheet in preheated oven for 25 to 30 minutes, or boil, cut side down and covered, in 2 inches (5 cm) of water for about 20 minutes.

2. In a skillet over medium-high heat, melt butter and cook mushrooms, green onion, celery and tomatoes for about 5 minutes or until tender. Stir in flour; gradually add milk. Cook, stirring constantly, until thickened. Stir in Cheddar cheese and seasonings until cheese is melted.

3. Pour sauce over squash; sprinkle with Parmesan cheese and serve.

> ▶ **Health Tip**
>
> In addition to having nutritional value, squash is a good source of dietary fiber in a useful and easy-to-tolerate form.

This recipe courtesy of Marlyn Ambrose-Chase.

Perfect Steamed Rice

Here is a simple recipe for that perfect complement to curries and other spiced dishes.

Tips

True basmati rice comes from the foothills of the Himalayas. There is rice available in the bulk bins of some supermarkets that is marked "basmati," but it is usually from California and will not work in this recipe. Be sure to use only Indian or Pakistani basmati rice.

Rice should always be transferred to a platter, never a bowl, as the weight of the freshly steamed rice causes the rice on the bottom to get mushy.

• **Large saucepan with tight-fitting lid**

2 cups	Indian basmati rice (see tip, at left)	500 mL
1 tbsp	oil	15 mL
2 tsp	salt (or to taste)	10 mL

1. Place rice in a bowl with plenty of cold water and swish vigorously with fingers. Drain. Repeat process 4 or 5 times until water is fairly clear. Cover with 3 to 4 inches (7.5 to 10 cm) cold water and soak for at least 15 minutes or up to 2 hours.

2. In a large saucepan, heat oil over medium-high heat. Drain rice and add to saucepan. Stir to coat rice. Add $3\frac{1}{2}$ cups (875 mL) cold water and salt.

3. Cover with a tight-fitting lid and bring to a boil over high heat. Reduce heat to as low as possible and cook, covered, without peeking, for 25 minutes.

4. Remove from heat and set lid slightly ajar to allow steam to escape. Let rest for 5 minutes. Gently fluff with a fork and carefully spoon onto platter to serve.

> ▶ **Health Tip**
>
> Rice is often considered a hypoallergenic food — that is, many people with food allergies do not react to rice in the way they react to wheat, dairy, soy and other foods.

Nutrients per serving	
Calories	156
Fat	3 g
Carbohydrate	31 g
Protein	3 g
Vitamin C	0 mg
Vitamin D	0 IU
Vitamin E	0 mg
Niacin	2 mg
Folate	119 mcg
Vitamin B$_6$	0.2 mg
Vitamin B$_{12}$	0.0 mcg
Zinc	0.5 mg
Selenium	9 mcg

Home-Style Skillet Rice with Tomato Crust

Skillet dishes are popular these days. Here is one with great natural seasonings where you can control the added salt.

Makes 6 servings

Tip

Lundberg sells a variety of brown rice mixes, all of which will work well in this recipe. Their Jubilee blend, which includes Wehani and Black Japonica, is particularly nice in this dish.

Nutrients per serving	
Calories	253
Fat	8 g
Carbohydrate	33 g
Protein	13 g
Vitamin C	39 mg
Vitamin D	14 IU
Vitamin E	2 mg
Niacin	3 mg
Folate	42 mcg
Vitamin B$_6$	0.5 mg
Vitamin B$_{12}$	0.5 mcg
Zinc	1.8 mg
Selenium	10 mcg

- **Preheat oven to 350°F (180°C)**

3 cups	cooked red or brown rice, or brown and wild rice mixture (see tip, at left)	750 mL
1 tbsp	olive oil	15 mL
8 oz	hot or mild Italian sausage, removed from casings	250 g
1	onion, finely chopped	1
4	stalks celery, diced	4
2	green bell peppers, finely chopped	2
4	cloves garlic, minced	4
1 tbsp	chili powder	15 mL
2 tsp	caraway seeds	10 mL
1 tsp	dried oregano	5 mL
½ tsp	salt (or to taste)	2 mL
	Freshly ground black pepper	
1½ cups	reduced-sodium tomato sauce	375 mL
2	large eggs, beaten	2
8 oz	sliced mozzarella cheese (optional)	250 g

1. In a cast-iron or other ovenproof skillet, heat oil over medium heat for 30 seconds. Add sausage, onion, celery and bell peppers and cook, stirring and breaking up sausage with a spoon, until vegetables are very tender and sausage is no longer pink, about 7 minutes. Add garlic, chili powder, caraway seeds, oregano, salt and black pepper to taste and cook, stirring, for 1 minute. Add cooked rice and cook, stirring, until heated through. Remove from heat.

2. In a bowl, beat tomato sauce and eggs until blended. Spread evenly over rice in skillet. Lay sliced mozzarella (if using) evenly over top. Place skillet in preheated oven and bake until top is crusty and cheese (if using) is melted, about 15 minutes.

> ▶ **Health Tip**
>
> Caraway is a natural digestive aid.

Fried Rice with Curry

Most fried rice dishes are gently seasoned, but this version has added curry paste and pepper. On its own it makes a good accompaniment for grilled fish or meat, but you can also add eggs and chicken for a more substantial dish.

Makes 4 servings

2 tbsp	vegetable oil	30 mL
1	onion, chopped	1
4	cloves garlic, chopped	4
1 tbsp	chopped gingerroot	15 mL
1½ cups	sliced mushrooms	375 mL
2 tsp	red curry paste	10 mL
1 tsp	granulated sugar	5 mL
¼ tsp	ground turmeric	1 mL
¼ tsp	freshly ground black pepper	1 mL
½ cup	finely sliced green beans	125 mL
4 cups	cooked rice	1 L
2 tbsp	fish sauce (nam pla)	30 mL
2 tbsp	chopped fresh cilantro leaves	30 mL
2	green onions, chopped	2

1. Heat a wok or large skillet over medium-high heat and add oil. Add onion, garlic and ginger and stir-fry for 1 minute or until soft and fragrant.

2. Add mushrooms and stir-fry for 2 minutes. Add curry paste, sugar, turmeric and pepper and stir-fry for 30 seconds.

3. Add beans and rice and toss for 3 to 4 minutes or until heated through. Add fish sauce, cilantro and green onions and toss to combine.

Nutrients per serving	
Calories	339
Fat	8 g
Carbohydrate	61 g
Protein	7 g
Vitamin C	6 mg
Vitamin D	2 IU
Vitamin E	1 mg
Niacin	5 mg
Folate	128 mcg
Vitamin B$_6$	0.3 mg
Vitamin B$_{12}$	0.1 mcg
Zinc	1.1 mg
Selenium	18 mcg

▶ **Health Tip**

Rice has the advantage of being a very tolerable grain that few people are allergic or sensitive to.

Desserts and Beverages

Perfect Chocolate Bundt

Here is a chocolate-lover's take on Bundt cake.

**Makes
16 servings**

Tip

Store the glazed cake at room temperature in a cake keeper, or loosely wrapped in foil or plastic wrap, for up to 3 days. Alternatively, wrap the cooled, unglazed cake in plastic wrap, then foil, completely enclosing cake, and freeze for up to 6 months. Let cake thaw at room temperature for 4 to 6 hours before glazing and serving.

- **10-inch (25 cm) Bundt pan, sprayed with nonstick baking spray with flour**

1 cup	semisweet chocolate chips	250 mL
¾ cup	unsweetened cocoa powder (not Dutch process)	175 mL
1 tsp	instant espresso powder	5 mL
¾ cup	boiling water	175 mL
2 cups	packed light brown sugar	500 mL
1 tsp	baking soda	5 mL
1 tsp	salt	5 mL
5	large eggs, at room temperature	5
1 cup	sour cream (see tip, opposite)	250 mL
¾ cup	unsalted butter, softened	175 mL
1 tbsp	vanilla extract	15 mL
1¾ cups	all-purpose flour	425 mL
	Chocolate Ganache Glaze (see recipe, opposite)	

1. In a large bowl, combine chocolate chips, cocoa powder and espresso powder. Add boiling water and whisk until chocolate is melted and mixture is smooth. Let cool for 20 minutes.

2. Meanwhile, preheat oven to 350°F (180°C).

3. Add brown sugar, baking soda, salt, eggs, sour cream, butter and vanilla to cocoa mixture. Using an electric mixer on high speed, beat for 2 minutes, until blended and fluffy. Add flour and beat on medium speed for 1 minute. Scrape sides and bottom of bowl with a spatula. Beat on high speed for 1 minute.

4. Spread batter evenly in prepared pan.

5. Bake in preheated oven for about 60 minutes or until a piece of uncooked spaghetti inserted in the center comes out with a few moist crumbs attached. Let cool in pan on a wire rack for 10 minutes, then invert cake onto rack to cool completely. Spoon glaze over top of cooled cake, letting it drizzle down the sides.

Nutrients per serving	
Calories	426
Fat	22 g
Carbohydrate	58 g
Protein	6 g
Vitamin C	0 mg
Vitamin D	22 IU
Vitamin E	1 mg
Niacin	1 mg
Folate	39 mcg
Vitamin B_6	0.1 mg
Vitamin B_{12}	0.2 mcg
Zinc	1.1 mg
Selenium	7 mcg

Tip

Use full-fat (not reduced-fat) sour cream. Reduced-fat sour cream will alter the taste and texture of the cake.

Variation

Mexican Chocolate Bundt: Add 1 1/2 tsp (7 mL) ground cinnamon and 1/4 tsp (1 mL) cayenne pepper with the brown sugar. Omit the glaze and dust the cooled cake with 2 tbsp (30 mL) confectioners' (icing) sugar.

> ▶ **Health Tip**
>
> Unsweetened chocolate and cocoa powder that have not been Dutch-processed have a higher concentration of the flavonols that are the key to this food's health benefits.

Makes about 1 cup (250 mL)

Chocolate Ganache Glaze

1/3 cup	heavy or whipping (35%) cream	75 ml
1 tbsp	light (white or golden) corn syrup	15 mL
1 1/4 cups	semisweet chocolate chips	300 mL
1/2 tsp	vanilla extract	2 mL

1. In a small saucepan, bring cream and corn syrup to a simmer over medium heat.

2. Place chocolate chips in a large heatproof bowl and pour in hot cream mixture. Let stand for 3 minutes or until chocolate chips are melted. Add vanilla and whisk until smooth. Let cool for 10 minutes, until slightly thickened.

Nutrients per 1 tbsp (15 mL)	
Calories	80
Fat	6 g
Carbohydrate	9 g
Protein	1 g
Vitamin C	0 mg
Vitamin D	1 IU
Vitamin E	0 mg
Niacin	0 mg
Folate	2 mcg
Vitamin B_6	0.0 mg
Vitamin B_{12}	0.0 mcg
Zinc	0.2 mg
Selenium	1 mcg

Cinnamon Cake with Whipped Mocha Frosting

Here is a delicious cinnamon-based cake, with an energizing mocha frosting to boot.

**Makes
16 servings**

Tips

If using a stand mixer, decrease the high-speed beating time by 1 minute.

Store the frosted cake in the refrigerator in a cake keeper, or loosely wrapped in foil or waxed paper, for up to 3 days. Alternatively, wrap the cooled, unfrosted cake layers individually in plastic wrap, then foil, and freeze for up to 6 months. Let cake layers thaw at room temperature for 2 to 3 hours before frosting and serving.

Nutrients per serving	
Calories	447
Fat	26 g
Carbohydrate	49 g
Protein	5 g
Vitamin C	0 mg
Vitamin D	34 IU
Vitamin E	1 mg
Niacin	1 mg
Folate	38 mcg
Vitamin B$_6$	0.0 mg
Vitamin B$_{12}$	0.3 mcg
Zinc	0.5 mg
Selenium	5 mcg

- **Preheat oven to 350°F (180°C)**
- **Two 9-inch (23 cm) round metal baking pans, sprayed with nonstick baking spray with flour**

2 cups	all-purpose flour	500 mL
2 cups	granulated sugar	500 mL
2 tsp	ground cinnamon	10 mL
1 tsp	baking soda	5 mL
1 tsp	baking powder	5 mL
½ tsp	salt	2 mL
4	large eggs, at room temperature	4
1 cup	unsalted butter, softened	250 mL
1 cup	sour cream	250 mL
2 tsp	vanilla extract	10 mL
½ cup	milk	125 mL
	Whipped Mocha Frosting (see recipe, opposite)	

1. In a large bowl, whisk together flour, sugar, cinnamon, baking soda, baking powder and salt.

2. Add eggs, butter, sour cream and vanilla to flour mixture. Using an electric mixer on medium-low speed, beat for 1 minute, until blended. Scrape sides and bottom of bowl with a spatula. Beat on high speed for 2 minutes. Add milk and beat on low speed for 15 to 30 seconds, until just blended.

3. Spread batter evenly in prepared pans, dividing equally.

4. Bake in preheated oven for 27 to 32 minutes or until a toothpick inserted in the center comes out with a few moist crumbs attached. Let cool in pans on a wire rack for 10 minutes. Run a knife around edges of pans, then invert cakes onto rack to cool completely.

5. Place one cake layer, flat side up, on a cake plate or platter. Spread ¾ cup (175 mL) of the frosting evenly over layer. Top with the second cake layer, flat side down. Spread the remaining frosting over top and sides of cake. Refrigerate for at least 1 hour before serving.

Tip

Select natural cocoa powder, which has a deep, true chocolate flavor.

Whipped Mocha Frosting

1 cup	confectioners' (icing) sugar	250 mL
1/2 cup	unsweetened cocoa powder (not Dutch process)	125 mL
1/8 tsp	salt	0.5 mL
1/4 cup	milk	60 mL
2 tsp	instant espresso powder	10 mL
2 tsp	vanilla extract	10 mL
2 cups	heavy or whipping (35%) cream	500 mL

1. In a large bowl, whisk together confectioners' sugar, cocoa powder, salt, milk, espresso powder and vanilla until blended and smooth. Cover and refrigerate for 1 hour.

2. Add cream to chilled cocoa mixture. Using an electric mixer on medium-high speed, beat, stopping to scrape the bowl occasionally, until stiff peaks form. Use immediately.

▶ **Health Tip**

Cinnamon has been shown to have a regulating effect on blood sugar — which is beneficial when incorporated into a sweet dessert like this one.

**Nutrients
per 1 tbsp (15 mL)**

Calories	138
Fat	11 g
Carbohydrate	10 g
Protein	1 g
Vitamin C	0 mg
Vitamin D	9 IU
Vitamin E	0 mg
Niacin	0 mg
Folate	1 mcg
Vitamin B$_6$	0.0 mg
Vitamin B$_{12}$	0.1 mcg
Zinc	0.1 mg
Selenium	0 mcg

Chocolate Chile Cupcakes

Chocolate and chile blend wonderfully here. If you're looking for a cupcake with zing, this is the one.

Makes 12 cupcakes

Tip

These are best served the day that they're made.

- **Preheat oven to 350°F (180°C)**
- **12-cup muffin pan, lined with paper liners**

1¼ cups	all-purpose flour	300 mL
½ cup	unsweetened cocoa powder, sifted	125 mL
1 tbsp	ancho chile powder (or 1 tsp/5 mL chipotle chile powder)	15 mL
2 tsp	finely ground espresso or French-roast coffee	10 mL
¾ tsp	baking soda	3 mL
¼ tsp	salt	1 mL
1 cup	granulated sugar	250 mL
⅓ cup	vegetable oil	75 mL
1	large egg	1
1 tsp	vanilla extract	5 mL
¾ cup	buttermilk	175 mL
1 tbsp	instant coffee granules	15 mL
½ cup	semisweet chocolate chips	125 mL
	Chocolate Fudge Frosting (see recipe, opposite)	

1. In a small bowl, mix together flour, cocoa powder, chile powder, ground coffee, baking soda and salt.

2. In a large bowl, whisk together sugar, oil, egg and vanilla until smooth. In a separate bowl, stir together buttermilk and instant coffee.

3. Alternately whisk flour mixture and buttermilk mixture into oil mixture, making three additions of flour mixture and two of buttermilk mixture, beating until smooth. Mix in chocolate chips.

4. Scoop batter into prepared muffin cups. Bake for 22 to 27 minutes or until tops of cupcakes spring back when lightly touched. Let cool in pan on rack for 10 minutes. Remove from pan and let cool completely on rack. Top cooled cupcakes with frosting.

Nutrients per cupcake	
Calories	397
Fat	18 g
Carbohydrate	55 g
Protein	5 g
Vitamin C	0 mg
Vitamin D	9 IU
Vitamin E	1 mg
Niacin	1 mg
Folate	29 mcg
Vitamin B$_6$	0.1 mg
Vitamin B$_{12}$	0.1 mcg
Zinc	0.3 mg
Selenium	2 mcg

Tip

Extra frosting will keep in an airtight container in the refrigerator for several days. Let soften and stir until smooth before spreading.

Variations

If you prefer your frosting a little less sweet, you can reduce the confectioners' sugar by 1/2 cup (125 mL).

To make this frosting vegan, substitute margarine for the butter and replace the chocolate cream liqueur with chocolate liqueur or rum.

Nutrients per 1 tbsp (15 mL)	
Calories	75
Fat	4 g
Carbohydrate	9 g
Protein	1 g
Vitamin C	0 mg
Vitamin D	3 IU
Vitamin E	0 mg
Niacin	0 mg
Folate	0 mcg
Vitamin B$_6$	0.0 mg
Vitamin B$_{12}$	0.0 mcg
Zinc	0.0 mg
Selenium	0 mcg

Chocolate Fudge Frosting

- **Food processor**

1 1/2 cups	confectioners' (icing) sugar	375 mL
3/4 cup	unsweetened cocoa powder, sifted	175 mL
1/2 cup	unsalted butter, at room temperature	125 mL
2 tbsp	chocolate cream liqueur	30 mL
1 tbsp	strong brewed coffee or milk	15 mL
Pinch	salt	Pinch

1. In food processor, process confectioners' sugar, cocoa powder, butter, chocolate liqueur, coffee and salt until smooth, scraping down sides as necessary.

2. Spread frosting on cooled cupcakes.

> ▶ **Health Tip**
>
> The beneficial compounds in chocolate can interrupt some of the chemical processes that drive atherosclerosis, a degenerative process that ages arteries.

Meringue Crowns with Ricotta Lemon Curd and Blueberries

Creamy lemon curd and sweet berries are happily nestled in these crisp meringue crowns.

Makes 8 servings

Tip
Room-temperature egg whites produce a better foam than cold egg whites.

- **Preheat oven to 400°C (200°F)**
- **2 baking sheets, lined with parchment paper**
- **Double boiler**

Meringue Crowns

2	large egg whites, at room temperature	2
1/4 tsp	cream of tartar	1 mL
Pinch	salt	Pinch
1/2 cup	granulated sugar	125 mL
1/2 tsp	lemon extract	2 mL

Ricotta Lemon Curd

4	large egg yolks	4
1/3 cup	granulated sugar	75 mL
2 tbsp	grated lemon zest	30 mL
1/3 cup	freshly squeezed lemon juice	75 mL
2 tbsp	non-hydrogenated margarine	30 mL
1 cup	light ricotta cheese	250 mL
2 cups	blueberries	500 mL
8	sprigs fresh mint	8

1. *Meringues:* On each prepared baking sheet, trace four 3-inch (7.5 cm) circles with a pen or pencil. Turn parchment over so marks are on the bottom. Set pans aside.

2. In a large bowl, using an electric mixer on high speed, beat egg whites, cream of tartar and salt until soft peaks form. Add sugar 2 tbsp (30 mL) at a time, beating for 30 seconds to 1 minute after each addition to ensure sugar is fully combined with egg whites, scraping sides of bowl occasionally. Beat until stiff, glossy peaks form. Fold in lemon extract.

3. Divide meringue evenly among circles on baking sheets, spreading to the entire width of each circle. With the back of a spoon, make a small indentation in the center of each (to hold the filling) and draw meringue upward on the outer edges, forming several peaks ("crown" tips).

Nutrients per serving	
Calories	207
Fat	8 g
Carbohydrate	29 g
Protein	6 g
Vitamin C	10 mg
Vitamin D	35 IU
Vitamin E	1 mg
Niacin	0 mg
Folate	21 mcg
Vitamin B_6	0.1 mg
Vitamin B_{12}	0.3 mcg
Zinc	0.7 mg
Selenium	12 mcg

4. Place baking sheets in preheated oven and immediately reduce oven temperature to 250°C (120°C). Bake for 30 minutes. Turn oven off and leave meringues in oven for at least 3 to 4 hours or overnight to dry completely.

5. *Curd:* In the top of double boiler set over simmering water, whisk egg yolks and sugar for 1 minute. Whisk in lemon zest and lemon juice. Cook, whisking constantly, for 3 to 4 minutes or until mixture is thick and coats the back of a spoon. Remove from heat and stir in margarine 1 tbsp (15 mL) at a time, letting the first blend in before adding the second. Let cool for 10 minutes.

6. Fold ricotta cheese into curd mixture. Transfer to a bowl, place plastic wrap directly on surface of curd and refrigerate for at least 4 hours, until chilled, or for up to 24 hours.

7. Place 1 meringue on each dessert plate. Divide curd among meringues and top each with berries and a mint sprig.

▶ Health Tip

Blueberries are a source of proanthocyanidins, pigments that have potent antioxidant properties and may promote the health of the retina (the back of the eye).

This recipe courtesy of dietitian Mary Sue Waisman.

Dark Chocolate Mousse

A mousse may sound like a sophisticated recipe that only accomplished French pastry chefs can master, but in fact an excellent dessert mousse can be easily made in your kitchen.

Makes 8 servings

Tips

Superfine sugar dissolves very quickly in liquid. It is sometimes labeled "instant dissolving fruit powdered sugar." If you can't find it, make your own by processing granulated sugar in a food processor until very finely ground.

Garnish mousse with fresh raspberries and sprigs of mint.

Variation

Substitute 1 tbsp (15 mL) orange-flavored liqueur for the vanilla extract.

8 oz	bittersweet chocolate, chopped	250 g
2½ cups	heavy or whipping (35%) cream, divided	625 mL
3 tbsp	superfine sugar (see tip, at left)	45 mL
2 tsp	vanilla extract	10 mL

1. In a microwave-safe bowl, combine chocolate and ½ cup (125 mL) cream. Microwave on High for 60 seconds or until cream is hot and chocolate is soft and almost melted. Stir until completely melted and smooth. Let cool slightly.

2. In a medium bowl, using electric mixer, whip remaining cream, sugar and vanilla until stiff peaks form. With a rubber spatula, fold melted chocolate mixture into whipped cream mixture.

3. Scoop mousse into small cups. Chill for several hours before serving.

> ▶ **Health Tip**
>
> The fats in chocolate are either heart-healthy or heart-neutral, but that's true only of chocolate that has not been mixed with other ingredients, such as caramel or hydrogenated fats.

Nutrients per serving	
Calories	422
Fat	43 g
Carbohydrate	15 g
Protein	5 g
Vitamin C	0 mg
Vitamin D	20 IU
Vitamin E	1 mg
Niacin	0 mg
Folate	11 mcg
Vitamin B_6	0.0 mg
Vitamin B_{12}	0.1 mcg
Zinc	2.9 mg
Selenium	3 mcg

Summertime Fruit Salad with Vanilla Maple Yogurt Dressing

Take advantage of the marvelous fresh, colorful and tasty berries available during the summer. This is an ideal breakfast treat, and perfect for a light dessert as well.

Makes 4 servings

Tip

This fantastic dressing can also be used as a dip for fruit, as a topping for cereal or as a light sauce for crêpes or pancakes. It works well with regular sour cream too.

1 cup	blueberries	250 mL
1 cup	raspberries	250 mL
1 cup	sliced strawberries	250 mL
1 cup	blackberries or Saskatoon berries	250 mL
¼ cup	toasted finely chopped hazelnuts (optional)	60 mL

Vanilla Maple Yogurt Dressing

¼ cup	low-fat vanilla yogurt	60 mL
¼ cup	light sour cream	60 mL
1 tbsp	pure maple syrup	15 mL
Pinch	ground cinnamon	Pinch

1. In a bowl, gently combine blueberries, raspberries, strawberries and blackberries.

2. *Dressing:* In a small bowl, combine yogurt, sour cream, maple syrup and cinnamon. Use immediately or cover and refrigerate for up to 3 days.

3. Place 1 cup (250 mL) berry mixture in each serving bowl. Top each with 2 tbsp (30 mL) dressing and 2 tsp (10 mL) hazelnuts (if using).

> ▶ **Health Tip**
>
> This recipe is a great way to get some of our daily servings of fruit.

This recipe courtesy of dietitian Mary Sue Waisman.

Nutrients per serving	
Calories	113
Fat	3 g
Carbohydrate	22 g
Protein	3 g
Vitamin C	44 mg
Vitamin D	8 IU
Vitamin E	1 mg
Niacin	1 mg
Folate	31 mcg
Vitamin B_6	0.1 mg
Vitamin B_{12}	0.2 mcg
Zinc	0.7 mg
Selenium	2 mcg

Super Antioxidant Smoothie

This simple smoothie provides a wide range of antioxidants and plenty of sweetness to balance and carry the spinach.

Makes 2 servings

Tip

Almond milk is available in a variety of flavors, but be sure to choose plain almond milk for this recipe.

- **Blender**

1 cup	loosely packed baby spinach	250 mL
1 cup	frozen cherries, blueberries or blackberries	250 mL
1 cup	plain almond milk	250 mL

1. In blender, purée spinach, cherries and almond milk until smooth. Pour into two glasses and serve immediately.

> ▶ **Health Tip**
>
> In addition to being high in protein, almond milk is an excellent source of vitamin E, an important antioxidant that plays a role in supporting normal heart and brain function, as well as in promoting a healthy complexion.

Nutrients per serving	
Calories	69
Fat	1 g
Carbohydrate	14 g
Protein	1 g
Vitamin C	5 mg
Vitamin D	50 IU
Vitamin E	6 mg
Niacin	1 mg
Folate	29 mcg
Vitamin B$_6$	0.0 mg
Vitamin B$_{12}$	0.0 mcg
Zinc	0.6 mg
Selenium	0 mcg

C-Blitz

This dynamic juice makes an effective eye-opener or a refreshing drink throughout the day.

Tip

To keep parsley fresh, wrap it in several layers of paper towels and place in a plastic bag. Store in the warmest part of your refrigerator — in the butter keeper, for example, or the door.

- **Juicer**

1	grapefruit, cut to fit juicer tube	1
2	oranges	2
6	sprigs fresh parsley	6
3	kiwifruit	3

1. Using juicer, process grapefruit, oranges, parsley and kiwis. Whisk and pour into one large or two smaller glasses.

> ▶ **Health Tip**
>
> Parsley packs a whopping amount of vitamin C and is one of the few fresh herbs widely available throughout the year.

Nutrients per 1 of 2 servings

Calories	171
Fat	1 g
Carbohydrate	43 g
Protein	3 g
Vitamin C	217 mg
Vitamin D	0 IU
Vitamin E	2 mg
Niacin	1 mg
Folate	85 mcg
Vitamin B_6	0.2 mg
Vitamin B_{12}	0.0 mcg
Zinc	0.4 mg
Selenium	1 mcg

Cherry Juice

This cherry-based juice incorporates two other fruits and digestion-friendly fennel.

Tip

Whole ripe cherries are best used immediately but will keep in the refrigerator for up to 2 days.

- **Juicer**

1 cup	pitted cherries	250 mL
1/4	bulb fresh fennel	1/4
1 cup	grapes	250 mL
1/2	lime	1/2

1. Using juicer, process cherries, fennel, grapes and lime. Whisk and pour into a glass.

> ▶ **Health Tip**
> Cherries contain numerous antioxidants that can help protect body tissues, including the brain.

Nutrients per serving	
Calories	187
Fat	1 g
Carbohydrate	48 g
Protein	3 g
Vitamin C	32 mg
Vitamin D	0 IU
Vitamin E	0 mg
Niacin	1 mg
Folate	26 mcg
Vitamin B$_6$	0.2 mg
Vitamin B$_{12}$	0.0 mcg
Zinc	0.3 mg
Selenium	1 mcg

Slippery Beet

This is a straight-ahead beet juice, with the power of garlic along for the ride.

Tip

Store unwashed beets in a plastic bag in the refrigerator for up to 10 days. Wash just before juicing.

- **Juicer**

2	beets	2
1	clove garlic	1
1	apple	1
1 tbsp	powdered slippery elm	15 mL

1. Using juicer, process beets, garlic and apple. Whisk together with slippery elm powder and pour into a glass.

> ▶ **Health Tip**
>
> The choline content of beets makes them a good support for the liver, while the addition of slippery elm make this juice an even better detox drink.

Nutrients per serving	
Calories	85
Fat	0 g
Carbohydrate	21 g
Protein	2 g
Vitamin C	9 mg
Vitamin D	0 IU
Vitamin E	0 mg
Niacin	0 mg
Folate	92 mcg
Vitamin B_6	0.1 mg
Vitamin B_{12}	0.0 mcg
Zinc	0.3 mg
Selenium	1 mcg

Dandelion Slam Dunk

Dandelion greens are becoming increasingly well known as a salad ingredient or simply cooked. In this recipe, you juice them along with other healthy ingredients.

Makes 1 serving

Tip

Look for fresh dandelion leaves from spring through fall at some supermarkets, farmers' markets and health food stores.

- **Juicer**

½ cup	fresh dandelion leaves	125 mL
¼	cabbage, cut to fit juicer tube	¼
2	apples	2
1	1-inch (2.5 cm) piece fresh dandelion root	1

1. Using juicer, process dandelion leaves, cabbage, apples and dandelion root. Whisk and pour into a glass.

> ▶ **Health Tip**
>
> Dandelion root supports liver function and the leaves are known to increase kidney activity; hence this juice is a good supporter of natural detoxification pathways.

Nutrients per serving	
Calories	260
Fat	1 g
Carbohydrate	66 g
Protein	5 g
Vitamin C	142 mg
Vitamin D	0 IU
Vitamin E	2 mg
Niacin	1 mg
Folate	148 mcg
Vitamin B_6	0.4 mg
Vitamin B_{12}	0.0 mcg
Zinc	0.7 mg
Selenium	2 mcg

Cell Support Juice

This is a nutritive boost with plenty of sweetness from apples.

Tip

Look for whole or cut dried alfalfa leaves at health food stores.

- **Juicer**

3	apples	3
1	handful fresh parsley	1
1	handful fresh alfalfa tops or 1 tbsp (15 mL) dried	1

1. Using juicer, process apples, parsley and, if using, fresh alfalfa. Whisk together and pour into a large glass. If using dried alfalfa, whisk into juice.

> ▶ **Health Tip**
>
> Alfalfa used to be given to convalescents who needed to put on weight. This plant has some phytoestrogen attributes as well, somewhat akin to soy.

Nutrients per serving	
Calories	291
Fat	1 g
Carbohydrate	77 g
Protein	2 g
Vitamin C	46 mg
Vitamin D	0 IU
Vitamin E	1 mg
Niacin	1 mg
Folate	42 mcg
Vitamin B_6	0.2 mg
Vitamin B_{12}	0.0 mcg
Zinc	0.5 mg
Selenium	0 mcg

Green Energy

This green energy drink can be a mid-afternoon pick-me-up or, later in the day, a serving of veggies.

Tip

Reduce the amount of soy milk to ¼ cup (60 mL) if using frozen spinach.

- **Blender**

2 cups	spinach, fresh or frozen	500 mL
½ cup	soy milk (see tip, at left)	125 mL
¼ cup	apricot milk or soy milk	60 mL
3 tbsp	chopped wheatgrass or barley grass	45 mL
1 tbsp	pumpkin seeds	15 mL
1 tsp	ginkgo (optional)	5 mL

1. In blender, process spinach, soy milk, apricot milk, grass, pumpkin seeds and ginkgo (if using), until smooth. Pour into a glass.

> ▶ **Health Tip**
>
> Getting the maximum number of servings of vegetables per day depends on taking opportunities to eat them. Using a vegetable-based (and low-sodium) drink is a great way to up your veggie intake.

Nutrients per serving	
Calories	257
Fat	7 g
Carbohydrate	38 g
Protein	13 g
Vitamin C	17 mg
Vitamin D	78 IU
Vitamin E	2 mg
Niacin	3 mg
Folate	144 mcg
Vitamin B$_6$	0.3 mg
Vitamin B$_{12}$	1.6 mcg
Zinc	2.3 mg
Selenium	18 mcg

Resources

Websites
Cambridge Brain Sciences:
www.cambridgebrainsciences.com

Happy Neuron:
www.happy-neuron.com

Lumosity:
www.lumosity.com

Multiple Intelligences for Adult Literacy and Education:
www.literacynet.org/mi/assessment/findyourstrengths.html

Psychology Today:
http://psychologytoday.tests.psychtests.com

Apps
Elevate: Your personal brain trainer (http://elevateapp.com/#/)

NeuroNation (www.neuronation.com)

Video Games
Echochrome (www. playstation.com/en-us/games/echochrome-ps3)

Minecraft (https://minecraft.net)

References

Books

Doidge, Norman. *The Brain That Changes Itself: Stories of Personal Triumph from the Frontiers of Brain Science.* New York: Penguin, 2007.

Katz, Lawrence C., and Manning Rubin. *Keep Your Brain Alive: 83 Neurobic Exercises to Help Prevent Memory Loss and Increase Mental Fitness.* New York: Workman, 1998.

Ratey, John J. *Spark: The Revolutionary New Science of Exercise and the Brain.* New York: Little, Brown and Company, 2008.

Smith, Fraser, and Ellie Aghdassi. *Keep Your Brain Young: A Health & Diet Program for Your Brain, Including 150 Recipes.* Toronto: Robert Rose, 2014.

Journals

Buschkuehl M, Hernandez-Garcia L, Jaeggi SM, et al. Neural effects of short-term training on working memory. *Cogn Affect Behav Neurosci,* 2014 Mar; 14 (1): 147–60. doi: 10.3758/s13415-013-0244-9.

Cassilhas RC, Lee KS, Fernandes J, et al. Spatial memory is improved by aerobic and resistance exercise through divergent molecular mechanisms. *Neuroscience,* 2012 Jan 27; 202: 309–17. doi: 10.1016/j.neuroscience.2011.11.029. Epub 2011 Dec 2.

Hindin SB, Zelinski EM. Extended practice and aerobic exercise interventions benefit untrained cognitive outcomes in older adults: A meta-analysis. *J Am Geriatr Soc,* 2012 Jan; 60 (1): 136–41. doi: 10.1111/j.1532-5415.2011.03761.x. Epub 2011 Dec 8.

Kiefer AW, Gualberto Cremades J, Myer GD. Train the brain: Novel electroencephalography data indicate links between motor learning and brain adaptations. *J Nov Physiother,* 2014 Apr; 4 (2). pii: 198

Mahncke HW, Bronstone A, Merzenich MM. Brain plasticity and functional losses in the aged: Scientific bases for a novel intervention. *Prog Brain Res,* 2006; 157: 81–109.

Mayas J, Parmentier FB, Andrés P, et al. Plasticity of attentional functions in older adults after non-action video game training: A randomized controlled trial. *PLoS One,* 2014 Mar 19; 9 (3): e92269. doi: 10.1371/journal.pone.0092269. eCollection 2014.

McDaniel MA, Maier SF, Einstein GO. "Brain-specific" nutrients: A memory cure? *Nutrition,* 2003 Nov–Dec; 19 (11–12): 957–75.

Melby-Lervåg M, Hulme C. Is working memory training effective? A meta-analytic review. *Dev Psychol,* 2013 Feb; 49 (2): 270–91. doi: 10.1037/a0028228. Epub 2012 May 21.

Morrison AB, Chein JM. Does working memory training work? The promise and challenges of enhancing cognition by training working memory. *Psychon Bull Rev,* 2011 Feb; 18 (1): 46–60. doi: 10.3758/s13423-010-0034-0.

Stepankova H, Lukavsky J, Buschkuehl M, et al. The malleability of working memory and visuospatial skills: A randomized controlled study in older adults. *Dev Psychol,* 2014 Apr; 50 (4): 1049–59. doi: 10.1037/a0034913. Epub 2013 Nov 11.

Weinberg L, Hasni A, Shinohara M, et al. A single bout of resistance exercise can enhance episodic memory performance. *Acta Psychol (Amst),* 2014 Nov; 153: 13–19. doi: 10.1016/j.actpsy.2014.06.011. Epub 2014 Sep 28.

Yurko-Mauro K. Cognitive and cardiovascular benefits of docosahexaenoic acid in aging and cognitive decline. *Curr Alzheimer Res,* 2010 May; 7 (3): 190–6.

Websites

Biel, Lindsey. Sensory diet activities. *Sensory Smarts*. Aug 2009, accessed June 2015, http://sensorysmarts.com/sensory_diet_activities.html.

Chapman, Alan. Puzzles, games, trivia questions and answers for quizzes, team building activities, training and motivation. *Businessballs*. Accessed June 2015, www.businessballs.com/games.htm.

Dewar, Gwen. Improving spatial skills in children and teens: Evidence-based activities and tips. *Parenting Science*. Nov. 2012, accessed June 2015, www.parentingscience.com/spatial-skills.html.

Harpold, Carol Leynse. Visual spatial awareness apps and games. *OT's with Apps and Technology*. 26 Jan. 2013, accessed June 2015, http://otswithapps.com/2013/01/26/visual-spatial-awareness-apps-and-games.

Janes, Jennifer. Ultimate guide to sensory integration activities. *Jennifer A. Janes Blog*. 8 Aug. 2012, accessed June 2015, http://jenniferajanes.com/ultimate-guide-to-sensory-integration-activities.

Katz, Larry, and Manning Rubin. Neurobotics: The unique new science of brain exercises. *Keep Your Brain Alive*. 2014, accessed June 2015, www.keepyourbrainalive.com/neurobics.

Lebowitz, Shana. 47 ways to boost brainpower now. *Greatist*. 23 July 2013, accessed June 2015, http://greatist.com/happiness/47-ways-boost-brainpower-now.

Payne, Tom. Linguistics challenge: Agta. *Linguistics Society of America*. 2005, accessed June 2015, http://lingclub.mycpanel.princeton.edu/challenge/agta.php.

Rynhart, Pavani. Learning rotation with pizza making activity. *Proactive Play*. 3 Aug. 2013, accessed June 2015, http://proactiveplay.com/learning-rotation-with-pizza-making-activity.

Sasson, Remez. Concentration exercises for training the mind. *Success Consciousness: Mental Tools for a Great Life*. Accessed June 2015, www.successconsciousness.com/index_000005.htm.

Sutherland, Stephani. How yoga changes the brain. *Scientific American*. 1 Mar. 2014, accessed June 2015, www.scientificamerican.com/article/how-yoga-changes-the-brain.

Contributing Authors

250 Best Beans, Lentils and Tofu Recipes
Recipes from this book are found on pages 224, 240, 259, 273, 285 and 316.

Alexandra Anca and Theresa Santandrea-Cull
Complete Gluten-Free Diet and Nutrition Guide
Recipes from this book are found on pages 213, 218, 233, 250, 258, 264, 305 and 307.

Byron Ayanoglu with contributions from Algis Kemezys
125 Best Vegetarian Recipes
Recipes from this book are found on pages 228, 254, 256 and 262.

Byron Ayanoglu and Jennifer MacKenzie
Complete Curry Cookbook
Recipes from this book are found on pages 236, 281 and 322.

Johanna Burkhard
500 Best Comfort Food Recipes
Recipes from this book are found on pages 212, 226, 318, 320 and 334.

Johanna Burkhard
The Comfort Food Cookbook
Recipes from this book are found on pages 263 and 336.

Pat Crocker
The Juicing Bible
Recipes from this book are found on pages 359–64.

Pat Crocker
The Vegan Cook's Bible
Recipes from this book are found on pages 223, 234, 253, 266 and 293.

Dietitians of Canada
Cook!
Recipes from this book are found on pages 203, 290, 303, 312, 329, 331, 354 and 357.

Dietitians of Canada
Cook Great Food
Recipes from this book are found on pages 241, 274–78, 296, 304, 323, 328 and 343.

Dietitians of Canada
Simply Great Food
Recipes from this book are found on pages 308, 339 and 342.

Maxine Effenson-Chuck and Beth Gurney
125 Best Vegan Recipes
Recipes from this book are found on pages 275, 296 and 341.

Judith Finlayson
150 Best Slow Cooker Recipes
A recipe from this book is found on page 327.

Judith Finlayson
The Complete Gluten-Free Whole Grains Cookbook
Recipes from this book are found on pages 205, 284, 310, 324, 332 and 345.

Judith Finlayson
The Vegetarian Slow Cooker
Recipes from this book are found on pages 204, 206, 267, 268, 272 and 340.

Julie Hasson
300 Best Chocolate Recipes
Recipes from this book are found on pages 352 and 356.

Lynn Roblin, Nutrition Editor
500 Best Healthy Recipes
Recipes from this book are found on pages
251, 252, 292 and 302.

Deb Roussou
350 Best Vegan Recipes
Recipes from this book are found on pages
209, 210, 231, 232, 270 and 288.

Camilla V. Saulsbury
5 Easy Steps to Healthy Cooking
Recipes from this book are found on pages
200, 201, 207, 208, 216, 222, 255, 257 and 358.

Camilla V. Saulsbury
500 Best Quinoa Recipes
Recipes from this book are found on pages
202, 230, 269, 279 and 333.

Camilla V. Saulsbury
750 Best Muffin Recipes
Recipes from this book are found on pages
219 and 220.

Camilla V. Saulsbury
Piece of Cake!
Recipes from this book are found on pages
348–51.

Kathleen Sloan-McIntosh
300 Best Potato Recipes
Recipes from this book are found on pages
214, 260, 300 and 306.

Carla Snyder and Meredith Deeds
300 Sensational Soups
Recipes from this book are found on pages
238 and 242–48.

Linda Stephen
Complete Book of Thai Cooking
Recipes from this book are found on pages
294, 298, 313, 314, 321, 326, 338 and 346.

Suneeta Vaswani
Complete Book of Indian Cooking
Recipes from this book are found on pages
282, 283 and 344.

Suneeta Vaswani
Easy Indian Cooking
Recipes from this book are found on pages
280, 297, 319 and 337.

Katherine E. Younker, Editor
America's Complete Diabetes Cookbook
Recipes from this book are found on pages
309 and 330.

Library and Archives Canada Cataloguing in Publication

Smith, Fraser, 1968-, author
    The complete brain exercise book : train your brain! : improve memory, language,
motor skills & more + a health & diet plan with 125 recipes / Dr. Fraser Smith, BA, MATD, ND.

Includes index.
ISBN 978-0-7788-0515-1 (paperback)

    1. Brain—Diseases—Prevention—Popular works. 2. Brain—Diseases—Nutritional aspects—
Popular works. 3. Brain—Diseases—Diet therapy—Recipes. I. Title.

RC386.2.S64 2015   616.805   C2015-904953-9

Index

A

acetylcholine, 14
aerobic exercise, 155
aging, 10–12, 21, 22–24, 159
alcohol, 166
allergies, 189–90
alpha-linolenic acid (ALA), 177
Alzheimer's disease, 21. *See also* dementia
amino acids, 14, 174
amygdala, 16
amylase, 186
antioxidants, 162, 167, 183–84
appetizers, 223–28
apples
  Cell Support Juice, 363
  Cinnamon Apple Chips, 222
  Curry-Roasted Squash and Apple Soup, 236
  Dandelion Slam Dunk, 362
  Hot Multigrain Cereal, 204
  Moroccan Pumpkin Soup, 234
  Open-Faced Salmon Salad Sandwich with Apple and Ginger, 303
  Potato Pancakes with Cinnamon Apples and Yogurt Cheese, 214
  Slippery Beet, 361
  Sweet Cinnamon Waldorf Salad, 252
arachidonic acid (AA), 175, 177
Artichoke Hearts and Parmesan, Shrimp Risotto with, 309
aspartame, 166
atherosclerosis, 20, 21, 158
avocado
  Avocado and Egg Breakfast Wraps, 208
  Avocado Salad, 254
  Chunky Guacamole, 225

B

Barbecued Lemongrass Pork, 326
basil
  Couscous Salad with Basil and Pine Nuts, 263
  Insalata Caprese, 256
  Spaghetti with Sun-Dried Tomatoes and Broccoli, 292
  Tomato Basil Soup, 232
BDNT (brain-derived neurotrophic factor), 25
beans. *See also* beans, green; bean sprouts
  Fragrant Rice-Stuffed Peppers (variation), 288
  Jerusalem Artichoke Stew, 266
  Minestrone, 233
  Navy Bean and Ham Soup, 248
  Quinoa Chili, 284
  Salmon over White and Black Bean Salsa, 302
  Southwest Butternut Squash Tortilla Bake, 285
  Three-Bean Chili, 286
  Three-Pepper Tamale Pie, 270
beans, green
  Cauliflower and Beans with Turmeric, 338
  Fried Rice with Curry, 346
  Green Bean, Pecan and Pomegranate Salad, 253
  Green Beans and Carrots with Aromatic Spices, 337
bean sprouts
  Egg Noodles with Vegetables, 294
  Pad Thai, 314
beef
  Beef and Quinoa Power Burgers, 334
  Beef with Broccoli, 328
  Blue Cheese–Stuffed Sweet and Spicy Meatloaf, 331
  Minestrone (variation), 233
  Orange Ginger Beef, 329
  Peppery Meatloaf with Quinoa, 332
  Saucy Swiss Steak, 327
  Shepherd's Pie with Creamy Corn Filling, 330
  Stuffed Cabbage Soup, 246